Medical Toxicology

Edited by Pınar Erkekoglu
and Tomohisa Ogawa

Published in London, United Kingdom

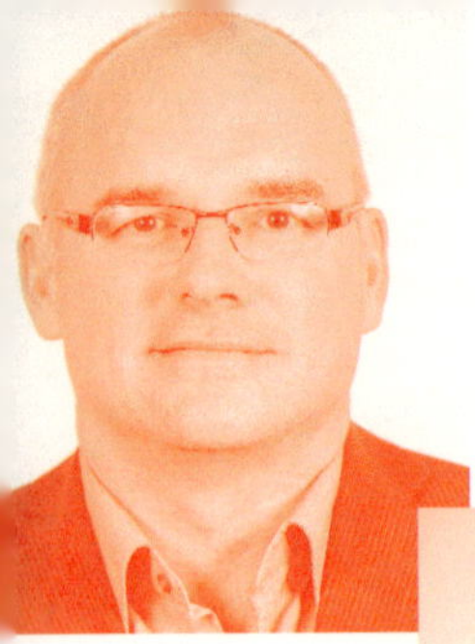

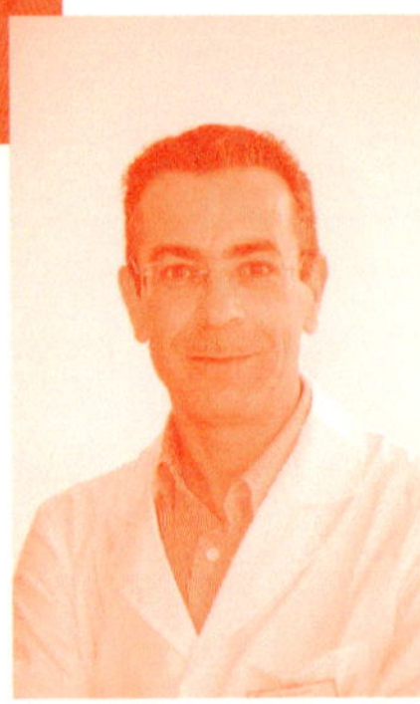

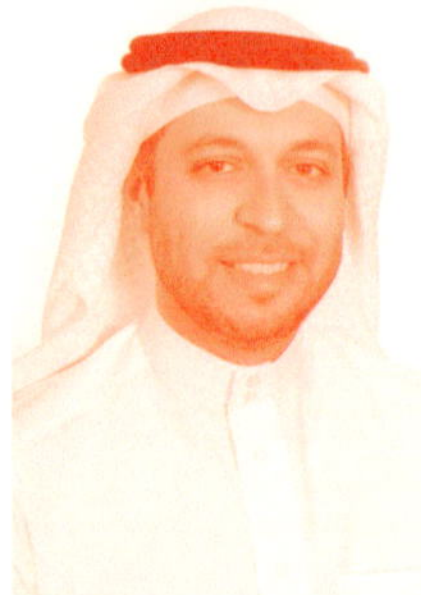

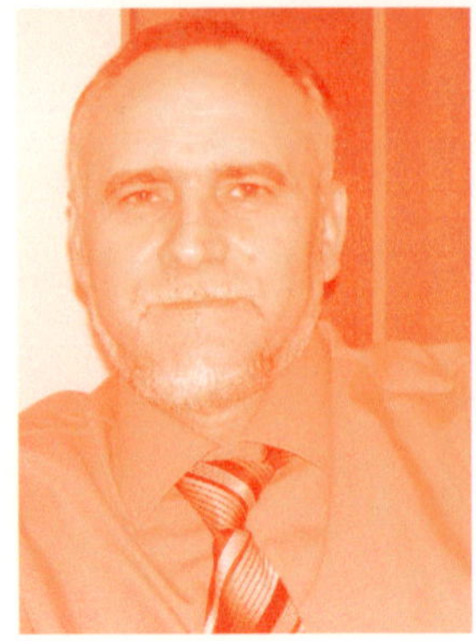

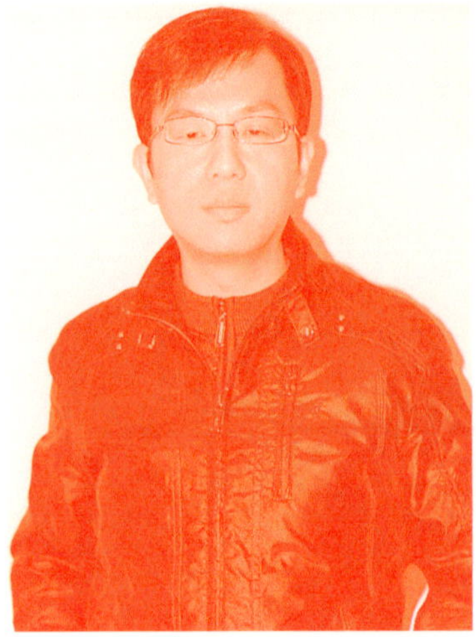

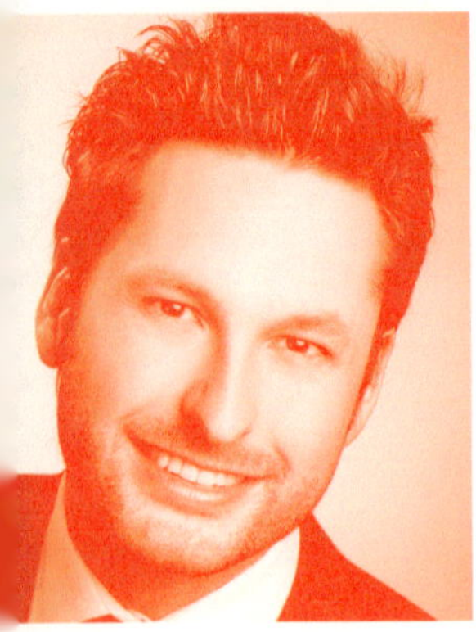

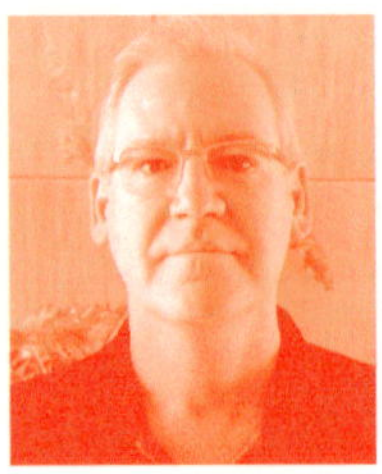

IntechOpen

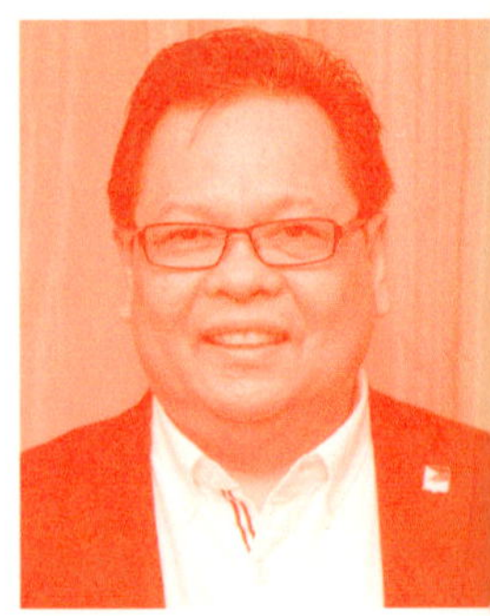

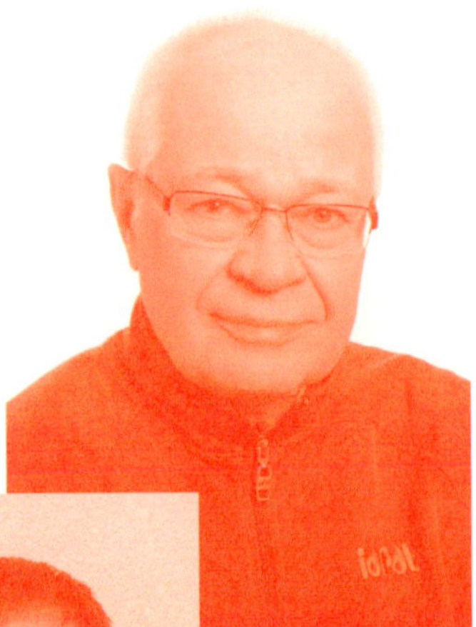

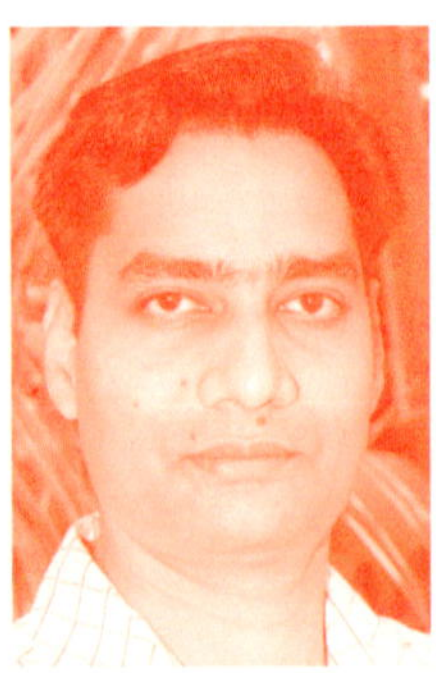

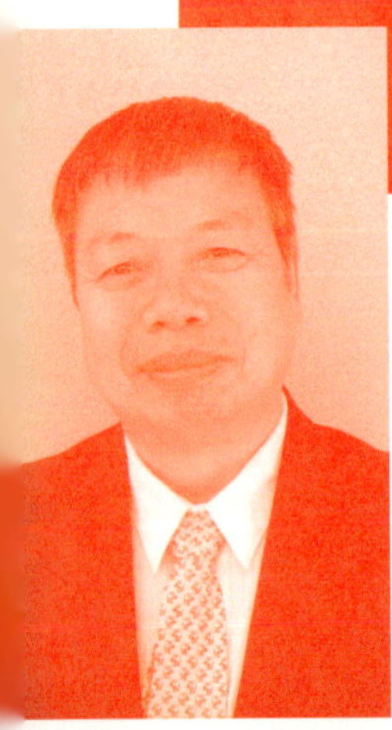

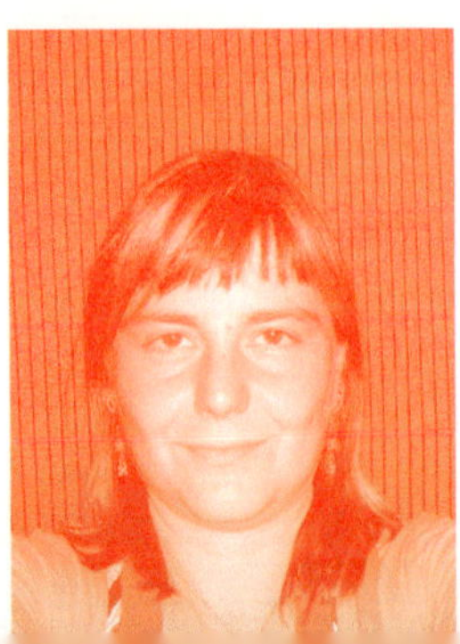

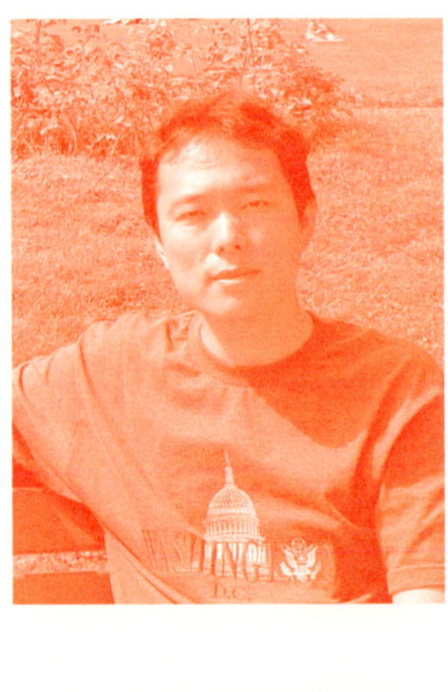

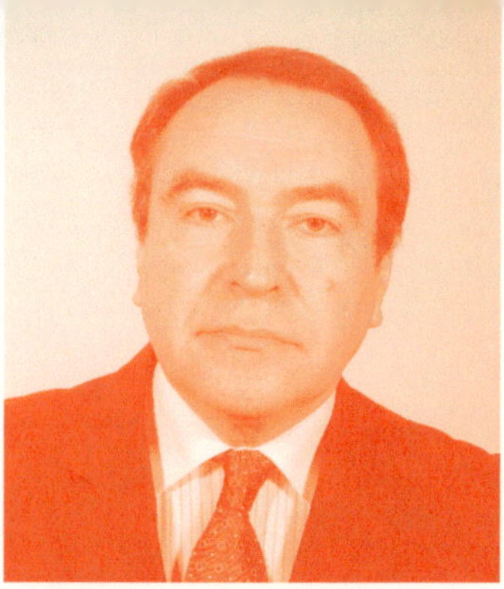
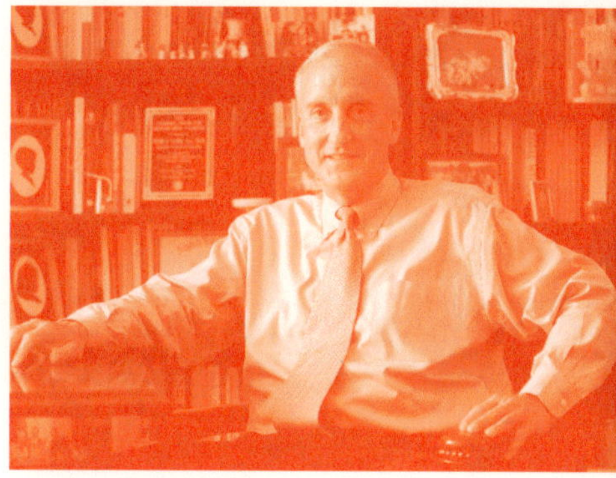
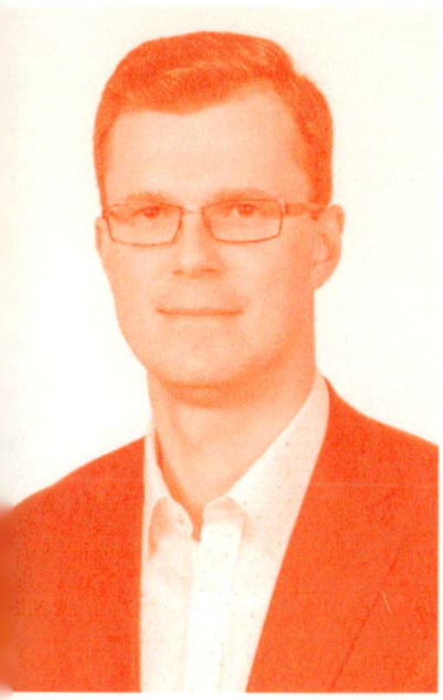
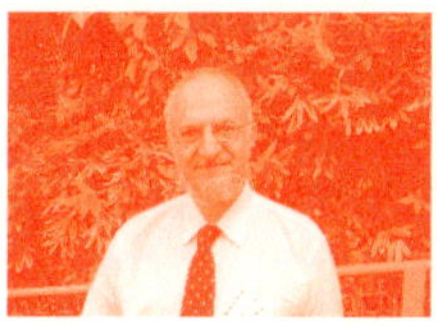
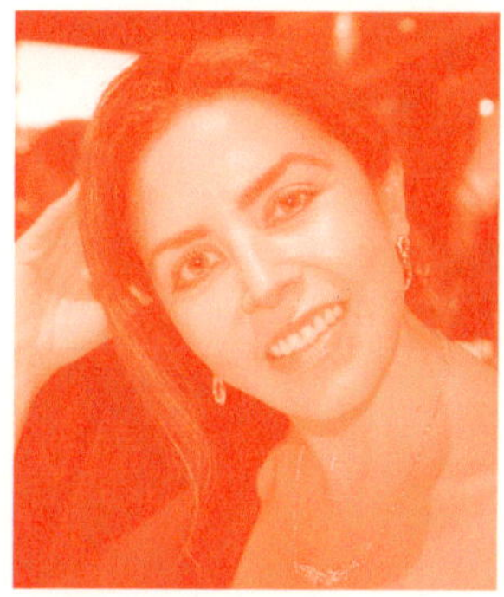

Supporting open minds since 2005

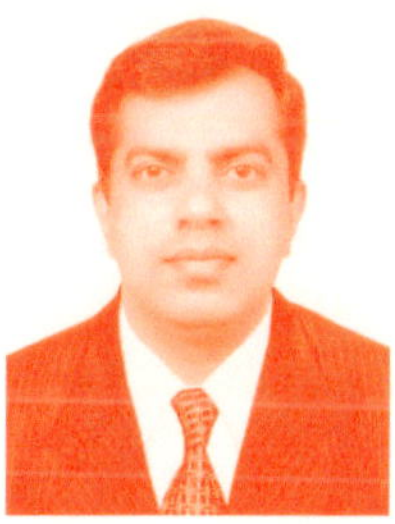
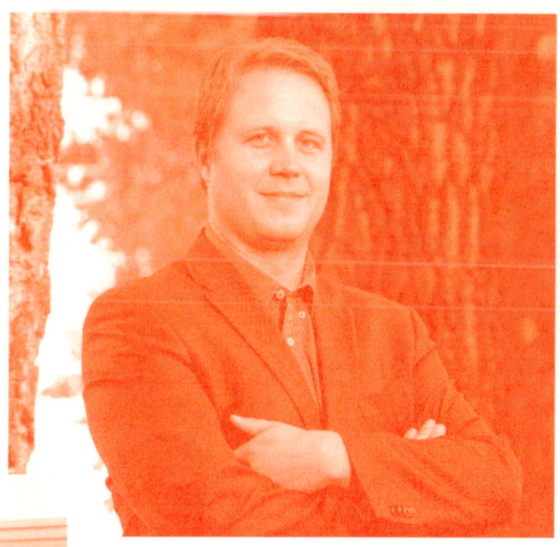
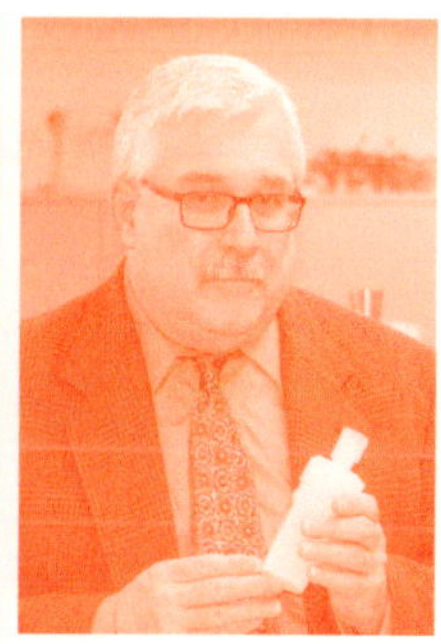
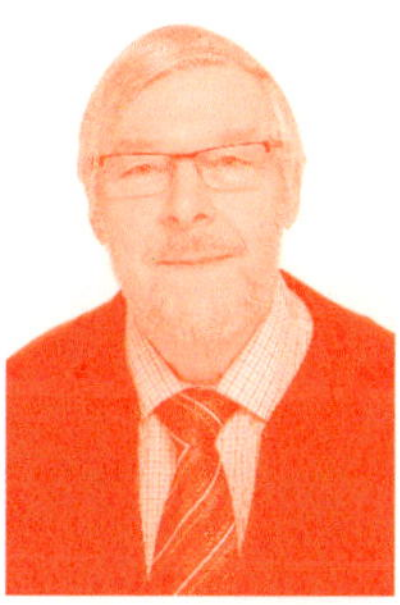
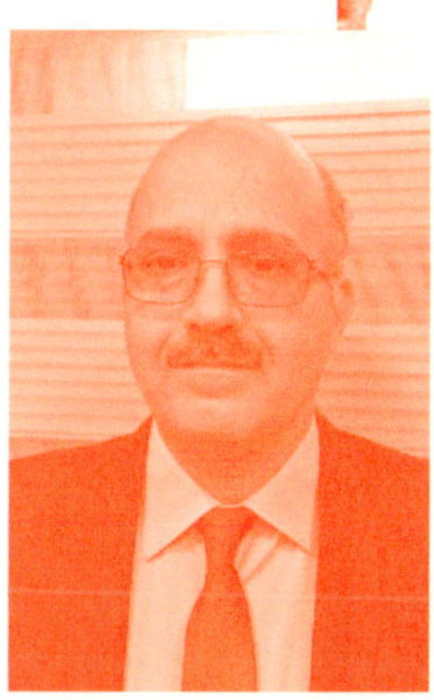
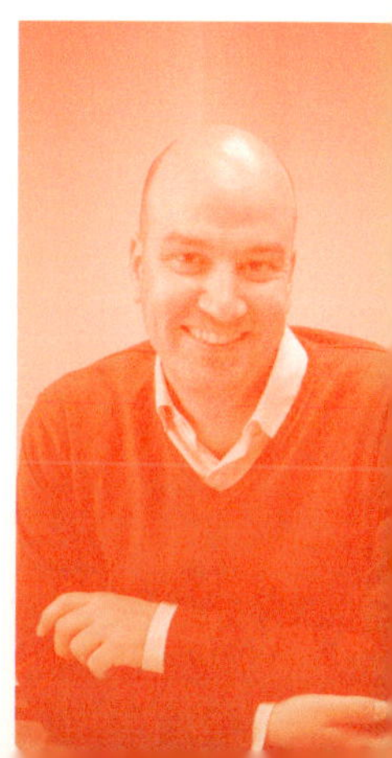
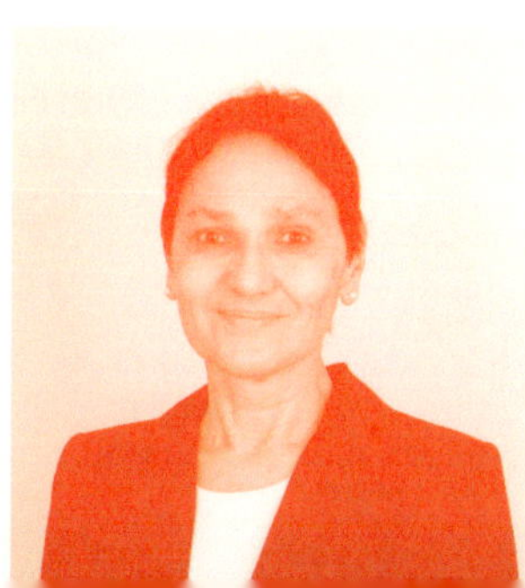

Medical Toxicology
http://dx.doi.org/10.5772/intechopen.77665
Edited by Pınar Erkekoglu and Tomohisa Ogawa

Contributors
Amarnath Mishra, Sreemoy Kanti Kanti Das, Alberto Frutos Pérez-Surio, Deyana Georgieva Vankova, Milena Gincheva Pasheva, Yoana Dimitrova Kiselova-Kaneva, Dobri Lazarov Ivanov, Diana Georgieva Ivanova, Saganuwan Alhaji Saganuwan, Verônica Farina Azzolin, Ivana Beatrice Mânica da Cruz, Fernanda Barbisan, Cibele Ferreira Teixeira, Euler Esteves Ribeiro, Ivo Emilio da Cruz Jung, Raquel de Souza Praia, Jie Tao, Xiaoli Wang, Zhiping Zhang, Yudan Zhu, Jiwei Cheng, Guoyi Li, Shuzhang Zhang, Mengyao Sun, Qian Xiao, Chia-Yi Tseng, Narumi Aoki-Shioi, Cassandra M. Modahl, Eva Petrovova, Vladimir Petrilla, Lenka Luptakova, Charlotte Peters, Tomohisa Ogawa, Hiroki Shibata, Kumbukani Nyirenda, Djafer Rachid, Mahluga Jafarova Demirkapu, Irem Tatli Cankaya, Zekiye Ceren Arituluk, Cigdem Kahraman, Pınar Erkekoglu, Suna Sabuncuoğlu

First published in London, United Kingdom, 2021 by IntechOpen
IntechOpen is the global imprint of INTECHOPEN LIMITED, registered in England and Wales, registration number: 11086078, 5 Princes Gate Court, London, SW7 2QJ, United Kingdom
Printed in Croatia

British Library Cataloguing-in-Publication Data
A catalogue record for this book is available from the British Library

Additional hard and PDF copies can be obtained from orders@intechopen.com

Medical Toxicology
Edited by Pınar Erkekoglu and Tomohisa Ogawa
p. cm.
Print ISBN 978-1-83880-277-6
Online ISBN 978-1-83880-278-3
eBook (PDF) ISBN 978-1-83969-155-3

Meet the editors

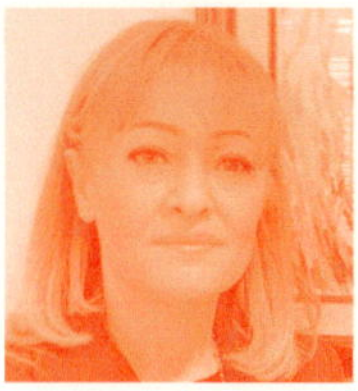

Pınar Erkekoglu was born in Ankara, Turkey. She graduated with a BS from Hacettepe University Faculty of Pharmacy. Later, she received an MSci and Ph.D. in Toxicology. She completed a part of her Ph.D. studies in Grenoble, France, at Universite Joseph Fourier and CEA/INAC/LAN after receiving a full scholarship from both the Erasmus Scholarship Program and CEA. She worked as a post-doc and a visiting associate in the Biological Engineering Department at Massachusetts Institute of Technology. She is currently working as a full professor at Hacettepe University, Faculty of Pharmacy, Department of Pharmaceutical Toxicology. Her main study interests are clinical and medical aspects of toxicology, endocrine-disrupting chemicals, and oxidative stress. She has published more than 150 papers in national and international journals. Dr. Erkekoglu has been a European Registered Toxicologist (ERT) since 2014.

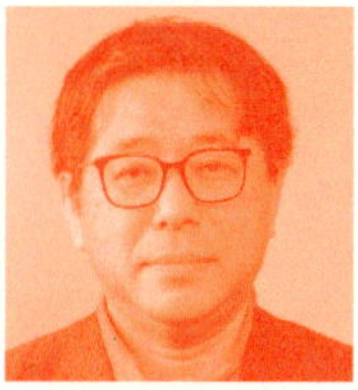

Dr. Tomohisa Ogawa obtained a Ph.D. in Chemistry from Kyushu University, Fukuoka, Japan, in 1991. After graduating, he was a postdoctoral research fellow for the Japan Society for the Promotion of Science (JSPS) and an assistant professor at the Faculty of Science, Kyushu University. In 1997, he became an associate professor at the Faculty of Agricultural Science, Tohoku University, Sendai, Japan. From 2001 to 2020, he was an associate professor at the Graduate School of Life Sciences, Tohoku University. Since then, Dr. Ogawa has been a professor at the Graduate School of Agricultural Science at the same university. He is active in the research fields of applied biochemistry (protein engineering), molecular biology (molecular evolution, venomics), and structural biochemistry. He has published a number of various reviews and original papers in renowned journals.

Contents

Preface

Medical toxicology focuses on the short- and long-term adverse effects of medications, including drug–drug, drug–herb, and drug–disease interactions and drug overdoses. It is involved in the diagnosis, management, and prevention of acute and chronic poisonings due to, among others, occupational, environmental, and industrial toxic chemicals.

Medical toxicologists are also interested in substance abuse, venoms, toxins, and antidotes. In the field of medical toxicology, practitioners are physicians. Their primary specialization is generally in emergency medicine, occupational medicine, or pediatrics. Medical toxicologists can provide direct treatment and bedside consultation of acutely poisoned patients, including children in emergency departments, intensive care units, and other inpatient and outpatient units/clinics.

Medical toxicologists can also provide advice in poison control centers, contribute to pharmaceutical research and drug safety, and deal with health policy issues. Therefore, medical toxicology has a wide variety of working fields. Medical Toxicology focuses on the prevention and treatment of poisonings with venoms and toxins, treatment of envenomation, interactions in clinics, antidotes, and forensic toxicology.

This volume provides the reader with a general overview of the treatment of acute/chronic poisonings including poisonings with drugs, venoms, and toxins, and the antidotes used in clinics.

Pınar Erkekoğlu
Department of Toxicology,
Faculty of Pharmacy,
Hacettepe University,
Ankara, Turkey

Tomohisa Ogawa
Graduate School of Agricultural Science Tohoku University,
Japan

Section 1

Introduction

Chapter 1

Introductory Chapter: Medical Toxicology

Pınar Erkekoğlu and Suna Sabuncuoğlu

1. Introduction

Toxicology is "the study of the occurrence, properties, detection, adverse effects, and regulation of biological, chemical or physical agents on living organisms." Modern toxicology focuses on the adverse effects of toxic substances (including toxins, venoms, and toxicants) at molecular level [1, 2].

Since toxicology is a multidisciplinary science, the contributions and activities of toxicologists are widespread and diverse. Toxicologists are mainly concerned with the mechanisms of action of different agents as, we now know, all agents can lead to toxicity due to the exposure period and dose. However, for even the most known and oldest agents, the pathways or endogenous molecules they affect to create toxicity are still being investigated by scientists. As toxicologists, we also contribute to other scientific areas including medicine, physiology, and pharmacology while we receive the help from several branches of science. Toxicologists mainly recognize, identify, and quantify the hazards of foods, pharmaceuticals, workplace chemicals, household products, cosmetics, and personal care products along with toxins and venoms. Furthermore, toxicologists who work as members of academic, industrial, and governmental organizations can also develop the standards and regulations in order to protect human and animal health as well as the environment from the adverse effects of microorganisms, chemicals, or physical agents. In the modern era, toxicologists share methodologies and scientific knowledge to obtain accurate data about the unwanted effects of different agents [1, 3, 4].

2. Poison, toxin, toxicant, and venom

Poison is any substance that leads to harmful effect/s to a living organism when taken by any route, either by accident or design. The history of poisons and poisoners has a long record dating back to the ancient times. In Homer's *Odyssey*, the first use of a specific antidote was documented. In three books (*De Antidotis I*, *De Antidotis II*, and *De Theriaca ad Pisonem*) written by Galen (AD 129–200), the development of a universal antidote was described in detail. Later, Nicander (197–170 BC) focused on the prevention of the gastrointestinal absorption of poisons, emesis induction by using an emetic agent and the mechanical stimulation of the hypopharynx. Greeks and Romans used oral wood charcoal to treat diseases such as anthrax and epilepsy. After 1960s, the use of activated charcoal was routinely recommended in many poisonings [5].

Paracelsus (1493–1541), the "Father of Toxicology," was a physician-alchemist. He formulated many revolutionary ideas that form the basic structure of toxicology, pharmacology, and medicine today. The scientist indicated "*Dosis facit venenum*," which simply means "All substances are poisons; there is none which is not a poison.

It is the dose that differentiates between a poison and a medicine." Therefore, poisoning is a quantitative concept, and we now know that the right dose distinguishes "a poison" from "a remedy." It can be stated that "Almost any substance, including water, can lead to toxicity at high doses without causing any harmful effects at lower doses." However, we also know that some chemicals can also lead to toxicity at lower doses and the harmful effect will not significantly increase at higher doses. The toxicity of some endocrine disruptors, particularly bisphenol A (BPA), is an example [1].

There is a certain difference between "a toxicant" and "a toxin" and they are not used as synonyms. Many people do not clearly know the difference and instead they refer every harmful substance as "a toxin." Toxicants are synthetic, human-made, and toxic chemicals which are capable of causing deleterious effects on living organisms. Toxicants are significantly different from toxins not only because of their synthetic origins but also because of their production volumes and masses, distribution processes, and structural heterogeneity. They can be present in houses, workplaces, living organisms, and environment. On the other hand, toxins are small molecules, peptides, or proteins that are produced by living organisms. In general, toxins are metabolic products, which are parts of the defense mechanisms of animals, plants, insects, microbes, etc. against other living forms. The term "biotoxin" is occasionally used to explicitly confirm the biological origin. The organisms produce them in order to predate or repel (such as in the snake, scorpion, spider, jellyfish, and wasp toxins) or defense (honeybee, bee, ant, wasp, termite, and dart frog toxins) [6, 7].

The action of toxins has long been recognized and understood throughout human history. Toxins from plants are associated with murder, assassination, and suicide. The deaths of several famous historical figures have directly or indirectly involved toxins from poisonous plants. Socrates was forced suicide with a toxic alkaloid from poison hemlock (*Conium maculatum*), while the many victims of Livia (wife of Emperor Augustus) and Agrippina (wife of Claudius) succumbed to the toxic tropane alkaloids of the deadly nightshade (*Atropa belladonna*) [7–9].

A common characteristic of natural toxins is to cause deleterious effects with small quantities on the metabolic and physiologic functions of a living organism. Toxins usually interact with biological macromolecules like enzymes or with cellular receptors. Toxins vary greatly in structure. Moreover, their harmful effects can range from minor (such as a bee sting) to almost immediately deadly (such as botulinum toxin). A systemic toxin affects the entire body or many organs rather than a specific site. An organ toxin affects only specific tissues or organs [10].

A "venom" is a secretion of an animal (like snake, spider, and scorpion) that contains one or more toxins. Venoms usually are classified into four major groups according to their mechanisms of action: (i) *Necrotoxins*, which cause necrosis in the cells they encounter (e.g., viper venoms), (ii) *Neurotoxins*, which primarily act on the nervous system of the exposed living organisms (e.g., box jellyfish, scorpion, octopus, cone snail, centipede, and black widow spider venoms), (iii) *Cytotoxins*, which kill the exposed individual cells (e.g., black widow spider venoms), and (iv) *Myotoxins*, which damage muscle cells by binding to a receptor (e.g., snake and lizard venoms). Due to the highly specific and potent effects of venoms, they often serve as excellent candidates from which therapeutic drugs may be developed. As venom peptides and proteins affect the mammalian physiological processes, these structures can assist in creating targeted libraries of potential drug candidates. They are extremely site-specific in their actions and this specificity can provide a value as a lead therapeutic or biological probe [11, 12].

3. Medical toxicology

Medical toxicology is a subbranch of toxicology, which is concerned with providing the diagnosis, management, and prevention of poisoning and other adverse effects of drugs, cosmetics, personal care products, occupational and environmental toxicants, and biological agents. Medical toxicology mainly deals with the prognostic indicators of poisoning severity and predictors for the treatment. For practical reasons, much of this work has been retrospective in nature; however, it has resulted in significant aids to guide the treatment rendered by clinical toxicologists. Medical toxicologists are involved in the assessment and treatment of a wide variety of problems, including acute or chronic poisoning, substance abuse, adverse drug reactions (ADRs), drug overdoses, envenomations, industrial accidents, and other chemical exposures. Generally, physicians who are specialized in emergency medicine, poison management, and pediatrics can become medical toxicologists. Medical toxicologists work on finding new and effective antidotes and treatments in order to prevent poisonings and xenobiotic injuries. Medical toxicology is closely related to clinical toxicology, with the latter discipline encompassing nonphysicians (generally pharmacists) as well [13–16].

Poisoning is a significant global public health problem. Childhood poisonings were recognized as a significant component of pediatric practice and patient morbidity in the 1930. However, little information was present on the toxicity of household products and management recommendations at that time. A Duke University pediatrician, Jay Arena, tried to systematically collect, analyze, and distribute the clinical information to physicians about childhood poisonings. In a case series, the researcher described the clinical outcome of 50 lye-poisoning cases. This was one of the first reports on the hazards of household products to children [17].

Medical toxicology has been improved by the evolution of poison control centers. Poison control centers were established to provide drug and chemical toxicity information and patient management guidance to physicians. These services were expanded to handle telephone calls from laypersons in the 1960s. Arising out of a growing concern over the rising incidence of poisoning worldwide, coupled with a lack of public awareness about its seriousness, poison control centers mainly serve for the public in order to direct information to patients and health-care professionals today. A poison control center is usually managed by a medical toxicologist who specializes in poisonings. These centers also recruit educators for poison prevention programs and provide education activities for health-care personnel and poison prevention organizations [18–20].

In 2017, 84% of poison exposures reported to US poison centers were nontoxic, minimally toxic, or had at most a minor effect. Intentional exposures were significantly more serious, with a 30-fold greater percentage of serious outcomes (major or fatal effects) compared to unintentional exposures. Exposures in teens and adults were also considerably more serious, with 19.09% of teens and 17.91% of adults having a moderate, major, or fatal effect compared to 1.10% of children younger than 6 years. In 2018, 12.1% of poisonings in the USA arose from cosmetics/personal care products, while cleaning substances (household) and analgesics caused 10.7% and 9.0% of the poisonings, respectively. In the same year, analgesics were responsible for 10.9% of all drug poisonings followed by sedatives/hypnotics/antipsychotics (9.3%), antidepressants (7.3%), and cardiovascular drugs (6.5%) [21]. According to data obtained from World Health Organization (WHO), unintentional poisonings claimed the lives of an estimated 193,460 people worldwide in 2012, and the majority of the deaths (84%) were in low- and middle-income countries. Suicide causes the loss of a million people each year and environmental chemicals such as pesticides lead to a significant number deaths annually. It is estimated that deliberate ingestion of pesticides causes 370,000 deaths each year. The problem is getting worse with time as newer drugs and chemicals are developed in vast numbers. On the other hand, snakebites are a largely underappreciated public health problem in many countries and they lead to significant challenges for medical care. While reliable data are hard to obtain, WHO estimated that about 5 million snakebites and 2.5 million envenomings occur each year. As antivenoms are not present in many parts of the world, snake venoms cause at least 100,000 deaths, 300,000 amputations, and many permanent disabilities [22].

Poisoning due to accidental or deliberate ingestion or inhalation of drugs or chemicals is a common, acute medical emergency. For a seriously poisoned patient, a hospital emergency room serves as the initial phase of treatment. For optimal care and treatment of a poisoned patient, clinical toxicologists usually recommend a methodically executed and stepwise approach. The six main steps of the initial clinical encounter for a poisoned patient are: (i) stabilization, (ii) clinical evaluation, (iii) prevention of absorption, (iv) enhancement of elimination, (v) administration of antidote, and (vi) supportive care and clinical follow-up [23–26].

4. Antidotes

An antidote is a substance that can counteract a form of poisoning. There is relatively small number of specific antidotes available for clinical use as it is difficult to develop a specific antidote and the market is very narrow. Furthermore, performing clinical trials in overdose patients have also practical difficulties. Although the Food and Drug Administration (FDA) forces drug companies to develop antidotes through the Orphan Drug Act, there is still need for safer and more specific antidotes today as many antidotes in use have a relatively low margin of safety or therapeutic index [27].

Antidotes have various modes of actions. Some are competitive receptor antagonists (e.g., naloxone, and flumazenil), while some are competitive receptor agonists (e.g., adrenaline and physostigmine). Some antidotes act as competitive enzyme antagonists (e.g., ethanol). Some act as chelating agents and they are mostly used against intoxication with metals [British anti-Lewisite (BAL) and succimer for lead, desferrioxamine for iron, cobalt edetate for cyanide, and calcium for fluoride]. Some antidotes reverse toxic effects on target molecules (glucagon and octreotide), while some use physiological antagonism (benzodiazepines). In some cases, antidotes pharmacologically antagonize the effects of the toxin/toxicant. Antidotes that bind to venoms or toxins are called "antivenoms." The antidote can also facilitate the body clearance of the toxin/toxicant and it is possible for certain chemicals to exert their antidote effects by chemically reacting with biological systems in order to increase the detoxifying capacity for the toxin/toxicant. In order to optimize the treatment of the poisoned patient, medical toxicologists must have detailed knowledge on the therapeutic use of antidotes and when to use them [28, 29].

5. Conclusion

Medical toxicology is an important field of medicine dedicated to the evaluation and treatment of poisoned and envenomated patients. Medical toxicologists mainly investigate the adverse health effects of medications, occupational and environmental toxins, and biological agents and specialize in the preventing, evaluating, treating, and monitoring an injury or illness from toxic exposure.

Medical toxicologists can work in a variety of settings including emergency departments, inpatient units, outpatient clinics, occupational health settings, national and regional poison control centers, academic institutions, industry, commerce, governmental agencies, and clinical and forensic laboratories to serve for public health. Medical toxicology will a more important area of toxicology in the future, as FDA has approved 20–25 new drugs per year in the past two decades and annual approvals in the past 5 years have been in the range of 40–50 new drugs, except for a dip in 2016. Moreover, thousands of chemicals, household products, and cosmetics are introduced to the market every year. Newer, safer, and more effective antidotes should be available. Therefore, medical toxicologists should also put effort on finding antidotes for both old and new drugs as well as for environmental chemicals, toxins, and venoms. Poison control centers should also be more active and effective, particularly in developing countries, in order to reduce emergency hospitalizations and increase the quality of life.

Author details

Pınar Erkekoğlu* and Suna Sabuncuoğlu
Department of Toxicology, Faculty of Pharmacy, Hacettepe University, Ankara, Turkey

*Address all correspondence to: erkekp@yahoo.com; erkekp@hacettepe.edu.tr

References

[1] Klaassen CD, editor. Casarett & Doull's Toxicology – The Basic Science of Poisons. 7th ed. New York: McGraw-Hill Medical Publishing Division; 2008

[2] Schrager TF. Toxicology Source. What is Toxicology? Ph.D. Available from: https://web.archive.org/web/20070310233247/; http://www.toxicologysource.com/whatistoxicology.html [Accessed: 20 July 2020]

[3] National Institute of Environmental Health Sciences (NIEHS). Toxicology. Available from: https://www.niehs.nih.gov/health/topics/science/toxicology/index.cfm [Accessed: 20 July 2020]

[4] Hodgson E, editor. A Textbook of Modern Toxicology. New York: John Wiley and Sons

[5] Anderson AH. Adsorption from gastro-intestinal contents. Experimental studies on the pharmacology of activated charcoal. Acta Pharmaceutica. 1948;**4**:275-284

[6] Tu AT, Gaffield W, editors. Natural and Selected Synthetic Toxins. Biological Implications. Colorado: American Chemical Society Publications; 1999

[7] Tu AT, Sing B, editors. Natural Toxins 2. Structure, Mechanism of Action, and Detection. Colorado: American Chemical Society Publications; 1999

[8] Centers for Disease Control and prevention (CDC). Toxins. Available from: https://www.cdc.gov/biomonitoring/toxins.html [Accessed: 20 July 2020]

[9] U.S. Department of Agriculture. Poisonous Plant Research. Poison Hemlock (*Conium maculatum*). Available from: https://www.ars.usda.gov/pacific-west-area/logan-ut/poisonous-plant-research/docs/poison-hemlock-conium-maculatum/ [Accessed: 20 July 2020]

[10] Keeeler RF, Tu AT. Handbook of Natural Toxins: Toxicology of Plant and Fungal Compounds. Vol. 6. New York: Marcel Decker, Inc; 1991

[11] Kordiš D, Gubenšek F. Adaptive evolution of animal toxin multigene families. Gene. 2000;**261**(1):43-52

[12] Harris JB. Animal poisons and the nervous system: What the neurologist needs to know. Journal of Neurology, Neurosurgery and Psychiatry. 2004;**75**(suppl_3):iii40-iii46

[13] Barceloux DG, editor. Medical Toxicology of Natural Substances: Foods, Fungi, Medicinal Herbs, Plants, and Venomous Animals. 1st ed. USA: John Wiley & Sons Inc; 2008

[14] American College of Medical Toxicology. Becoming a Medical Toxicologist. Available from: https://www.acmt.net/becoming-a-med-tox.html [Accessed: 20 July 2020]

[15] Nelson LS, Neal L, Howland MA, Hoffman RS, Goldfrank LR, Flomenbaum N, editors. Goldfrank's Toxicologic Emergencies. 9th ed. New York: McGraw-Hill Medical Publishing Division; 2010

[16] Dart RC, editor. Medical Toxicology. Philadelphia: Lippincott, Williams & Wilkins; 2003

[17] Martin JM, Arena JM. Lye poisoning and stricture of the esophagus. Southern Medical Journal. 1939;**32**:289-290

[18] Grayson R. The poison control movement in the United States. Indian Medical Surgery. 1962;**31**:296-297

[19] Miller T, Lestina D. Costs of poisoning in the United States

and savings from poison control centers: A benefit-cost analysis. Annals of Emergency Medicine. 1997;**29**(2):239-245

[20] Proudfoot A. Clinical toxicology—Past, present and future. Human Toxicology. 1988;**7**(5):481-487

[21] National Capital Poison Center. Poison Statistics. National Data 2018. Available from: https://www.poison.org/poison-statistics-national [Accessed: 20 July 2020]

[22] World Health Organisation (WHO). Poisoning Prevention and Management. Available from: https://www.who.int/ipcs/poisons/en/ [Accessed: 20 July 2020]

[23] National Health Services (NHS). Treatment. Poisoning. Available from: https://www.nhs.uk/conditions/poisoning/treatment/ [Accessed: 20 July 2020]

[24] Mayo Clinic. Poisoning: First Aid. Available from: https://www.mayoclinic.org/first-aid/first-aid-poisoning/basics/art-20056657 [Accessed: 02 July 2020]

[25] WebMD. Poisoning Treatment. Available from: https://www.webmd.com/first-aid/poisoning-treatment [Accessed: 20 July 2020]

[26] Chandran J, Krishna B. Initial management of poisoned patient. Indian Journal of Critical Care Medicine. 2019;**23**(Suppl 4): S234-S240

[27] Marcus SM, editor. Medical Toxicology: Antidotes and Anecdotes. 1st ed. New Jersey: Springer; 2017

[28] Chacko B, Peter JV. Antidotes in poisoning. Indian Journal of Critical Care Medicine. 2019;**23**(Suppl 4): S241-S249. DOI: 10.5005/jp-journals-10071-23310

[29] World Health Organization (WHO). International Programme on Chemical Safety II. Technical Guidance - 7. Antidotes and Their Availability. Available from: https://www.who.int/ipcs/publications/training_poisons/guidelines_poison_control/en/index7.html [Accessed: 20 July 2020]

Section 2

Venoms

Chapter 2

Venomics Study of *Protobothrops flavoviridis* Snake: How Venom Proteins Have Evolved and Diversified?

Tomohisa Ogawa and Hiroki Shibata

Abstract

Venomics projects have been conducted to disclose the divergent profiles and evolution of various venomous animals. Here, we describe the venomics project including genome and transcriptome of habu snake, leading to drug discovery. Venomics project including the decoding of their whole genomes revealed partly a producing mechanism of various venom proteins including accelerated evolution and alternative splicing and how the toxic organisms have evolved from the nontoxic ones. In addition, the venomics analysis of transcriptomes and proteomes beyond species reveals the relationship between the geographical distribution and evolution of toxic organisms. The abundance of different gene products within a gene family caused by accelerated evolution and alternative splicing may contribute to expand the repertoire of effective weapons to prey capture accompanied with neofunctionalization.

Keywords: alternative splicing, evolution, snake, venomics, whole genome analysis

1. Introduction

A wide variety of creatures, bio-diversified life, have been evolved over 3.8 billion years on earth. Some organisms can produce the biological weapons called "toxins." How have these poisonous organisms evolved to become poisonous? Recent progress on genome sequencing technology has made it possible to analyze the whole genomes of non-model organisms other than model ones and become an important tool for understanding their evolutionary history [1, 2]. "Venomics project" has been undertaken, in which the genomes of a venomous animals are deciphered, and their entire contents of venom are revealed by proteomics and transcriptomics in addition to genome analysis.

2. Toxin-producing organisms

There are various creatures with "toxins" in nature. Toxin derived from living organisms are originally toxic organic compounds such as alkaloids and polyethers produced by plants and phytoplankton and then accumulated through the food chain. On the other hand, the toxins produced by venomous animals are called "venom" and mainly consist of "cocktails" of various bioactive peptides and proteins. In nature, various poisonous animals such as spider (~38,000 species), scorpions (~1400 species), cone snail (~3200 species), and snakes (~800 species) exist. These peptide/protein toxins act specifically on various target sites as a mixture, disrupting the biological function of prey species.

Since each toxic component have been shown to be very selective, specific, and potent, they represent the lead compounds for the development of new drugs, pharmaceutical lead with few side effects, and useful tool which reveals complex mechanisms of life such as central and peripheral nervous, cardiovascular, blood coagulation, complement, and immune systems. In fact, some successful examples of venom-derived peptides and proteins have been already developed and in practical use such as Prialt and ziconotide. Ziconotide is a 25-amino acid peptide ω-conotoxin M isolated from *Conus magus* and blocks neuronal N-type voltage-gated calcium channels, causing a potent analgesic effect for chronic severe pain with 1000 times more effective than morphine. Captopril is also a notable example of pharmaceutical drug derived from toxins as a bradykinin-potentiating peptide isolated from the venom of *Bothrops jararaca* snake and widely used as an anti-hypotensive by inhibition of angiotensin-converting enzyme (ACE). Thus, a variety of toxins are useful as pharmaceutical leads.

3. Venomics projects

The "venomics projects," international joint research projects on various venomous animal genome, transcriptome, and proteome analyses, were proposed at the 14th International Society on Toxinology (IST) held in Adelaide, Australia, in 2003 [3]. These projects aim to obtain the common information to toxic organisms such as snakes, scorpions, spiders, bees, poisonous frogs, cone snails, sea anemones, jellyfishes, etc. They also provided new knowledge that leads to understanding the venom production and transport systems, molecular mechanisms of diversity of venomous proteins, search for new toxic components related to the drug discovery and pharmacological agents that directly relate to unmet medical needs for diseases, and new therapeutic treatments for venom animal bites. For example, the European Venomics Project (completed in October 2015) was based on the several omics analyses (mainly proteome and transcriptome analyses) of 203 venomous animal species ranging from scorpions, corn snails, poisonous spiders, snakes, and lizards, resulting in the identification of 25,000 toxic protein/peptide sequences, of which 4000 were functionally analyzed [4].

In Japan, to elucidate the novel toxins and the diversification mechanism of venom proteins by accelerated evolution, we deciphered the whole genome sequence of habu snake (*Protobothrops flavoviridis*).

To date, genome analysis of venomous animals including sea anemones [5], mites [6], scorpions [7], poisonous frogs [8], and bees [9] has been performed. Furthermore, whole genome sequence analyses of several venomous snakes that include king cobra [10], pygmy rattlesnake [11], saw-scaled viper [12], five-pacer viper [13], Taiwan habu [14], habu [15], hot-spring snake [16], and some sea snakes [17] have been reported in addition to nontoxic snakes such as python [18], boa [11], corn snake [19], and common garter snake [20] (**Table 1**). More recently, near chromosome-level assembly has been also achieved for Indian cobra [21] and garter snake (**Table 1**).

Here, we describe what we have learned from the venomics analyses on the genome and transcriptome decoding of habu snake (*P. flavoviridis*).

	Spiecies	Common name	Accession	ID	Total length (Mb)	GC%	Assembly	Number of genes	Registration date	Ref.	Remarks
1	*Ophiophagus hannah*	King cobra	PRJNA73575	73575	1594.07	40.6	GCA_000516915.1; OphHan1.0; scaffolds: 296,399; contigs: 816,633; N50: 5,201; L50: 71,224	18,445	26-Sep-11	Vonk FJ et al. (2013) [10]	
2	*Python bivittatus*	Burmese python	PRJNA61243	61243	1435.04	39.8	GCA_000186305.2; Python_molurus_bivittatus-5.0.2; scaffolds: 39,113; contigs: 274,244; N50: 10,658; L50: 38,694	25,385	9-Sep-13	Castoe TA et al. (2013) [18]	Non-venomous
3	*Boa constrictor*	Boa constrictor	PRJNA210004	210004	1415.23		scaffolds: 144,256; N50: 16,487	10,793	28-Jun-13	Vicoso B et al., (2013) [11]	Non-venomous
4	*Sistrurus miliarius*	Pygmy rattlesnake	PRJNA210004	210004	1309.02		scaffolds: 187,303; N50: 12,501	11,939	28-Jun-13	Vicoso B et al., (2013) [11]	
5	*Echis coloratus*	Saw-scaled viper	PRJNA252690	252690	1717.11		scaffolds: 4,790,800; N50: 5,576; contig: 4,973,413; N50: 3,857		13-Jun-14	Hargreaves AD et al., (2014) [12]	
6	*Pantherophis guttatus*	Corn snake	PRJNA268069	268069	1404.22	38.3	GCA_001185365.1; PanGut1.0; scaffolds: 883,920; contigs: 1,320,171; N50: 2,394; L50: 138,295	24,258	21-Jul-15	Ullate-Agote A et al. (2014) [19]	Non-venomous
7	*Thamnophis sirtalis*	Common garter snake	PRJNA290790	290790	1424.9	41.8	GCA_001077635.2; Thamnophis_sirtalis-6.0; scaffolds: 7,930; contigs: 175,977; N50: 10,447; L50: 28,683		23-Jul-15	Castoe TA et al. (2011) [20]	Non-venomous TTX-resistance
8	*Deinagkistrodon acutus*	Five-pacer viper / Chinese moccasin	PRJNA314443	314443	1526.36/1473.4		Female: scaffolds: 183,158; N50: 2,018,329; contigs: 297,390; N50: 26,709; Male: scaffolds:160,256; N50: 2,122,253; contigs: 287,757; N50: 22,424	21,194	7-Mar-16	Yin W et al. (2016) [13]	
9	*Protobothrops mucrosquamatus*	Taiwan habu	PRJNA313429	313429	1673.88	40.6	GCA_001527695.3; P.Mucros_1.0; scaffolds: 52,280; contigs: 167,851; N50: 21,948; L50: 19,485	20,122	15-Jan-16	Aird SD et al (2017) [14]	
10	*Protobothrops flavoviridis*	Amami habu	PRJDB5507	484141	1413.2	38.2	GCA_003402635.1; HabAm_1.0; scaffolds: 84,502; contigs: 218,011; N50: 18,879; L50: 20,311	25,134	2-Aug-18	Shibata H et al.(2018) [15]	
11	*Thermophis baileyi*	Bailey's snake / hot-spring snake	PRJNA473624	473624	1747.68		GCA_003457575.1; DSBC_Tbai_1.0; scaffolds: 20,729; contigs: 179,554; N50: 18,227; L50: 25,622	20,995	5-Sep-18	Li JT et al.(2018) [16]	
12	*Laticauda colubrina*	Yellow-lipped sea krait	PRJDB7284	513505	2024.69	35.6	GCA_004320045.1; latCor_1.0; scaffolds: 62,906; contigs: 164,306; N50: 26,721; L50: 18,756		7-Jan-19	Kishida T et al.(2019) [17]	
13	*Hydrophis melanocephalus*	Slender-necked sea snake	PRJDB7271	513504	1402.64	34.8	GCA_004320005.1; hydMel_1.0; scaffolds: 122,022; contigs: 306,746; N50: 7,411; L50: 46,598		7-Jan-19	Kishida T et al.(2019) [17]	
14	*Laticauda laticaudata*	Blue-ringed sea krait	PRJDB7226	513503	1558.71	40.1	GCA_004320025.1; latLat_1.0; scaffolds: 83,587; contigs: 89,677; N50: 35,581; L50: 12,655		7-Jan-19	Kishida T et al.(2019) [17]	
15	*Emydocephalus ijimae*	Ijima's turtleheaded sea snake	PRJDB7221	513502	1625.2	40.3	GCA_004319985.1; emyIji_1.0; scaffolds: 157,858; contigs: 171,534; N50: 18,545; L50: 24,83		7-Jan-19	Kishida T et al.(2019) [17]	
16	*Naja naja*	Indian cobra	PRJNA527614	527614	1768.54	40.39	GCA_009733165.1; Nana_v5; scaffolds: 1,897; contigs: 13,805; N50: 302,474; L50: 1,397	23,248	5-Dec-19	Suryamohan K et al (2020) [21]	Chromosome-level assembly
17	*Thamnophis elegans*	Western terrestrial garter snake	PRJNA561997	561997	1672.19		GCA_009769535.1; rThaEle1; Scaffolds: 365; Contigs:1,883; N50: 4,620,601; L50: 83		19-Dec-19		Non-venomous/ Chromosome-level assembly
18	*Notechis scutatus*	Mainland tiger snake	PRJEB27871	483163	1665.53	40.2	GCA_900518725.1; TS10Xv2-PRI; scaffolds: 52,414; contigs: 131,885; N50: 31,763; L50: 13,462		27-Jul-18		
19	*Pseudonaja textilis*	Eastern brown snake	PRJEB27869	483162	1590.04	40.1	GCA_900518735.1; EBS10Xv2-PRI; scaffolds: 28,550; contigs: 88,019; N50: 50,443; L50: 8,240		27-Jul-18		
20	*Hydrophis cyanocinctus*	Asian annulated sea snake	PRJNA506024	506024	1389.86	37.6	GCA_004023725.1; ASM402372v1; scaffolds: 546,690; contigs: 1,037,439; N50: 3,626; L50: 96,206		19-Nov-18		
21	*Hydrophis hardwickii*	Hardwick's sea snake	PRJNA506024	506024	1296.39	37.2	GCA_004023765.1; ASM402376v1; scaffolds: 616,046; contigs: 1,057,848; N50: 2,852; L50: 115,477		19-Nov-18		

Table 1.
*Whole genome decoding project for habu snake (*P. flavoviridis*) is highlighted in orange color.*

4. What is habu snake, *P. flavoviridis*?

Habu snakes inhabiting in Nansei Islands (Southwest Islands) of Okinawa and Kagoshima prefectures are the most dangerous domestic snakes in Japan (**Figure 1**). Due to their relatively large body size, long attacking range, and a large amount of delivered venom, still many snakebites and envenoming occur especially during farming (about 80 to 100 cases per year). While habu snakes are specific animals designated by Japanese laws, they are subject to extermination as sanitary animals in many habitats, and some are also consumed commercially such as habu liquor and leather products including the Okinawan musical instrument, Sanshin.

Among the 14 species of *Protobothrops* (The Reptile Database: http://www.reptile-database.org/), three species, *P. flavoviridis* from the Amami and the Okinawa islands, *P. tokarensis* from the Tokara Islands, *P. elegans* from the Yaeyama Islands, are endemic to Japan (**Figure 2A**).

In addition to *Protobothrops*, *Ovophis okinavensis* (hime-habu) are distributed from the Amami and Okinawa islands. From the view of geographical history of the Nansei Islands of Japan and Taiwan, it was expected that these *Protobothrops* snakes including the Taiwan habu (*P. mucrosquamatus*), which are distributed in Taiwan, have been diversified from the beginning of the Quaternary Pleistocene to 2.0 million years ago when the islands began to be separated from the continent. Isolated environment on each island resulted in the differentiation and the

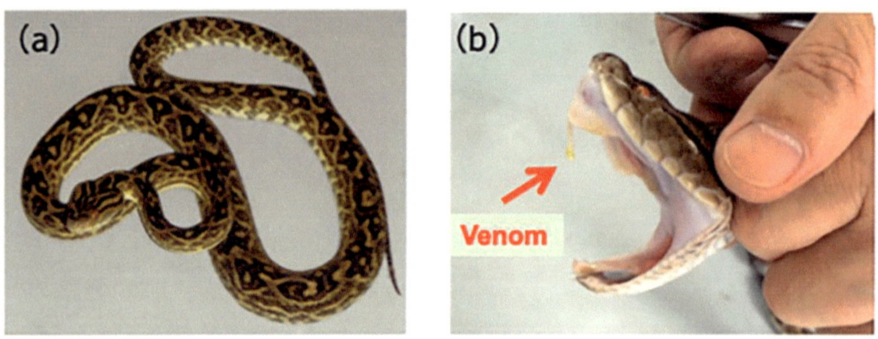

Figure 1.
Protobothrops flavoviridis *snake (a) and its venom (b).*

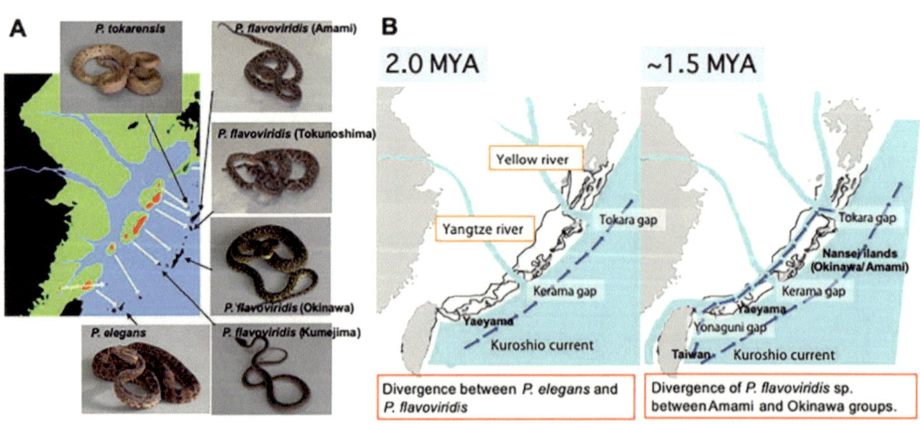

Figure 2.
Distribution of Protobothrops *snakes (a) and geological history of the Nansei Islands in Japan (B).*

speciation of *Protobothrops* species. Molecular phylogenetic analyses using the full-length mtDNA genome sequences of *Protobothrops* snakes showed that the habu snake (*P. flavoviridis*) is close to the Tokara habu (*P. tokarensis*) and Sakishima habu (*P. elegans*) is close to the Taiwan habu (*P. mucrosquamatus*), respectively [22]. These observations are consistent with the geographical history of the Nansei Islands, that is, Okinawa-Amami islands and Taiwan-Yaeyama islands were first separated by Yangtze River (corresponding to the Kerama Gap) and diverged into two groups, the habu (*P. flavoviridis*) and Tokara habu (*P. tokarensis*) species groups and the Sakishima habu (*P. elegans*) and Taiwan habu (*P. mucrosquamatus*) species groups. Further, a remarkable genetic gap between the Amami and Okinawa clades within *P. flavoviridis* was observed. Interestingly, the Tokara habu (*P. tokarensis*) was found to be genetically very close to the Amami clade of *P. flavoviridis* than the Okinawa clade. This indicates that some populations of the Amami clade of *P. flavoviridis* have distributed on the Tokara Islands (Takara and Kodakara islands) and become differentiated to the Tokara habu (*P. tokarensis*) after the divergence of Amami and Okinawa clades. In addition, the Sakishima habu and Taiwan habu diverged as the Yaeyama Islands are separated from Taiwan due to the Yonaguni Gap (**Figure 2B**). Due to the gap of the mouth of the old Yellow River (equivalent to the Tokara Gap), there is no *Protobothrops* snake in the mainland of Japan beyond the Tokara Gap. In summary, the evolutionary history of the speciation of *Protobothrops* in the Nansei Islands is closely associated with the geographical history of the islands.

Snake venoms are potentially lethal complex mixtures composed of proteins and peptides encoded by multigene families that function specific but synergistically to incapacitate the prey or opponent. Venom components can be classified based on their effects as neurotoxic, cardiotoxic, cytotoxic, and hemorrhagic. The viper venoms are known as hemorrhagic toxins that include a wide variety of physiological activities such as metalloproteases (MPs) that destroy blood vessels, phospholipase A_2 (PLA2) that causes inflammation and necrosis, C-type lectin-like proteins (CTLP) and serine proteases (SP) that effect on blood clotting, and so on. Since each of these peptide/protein toxins has very high specificity, it is expected to be a useful tool for clarifying the complex mechanism of life and as a pharmaceutical lead compound. To fully characterize snake venom repertoires and to understand the molecular mechanisms involved in evolution and physiological functions of snake venoms, "venomics studies" including whole genome decoding has been much anticipated.

5. Habu venomics: decoding of the habu genome reveals the evolutionary mechanism of venom-related genes that create a wide variety of venoms

The genome of habu (*P. flavoviridis*) consists of 8 pairs of macro-chromosomes including ZW sex chromosomes and 10 pairs of micro-chromosomes (total 2n = 36). The genome size was estimated to be approximately 1.8 Gb or 1.41 Gb in size by FACS and *k*-mer analysis, respectively [15]. Recently, we decoded the whole genome sequence of habu (*P. flavoviridis*) snake, that is, a total of 136 Gb of shotgun sequences were analyzed and successfully decoded with a sequencing depth of about 96-fold, resulting in the draft genome of habu snake, HabAm1, that include 25,134 protein-coding genes (**Table 1**) [15]. Among 20,540 annotated gene models of HabAm1, we validated 284 genes as venom-related genes, 60 toxic protein genes (SV), and 224 of their non-venom paralog genes (NV). Finally, 18 gene families can be identified as venom-related genes, that is, metalloprotease, serine protease, C-type lectin-like protein, phospholipase A_2, three-finger toxin (3FTX), aminopeptidase (APase), Cys-rich secreted protein (CRISP), 5 'nuclease (5Nase), hyaluronidase (Hyal), nerve growth factor (NGF), vascular endothelial growth factor (VEGF), L-amino acid oxidase (LAAO), bradykinin-enhancing peptide and C-type diuretic peptide (BPP and CNP), and so on (**Figure 3**).

Furthermore, the venom-related genes can be classified into three categories according to the degree of gene duplication (**Figure 3**). Category III consists of four gene families of MP, SP, CTLP, and PLA2, which are major components of venom and highly multiplexed in both SV gene copies and NV paralog. Category II includes 3FTX, APase, and CRISP, which showed moderate multiplexing in both SV gene copies and NV paralogs. Finally, category I, which consists of only 1 SV copy and 2 to 10 copies of NV paralogs, contained other venom-related genes such as LAAO, NGF, VEGF, Hyal, 5Nase, etc. Phylogenetic analyses of these venom-related genes revealed the unique evolutionary aspects of venomous proteins, that is, only one gene out of four copies have gained venom functions during two-round whole genome duplications (2R-WGD) that occurred in the early evolution of vertebrates.

The accelerated evolution phenomenon in venom proteins was first found in the habu snake PLA2 genes [23, 24] and was later found in other animal venom proteins and peptides such as conotoxin [25, 26], scorpion toxins [27, 28], and spider toxins [29]. Although accelerated evolution has been demonstrated in the genes involved in the biodefence molecule and reproduction in addition to the toxin genes [30], their mechanisms are unknown. Using the complete set of SV and NV gene families in the habu genome, molecular evolution rates analysis by computing numbers of synonymous (K_S) and non-synonymous (K_A) nucleotide substitutions per site for each pair suggested that accelerated evolution was observed only in category III and category II, such as SP, PLA2, and CTLP (K_A/K_S ratios: mean +/−SE =1.047 +/−0.438 for svMPs, 1.253 +/− 0.090 for svSPs,

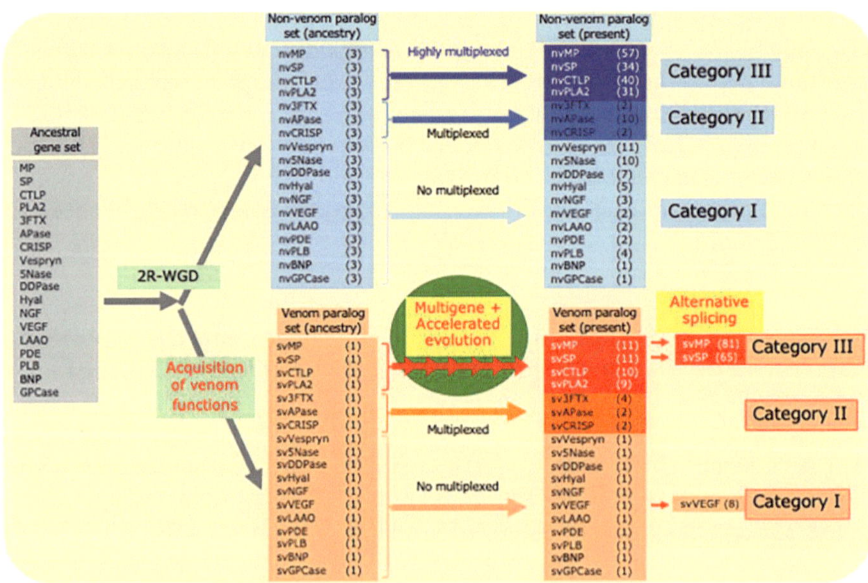

Figure 3.
Deduced evolutionary and diversification history of Protobothrops flavoviridis *snake venom proteins. Through two rounds of whole genome duplication, original set of 18 venom-related gene families (shown in a gray box) became 72 genes (four copies each). Then, a single copy of each family had been a co-option to gain toxic functions, resulting in one toxic gene (shown in an orange box) and three non-venom paralogs (shown in a blue box). Four families of major protein components in the venom (category III: MP, SP, CTLP, and PLA2) have experienced repeated duplication, resulting in complex configurations with 9–11 SV genes and 31–57 NV genes. SV genes in category III showed accelerated evolution. svMP, svSP, and svVEGF were also diversified by alternative splicing.*

0.871 +/− 0.071 for svCTLPs, and 1.093 +/− 0.062 for svPLA2s) [15]. On the other hand, the venom-related genes in category I and NV paralogs in all categories I–III showed no accelerated evolution (K_A/K_S ratios: 0.512 +/− 0.018).

Furthermore, RNA-seq (total of 1.7 billion read pairs, 348 Gb sequence, 1.11 million transcripts identified) from 18 tissues of habu snake and the comprehensive transcript analysis in the venom gland by using PacBio sequencing (~97,000 transcripts) were conducted [31]. Extensive alternative splicing was observed in three venom protein gene families, metalloproteinase (MP), serine protease, and vascular endothelial growth factors (VEGF) with a total of 81, 65, and 8 transcript variants, respectively (**Figure 3**). Especially, svMP showed that over 80 splice variants were transcribed from 11 genes diversified by gene duplication. MPs are key toxins that cause venom-induced pathogenesis such as hemorrhage, fibrinolysis, and apoptosis. According to their domain architecture, svMPs are classified into four groups (P-I to P-IV) (**Figure 4A**). P-I type MPs possess only the metalloproteinase domains and are largely non-hemorrhagic. P-II type MPs contain MP domains and disintegrin domains. P-III type MPs contain Cys-rich domains as well as MP and disintegrin domains. P-IV type MPs harbor lectin-like domains linked by disulfide bonds to the P-III-like structures. These different types of MP proteins can be produced from single MP genes not only by proteolytic processing but also alternatively splicing, resulting in a wider variety of svMPs and disintegrin peptides (**Figure 4B**).

Thus, the alternative splicing is involved in a mechanism for generating diversity of venom proteins in addition to the accelerated evolution [15, 31]. The abundance of different gene products within a gene family caused by accelerated evolution and alternative splicing may contribute to expand the repertoire of effective weapons to prey capture accompanied with neofunctionalization.

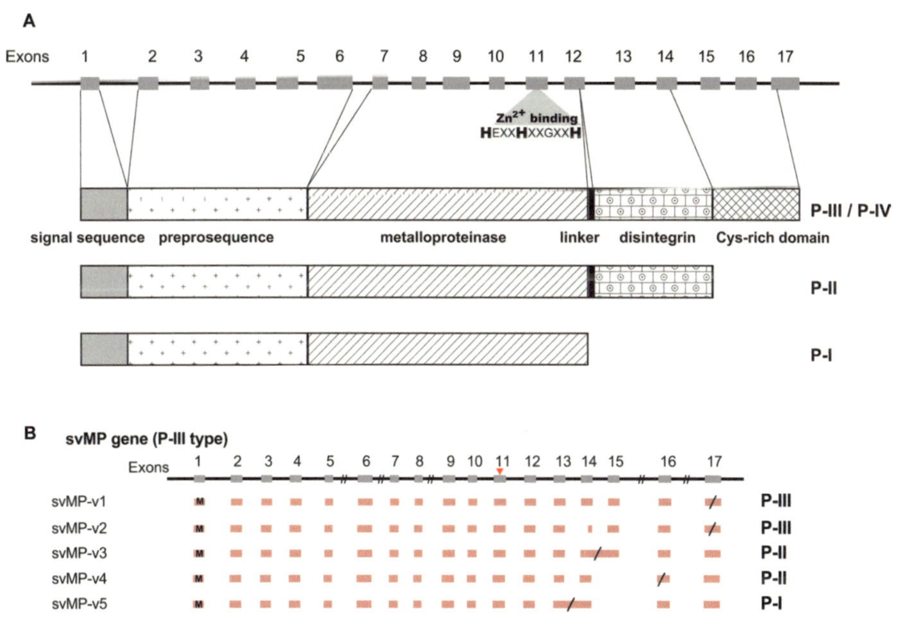

Figure 4.
Schematic structures (A) and alternative splicing (B) of metalloproteinase genes expressed in habu venom glands. (A) the gene structure is shown with 17 exons. A Zn-binding site is also shown in exon 11. Different domains in the three types of MP protein products (P-I, P-II, and P-III/P-IV) are shown as boxes. The active site is also shown by asterisk as "Zn-binding" motif, HEXGHNLGXXHD. P-IV contains lectin-like domain linked by disulfide bonds to the P-III structures. (B) Typical example of P-III type MP gene was shown with validated transcript variants verified in the venom gland, which encode P-I~III type MPs. Initiation and stop codons are marked with "M" and slashes, respectively. Red-colored arrowhead indicates Zn-binding site in exon 11.

6. What comes from venomics project

What did we learn from the "venomics" researches including the decoding of their whole genomes? It revealed partly a producing mechanism of various venom proteins including accelerated evolution and alternative splicing and how the toxic organisms have evolved from the nontoxic ones. In addition, the "venomics" analysis of transcriptomes and proteomes beyond species reveals the relationship between the geographical distribution and evolution of toxic organisms. Recent transcriptomic and proteomic analyses of several snake venoms have reconfirmed in detail that snake venom variation often occurs between individuals of not only interspecifically but also intra-specifically, of which distributions are different geographic locations, diverse environment, and eating habits [32]. For example, a proteomic analysis of 18 species of the genus *Micrurus* snakes in the American continent revealed that the toxic compositions of the major neurotoxins, PLA2, and 3FTX dramatically vary from species to species [32]. Terciopelo (*Bothrops asper*) inhabiting Costa Rica has been also shown to have different toxic compositions between populations from the Pacific coast and from the Caribbean coast. In addition another specie from the same genus, kaisaka (*Bothrops atrox*) inhabiting the same Latin America, also has been shown to have different venom components between Colombia and Brazil [33, 34]. These studies indicate that the composition and structure of the venom varies from region to region even within the same species and that the treatment with anti-venom for snakebites may not work in some areas due to the venom diversity. The envenoming by snakebites is estimated to be about 5 million people annually worldwide, of which about 125,000 die and 400,000 suffer from sequelae such as the loss of extremities [35]. Currently, although anti-venom is currently the only effective treatment for snakebites, there are some cases where the anti-venom production is discontinued due to the economical or political reasons. This serious situation was pointed out by the World Health Organization (WHO) as "neglected tropical disease" [36]. Venomics research is important to develop the anti-venom by using protein engineering techniques against unknown venom proteins, which are obtained by genome decoding, and to understand the mechanism of action of the venom. Venomics research will also lead to the discovery of new useful tools for clarifying the complex mechanisms of life and new functional molecules useful as pharmaceutical leads. For example, three-finger toxins, which have been known as major components of Elapidae and Hydrophiidae neurotoxins, were found in habu snake genome [15].

Whole genome analysis is a powerful tool to understand molecular mechanisms involved in snake venom evolution. We expect that the whole genome analyses of wider variety of venomous species will accelerate the acquisition of useful comprehensive information about different mixtures of venom proteins encoded by different sets of genes and the understanding of the evolutionary histories of venom systems and the common features of venomous animals.

Acknowledgements

This work was supported by Grants-in-Aid of MEXT, Japan (#25440214 and #18H02498 to H.S., #24651130 and #23107505 to T.O.). This work was partly supported by the Cooperative Research Project Program of the Medical Institute of Bioregulation, Kyushu University (T.O.).

Conflict of interest

The authors declare no conflict of interest.

Author details

Tomohisa Ogawa[1*] and Hiroki Shibata[2]

1 Graduate School of Agricultural Science, Tohoku University, Sendai, Japan

2 Division of Genomics, Medical Institute of Bioregulation, Kyushu University, Fukuoka, Japan

*Address all correspondence to: tomohisa.ogawa.c3@tohoku.ac.jp

References

[1] Ellegren H. Genome sequencing and population genomics in non-model organisms. Trends in Ecology & Evolution. 2014;**29**:51-63. DOI: 10.1016/j.tree.2013.09.008

[2] Gouin A, Legeai F, Nouhaud P, Whibley A, Simon J-C, Lemaitre C. Whole-genome re-sequencing of non-model organisms: Lessons from unmapped reads. Heredity. 2015;**114**: 494-501. DOI: 10.1038/hdy.2014.85

[3] Ménez A, Stöcklin R, Mebs D. 'Venomics' or: The venomous systems genome project. Toxicon. 2006; **47**(3):255-259. DOI: 10.1016/j. toxicon.2005.12.010

[4] Nzytech Genes & Tech News: The European VENOMIMCS Project Ends with the Creation of the Largest Database of Toxins in History [Internet]. 2015. Available from: https://www.nzytech.com/news/the-european-venomics-project-ends-with-the-creation-of-the-largest-database-of-toxins-in-history/ [Accessed: 30 January]

[5] Putnam NH, Srivastava M, Hellsten U, Dirks B, Chapman J, Salamov A, et al. Sea anemone genome reveals ancestral eumetazoan gene repertoire and genomic organization. Science. 2007;**317**(5834):86-94. DOI: 10.1126/science.1139158

[6] Grbić M, Leeuwen TV, Clark RM, Rombauts S, Rouzé P, Grbić V, et al. The genome of *Tetranychus urticae* reveals herbivorous pest adaptations. Nature. 2011;**479**:487-492. DOI: 10.1038/nature10640

[7] Cao Z, Yu Y, Wu Y, Hao P, Di Z, He Y, et al. The genome of Mesobuthus martensii reveals a unique adaptation model of arthropods. Nature Communications. 2013;**4**:2602. DOI: 10.1038/ncomms3602

[8] Sanggaard KW, Bechsgaard JS, Fang X, Duan J, Dyrlund TF, Gupta V, et al. Spider genomes provide insight into composition and evolution of venom and silk. Nature Communications. 2014;**5**:3765. DOI: 10.1038/ncomms4765

[9] Sadd BM, Barribeau SM, Bloch G, de Graaf DC, Dearden P, Elsik CG, et al. The genomes of two key bumblebee species with primitive eusocial organization. Genome Biology. 2015;**16**:76. DOI: 10.1186/s13059-015-0623-3

[10] Vonk FJ, Casewell NR, Henkel CV, Heimberg AM, Jansen HJ, McCleary RJR, et al. The king cobra genome reveals dynamic gene evolution and adaptation in the snake venom system. Proceedings of the National Academy of Sciences of the United States of America. 2013;**110**:20651-20656. DOI: 10.1073/pnas.1314702110

[11] Vicoso B, Emerson JJ, Zektser Y, Mahajan S, Bachtrog D. Comparative sex chromosome genomics in snakes: Differentiation, evolutionary strata, and lack of global dosage compensation. PLoS Biology. 2013;**11**(8):e1001643. DOI: 10.1371/journal.pbio.1001643

[12] Hargreaves AD, Swain MT, Hegarty MJ, Logan DW, Mulley JF. Genomic and transcriptomic insights into the regulation of snake venom production. bioRxiv 008474; 2014. DOI: 10.1101/008474

[13] Yin W, Wang Z, Li Q, Lian J, Zhou Y, Lu B, et al. Evolutionary trajectories of snake genes and genomes revealed by comparative analyses of five-pacer viper. Nature Communications. 2016;**7**:13107. DOI: 10.1038/ncomms13107

[14] Aird SD, Arora J, Barua A, Qiu L, Terada K, Mikheyev AS. Population genomic analysis of a pitviper reveals microevolutionary forces underlying

venom chemistry. Genome Biology and Evolution. 2017;**9**(10):2640-2649. DOI: 10.1093/gbe/evx199

[15] Shibata H, Chijiwa T, Oda-Ueda N, Nakamura H, Yamaguchi K, Hattori S, et al. The habu genome reveals accelerated evolution of venom protein genes. Scientific Reports. 2018;**8**(1):11300. DOI: 10.1038/s41598-018-28749-4

[16] Li JT, Gao YD, Xie L, Deng C, Shi P, Guan ML, et al. Comparative genomic investigation of high-elevation adaptation in ectothermic snakes. Proceedings of the National Academy of Sciences of the United States of America. 2018;**115**(33):8406-8411. DOI: 10.1073/pnas.1805348115

[17] Kishida T, Go Y, Tatsumoto S, Tatsumi K, Kuraku S, Toda M. Loss of olfaction in sea snakes provides new perspectives on the aquatic adaptation of amniotes. Proceedings of the Royal Society B. 2019;**286**:1828. DOI: 10.1098/rspb.2019.1828

[18] Castoe TA, de Koning APJ, Hall KT, Card DC, Schield DR, Fujita MK, et al. The Burmese python genome reveals the molecular basis for extreme adaptation in snakes. Proceedings of the National Academy of Sciences of the United States of America. 2013;**110**:20645-20650. DOI: 10.1073/pnas.1314475110

[19] Ullate-Agote A, Milinkovitch MC, Tzika AC. The genome sequence of the corn snake (Pantherophis guttatus), a valuable resource for EvoDevo studies in squamates. The International Journal of Developmental Biology. 2014;**58**: 881-888. DOI: 10.1387/ijdb

[20] Castoe TA, Bronikowski AM, Brodie ED III, Edwards SV, Pfrender ME, Shapiro MD, et al. A proposal to sequence the genome of a garter snake (*Thamnophis sirtalis*). Standards in Genomic Sciences. 2011;**4**:257-270. DOI: 10.4056/sigs.1664145

[21] Suryamohan K, Krishnankutty SP, Guillory J, et al. The Indian cobra reference genome and transcriptome enables comprehensive identification of venom toxins. Nature Genetics. 2020;**52**:106-117. DOI: 10.1038/s41588-019-0559-8

[22] Shibata H, Chijiwa T, Hattori S, Terada K, Ohno M, Fukumaki Y. The taxonomic position and the unexpected divergence of the Habu viper, Protobothrops among Japanese subtropical islands. Molecular Phylogenetics and Evolution. 2016;**101**:91-100. DOI: 10.1016/j.ympev.2016.04.027

[23] Nakashima K, Ogawa T, Oda N, Hattori M, Sakaki Y, Kihara H, et al. Accelerated evolution of Trimeresurus flavoviridis venom gland phospholipase A2 isozymes. Proceedings of the National Academy of Sciences of the United States of America. 1993;**90**:5964-5968. DOI: 10.1073/pnas.90.13.5964

[24] Nakashima K, Nobuhisa I, Deshimaru M, Nakai M, Ogawa T, Shimohigashi Y, et al. Accelerated evolution in the protein-coding regions is universal in crotalinae snake venom gland phospholipase A2 isozyme genes. Proceedings of the National Academy of Sciences of the United States of America. 1995;**92**:5605-5609. DOI: 10.1073/pnas.92.12.5605

[25] Duda TF, Palumbi SR. Molecular genetics of ecological diversification: Duplication and rapid evolution of toxin genes of the venomous gastropod Conus. Proceedings of the National Academy of Sciences of the United States of America. 1999;**96**(12):6820-6823. DOI: 10.1073/pnas.96.12.6820

[26] Phuong MA, Mahardika GN. Targeted sequencing of venom genes from cone snail genomes improves understanding of Conotoxin molecular evolution. Molecular Biology and Evolution. 2018;**35**(5):1210-1224. DOI: 10.1093/molbev/msy034

[27] Gao B, Zhu S. Accelerated evolution and functional divergence of scorpion short-chain K+ channel toxins after speciation. Comp. Biochem. Phys. Part B, Biochem & Mol Biol. 2012;**163**(2):238-245. DOI: 10.1016/j.cbpb.2012.06.002

[28] Zhang S, Gao B, Zhu S. Target-driven evolution of scorpion toxins. Scientific Reports. 2015;**5**:14973. DOI: 10.1038/srep14973

[29] Pineda SS, Sollod BL, Wilson D, et al. Diversification of a single ancestral gene into a successful toxin superfamily in highly venomous Australian funnel-web spiders. BMC Genomics. 2014;**15**:177. DOI: 10.1186/1471-2164-15-177

[30] Ogawa T. Molecular diversity of proteins in biological offense and defense systems. Molecular Diversity. 2006;**10**(4):511-514. DOI: 10.1007/s11030-006-9048-y

[31] Ogawa T, Oda-Ueda N, Hisata K, Nakamura H, Chijiwa T, Hattori S, et al. Alternative mRNA splicing in three venom families underlying a possible production of divergent venom proteins of the Habu Snake, Protobothrops flavoviridis. Toxins. 2019;**11**(10):581. DOI: 10.3390/toxins11100581

[32] Lomonte B, Rey-Suárez P, Fernández J, Sasa M, Pla D, Vargas N, et al. Venoms of micrurus coral snakes: Evolutionary trends in compositional patterns emerging from proteomic analyses. Toxicon. 2016;**122**:7-25. DOI: 10.1016/j.toxicon.2016.09.008

[33] Alape-Girón A, Sanz L, Escolano J, Flores-Díaz M, Madrigal M, Sasa M, et al. Snake venomics of the lancehead pitviper Bothrops asper: Geographic, individual, and ontogenetic variations. Journal of Proteome Research. 2008;**7**(8):3556-3571. DOI: 10.1021/pr800332p

[34] Núñez V, Cid P, Sanz L, Torre PD, Angulo Y, Lomonte B, et al. Snake venomics and antivenomics of Bothrops atrox venoms from Colombia and the Amazon regions of Brazil, Perú and Ecuador suggest the occurrence of geographic variation of venom phenotype by a trend towards paedomorphism. Journal of Proteomics. 2009;**73**(1-2):57-78. DOI: 10.1016/j.jprot.2009.07.013

[35] The Lancet. Snake bite- the neglected tropical disease. Lancet. 2015;**386**(9999):1110

[36] WHO Fact sheets, Snakebite Envenoming Available from: https://www.who.int/en/news-room/fact-sheets/detail/snakebite-envenoming

Chapter 3

Snakebite Therapeutics Based on Endogenous Inhibitors from Vipers

Narumi Aoki-Shioi and Cassandra M. Modahl

Abstract

Venomous snakebite is a major human health issue in many countries and has been categorized as a neglected tropical disease by the World Health Organization. Venomous snakes have evolved to produce venom, which is a complex mixture of toxic proteins and peptides, both enzymatic and nonenzymatic in nature. In this current era of high-throughput technologies, venomics projects, which include genome, transcriptome, and proteome analyses of various venomous species, have been conducted to characterize divergent venom phenotypes and the evolution of venom-related genes. Additionally, venomics can also inform about mechanisms of toxin production, storage, and delivery. Venomics can guide antivenom and therapeutic strategies against envenomations and identify new toxin-derived drugs/tools. One potentially promising drug development direction is the use of endogenous inhibitors present in snake venom glands and serum that could be useful for snakebite therapeutics. These inhibitors suppress the activity of venom proteases, enzymatic proteins responsible for the irreversible damage from snakebite. This book chapter will focus on insights from venomous snake adaptations, such as the evolution of venom proteases to generate diverse activities and snake natural resistance to inhibit activity, and how this information can inform and have applications in the treatment of venomous snakebite.

Keywords: venomous snake, snake venom metalloprotease, hemorrhagic, nonhemorrhagic, toxin resistance, natural inhibitor, endogenous inhibitor

1. Introduction

There are over 3700 extant snake species, but only approximately 200 in 600 venomous snake species, belonging to families Viperidae, Elapidae, Atractaspididae, and some of Colubridae, are considered medically important on public health aspects of snakebite [https://www.who.int/snakebites/disease/en/; http://www.reptile-database.org/, Accessed: 2019-11-22]. The World Health Organization (WHO) has recognized snakebite envenomation as a neglected tropical disease and has characterized a subset of venomous snake species as being of higher medical importance in the four geographical areas of the world snakebite is most frequent. The definition of highest medical importance to human public health (category 1) is "highly venomous snakes which are common or widespread and cause numerous snakebites, resulting in high levels of morbidity, disability, or mortality" [1]. These species are predominately from Elapidae and Viperidae families, but the majority of these species are from the family Viperidae (vipers and pit vipers). Viperidae species consist of approximately 50–100% of listed species in each geographical area and make up just over 60% of the entire list (**Table 1**).

Venom variation results in pharmacological and clinical symptomology differences across venomous snake species, primarily varying in the extent of snakebite tissue damage and toxicity. In recent years, venom has been investigated using comprehensive venomics approaches, combining proteomics, transcriptomics, and genomics, in an attempt to better understand venom components responsible for variation. Next-generation sequencing (NGS) has greatly accelerated the pace of

Geographical regions		Species	Total
Africa and the Middle East	Atractaspididae	*Atractaspis andersonii*	1
	Elapidae	*Dendroaspis viridis, Dendroaspis angusticeps, Dendroaspis jamesoni, Dendroaspis polylepis; Naja anchietaea, Naja annulifera, Naja asheia, Naja arabica, Naja haje, Naja katiensis, Naja melanoleuca, Naja mossambica, Naja nigricollis, Naja nigricincta, Naja nivea, Naja oxiana, Naja senegalensis*	17
	Viperidae	*Bitis arietans, Bitis gabonicaa, Bitis nasicornis, Bitis rhinocerosa; Cerastes cerastes, Cerastes gasperettii; Daboia mauritanicaa, Daboia palaestinaea; Echis borkini, Echis carinatus, Echis coloratus, Echis jogeri, Echis leucogaster, Echis ocellatus, Echis omanensisa, Echis leucogaster, Echis pyramidum; Macrovipera lebetina, Montivipera xanthina1; Pseudocerastes persicus,*	20
Asia and Australasia	Elapidae	*Acanthophis laevisa; Bungarus caeruleus, Bungarus candidus, Bungarus niger, Bungarus magnimaculatus, Bungarus multicinctus, Bungarus sindanus, Bungarus walli; Naja atra, Naja kaouthia, Naja naja, Naja mandalayensis, Naja philippinensis, Naja samarensis, Naja siamensis, Naja sumatrana, Naja sputatrix, Naja oxiana; Notechis scutatus; Oxyuranus scutellatus; Pseudonaja affinis, Pseudechis australisb, Pseudonaja mengdeni, Pseudonaja nuchalis, Pseudonaja textilis.*	25
	Viperidae	*Cryptelytrops albolabrisa, Cryptelytrops erythrurusa, Cryptelytrops insularisa, Calloselasma rhodostoma; Deinagkistrodon acutus, Daboia russeliia, Daboia siamensisa; Deinagkistrodon acutu; Echis carinatus; Gloydius blomhoffii, Gloydius brevicaudus, Gloydius halys; Hypnale hypnale; Macrovipera lebetina, Protobothrops flavoviridis, Protobothrops mucrosquamatus; Viridovipera stejnegeria,*	17
Europe	Viperidae	*Vipera ammodytes, Vipera berus, Vipera aspis,*	3
the Americas	Viperidae	*Agkistrodon bilineatus, Agkistrodon contortrix, Agkistrodon piscivorus, Agkistrodon tayloria; Bothrops asper, Bothrops atrox, Bothrops cf. atrox (Trinidad), Bothrops bilineatus, Bothrops alternatus, Bothrops brazili, Bothrops caribbaeus (St Lucia), Bothrops lanceolatus (Martinique), Bothrops diporusa, Bothrops jararaca, Bothrops jararacussu, Bothrops leucurus, Bothrops mattogrossensisa, Bothrops moojeni, Bothrops pictus, Bothrops venezuelensis; Crotalus adamanteus, Crotalus atrox, Crotalus durissus, Crotalus durissus (Aruba), Crotalus horridus, Crotalus oreganusa, Crotalus simus, Crotalus scutulatus, Crotalus totonacusa, Crotalus viridis, Lachesis muta*	31

Table 1.
Venomous snakes of highest medical importance (category 1); The table was modified classified sub-area in each of four broad geographical regions in tables 3-6 of Fifty-ninth report/WHO Expert Committee.

venomics, making high-throughput outputs possible; several venom gland transcriptomes can be sequenced together using multiplexed barcoded libraries, with little difference in cost, and third-generation longer read technologies, such as Oxford Nanopore (minION), are now available to correct transcriptome assembly errors [2]. Venom characterization that integrates both transcriptomics with proteomics has optimized proteomics by providing a species-specific database (venom gland transcriptome) for toxin identification, an ideal method to better distinguish unique toxins present in each species [3]. Current venom gland transcriptomes, completed using NGS technologies (Illumina and Roche) and *E. coli*, generated cDNA clone libraries, and assembled genomes of venomous snakes categorized as of highest medical importance are listed in **Table 2**. In our investigation, completed

	Venom gland transcriptomes		Venomous snake genomes	
	Species	**Reference**	**Species**	**Reference**
Elapidae	*Naja kaouthia,*	[4, 5]	*Notechis scutatus*	Unpublished
	Dendroaspis angusticeps,	[6]	*Pseudonaja textilis*	Unpublished
	Dendroaspis jamesoni,	[6]		
	Dendroaspis polylepis,	[6]		
	Dendroaspis viridis	[6]		
	Pseudonaja nuchalis	[7]		
	Pseudonaja textilis	[7]		
Viperidae	*Agkistrodon piscivorus*	[2, 8]	*Deinagkistrodon acutus*	[33]
	leucostoma	[9]	*Protobothrops mucrosquamatus*	[34]
	Bitis gabonica	[10]	*Protobothrops flavoviridis*	[35]
	Bothrops alternatus	[11, 12]	*Vipera berus*	[36]
	Bothrops asper	[13, 14]	*Crotalus viridis*	[37]
	Bothrops atrox	[4, 13, 15–17]	*Crotalus horridus*	[38]
	Bothrops jararaca,	[18]		
	Bothrops jararacussu	[19–21]		
	Bothrops moojeni	[19, 20, 22, 23]		
	Crotalus adamanteus	[24, 25]		
	Crotalus durissus terrificus	[12, 24]		
	Crotalus horridus	[26]		
	Crotalus oreganus helleri	[26]		
	Crotalus scutulatus,	[11, 27, 28]		
	Crotalus simus	[29]		
	Echis carinatus shochureki	[29, 30]		
	Echis coloratus	[66, 31]		
	Echis ocellatus	[29]		
	Echis pyramidum leakeyi	[32]		
	Lachesis muta	[11]		
	Protobothrops flavoviridis			

Table 2.
Venom gland transcriptomes and currently completed snake genomes of species in category 1.

transcriptomes in snake species in category 1 are only about 20% despite the advance in increasing sequencing data. Additionally, on the completed snake genome, sequences are also less than 10% limited number.

Transcriptome and proteome analyses of Viperidae species have consistently found that snake venom metalloproteinases (SVMPs), phospholipases A_2 (PLA_2s), serine proteinases, and L-amino acid oxidases are the most abundant toxins in these venoms [39]. These toxins are all enzymatic, providing immobilization and digestive roles in prey capture. Snakebites from these species result in local tissue damage, hemorrhage, and impaired coagulation symptoms in humans, which can lead to disability and mortality [40].

To date, the only effective snakebite treatment is intravenous administration of antibodies (often called antivenom), which come from animals immunized with toxins. However, using heterologous antibodies generated from numerous venom components has inherent weaknesses, such as an increased likelihood of an allergic reaction or life-threatening anaphylactic shock. Further, antivenom does not abolish local tissue damage, as it is intravenous and is usually not administered quickly enough. Thus, there is the issue of incomplete neutralization because of geographic venom variation, and high manufacturing costs and regulations have resulted in a struggle to properly match antivenom to venomous snakes of each locality and maintain antivenom stock [40]. To alleviate these issues, specific toxin inhibitors are actively being characterized and evaluated that neutralize snake venom toxicity and would work as an alternative antivenom snakebite therapy [41–43]. The challenge still remains to investigate the safety and efficiency of these toxin inhibitors to treat snakebite envenoming in humans.

Venomous snakes have endogenous inhibitors circulating in their plasma that provide resistance to their own venoms. These inhibitors can suppress the activity of enzymatic venom components, such as SVMPs, with high specificity. SVMPs are key venom components in viper venoms that contribute to hemorrhage and tissue damage; therefore, targeting these enzymes would greatly reduce human morbidity and mortality from snakebite. In this review, an overview of SVMPs is provided, with a focus on structure-function relationships within the various classes of SVMPS across snake families, and is followed by insights into how snake endogenous inhibitors function to abolish SVMP activity. The goal of our group is to design peptide inhibitors that bind to hemorrhagic SVMPs with high affinity and effectively neutralize these toxins. This chapter deeply understands the target SVMP behaviors on the snakebite issue and is a summary of our current work with historical studies in endogenous inhibitor of venomous snake.

2. Metalloproteinases

Metalloproteinases (MPs) are one of the most functionally diverse proteases in more than 50 families characterized in the MEROP database [44]. MPs play a significant role in organism homeostasis, and are involved in, cell invasion, cell fertilization, self-defense, and reproduction. Metalloproteinases are classified into two subgroups known by their enzyme commission numbers (ECNs), exopeptidases (ECN 3.4.17), and endopeptidases (ECN 3.4.24). The second group are enzymes from the metzincin family and include serralysins, astacins, adamalysins (a disintegrin and metalloproteinase domain; ADAMs), and matrix metalloproteinases (MMPs). There have been many studies documenting endogenous metalloproteinase dysregulation in cancer cells [45], especially mammalian ADAMs. ADAM proteins and SVMPs belonged to the same M12 family [46], and similar domain features are present for both. For SVMPs, three-dimensional structures and well-characterized effects on animal models in vivo have been published. Thus, the functional and structural insights provided by SVMPs have been useful for human ADAM inferences.

2.1 Structural classification of snake venom metalloproteinases (SVMPs)

All SVMP genes exhibit a conserved signal peptide region and a pro-(pre) domain. The number of domains following these conserved N-terminal regions varies, and the arrangements of the domains have resulted in the categorization of SVMPs into three main classes. SVMPs of the P-III class consist of the metalloproteinase domain (MD), disintegrin-like domain (DID), and cysteine-rich domain (CRD). P-IIs have a MD and DID, and P-I has only a MD. Further, each class has subclasses classified for different representation forms (P-Ia, P-IIa-e, P-IIIa-d). These subclasses include dimeric or truncate isoforms that have only been observed within the venom and are generated mainly by post-translational modifications.

There have been many observations of gene neofunctionalization generating large families of venom proteins with multiple functionalities, and the SVMP gene family is an example of this. SVMPs originated from the gene duplication of an ancestral ADAM gene. The ADAM 28 precursor gene is the closed SVMP homolog present in nonvenomous snakes and is also present in mammalian species [47, 48]. Sequence comparisons between the lizard (*Anolis carolinensis*) ADAM 28 gene and viper (*Echis ocellatus*) SVMP gene suggested that SVMPs originated from a nonsense mutation following ADAM gene duplication. This nucleotide substitution resulted in a chain-termination codon (STOP codon) at the end of exon 12, following the CRD. The modified gene precursor produced proteins that were devoid of the C-terminal membrane anchor and cytoplasmic region present in ADAMs [49]. As more snake genome sequences have become available, it has been hypothesized that the ancestral SVMP coded for the P-III class of SVMPs. Gene duplications of P-III SVMPs resulted in P-II and P-I SVMP genes, each generated by domain loss from splicing site mutations. These last two classes, P-II and P-I, are only found in Viperidae. The reason why a large number of different SVMPs are expressed in viper venoms is still unclear, even though some of these SVMPs are not primary lethal toxins.

SVMPs constitute more than 30% of the total venom proteins present in many Viperidae species. While these proteins are less abundant in the venoms of Elapidae, Atractaspididae, and Colubridae, they appear to be ubiquitously occurring [50, 51]. These observations suggest that P-III SVMP in Elapidae, Atractaspididae, and Colubridae venoms may have a conserve ancestral function and serve a common biological role in snake envenomation. Therefore, the functional roles of the diversified SVMPs are important for the clinical symptomology associated with Viperidae envenoming in humans. Domain structure, at least the topological shape, and sequence, especially the catalytic motif on the MD, are very similar among SVMPs, but SVMP activities vary, including their target substrates. Elucidating the structure-function relationships within this protein superfamily has applications for both protein evolution and snakebite treatment.

2.2 SVMP structure-function relationships and mechanism of action

Viperid snakebites are characterized by severe hemorrhagic, microvessel damage and inflammation, both local and systemic [52]. There is strong evidence from in vivo and in vitro studies of isolated SVMPs that these proteins are responsible for snakebite hemorrhage. Mitigating hemorrhage is critical in snakebite treatment; therefore studying the SVMP molecular mechanism of inducing hemorrhage is of critical importance. Hemorrhage results from SVMP proteolysis, targeted cleavage of extracellular matrix components, transmembrane receptors, and fibrinogen, mostly around microvessels. Interestingly, despite sharing similar catalytic activity, not all SVMPs induce hemorrhage in vivo. SVMP effects also include blood coagulation irregularities, platelet aggregation, cell infiltration, apoptosis-induced activity, and alternations in vascular permeability, even if these SVMPs do not show hemorrhagic activity [52]. These additional functionalities and targets likely result from C-terminal P-III SVMP binding, not only the catalytic activity of the N-terminally located MP domain [53]. To design inhibitors to neutralized hemorrhagic effects of SVMPs, we must first understand SVMP targets, as well as the tissue distribution and localization of SVMPs upon envenomation.

Both of P-III and P-I SVMPs have hemorrhagic activities, but P-III SVMPs tend to show greater hemorrhagic activity than P-I SVMPs [54, 55]. It has been proposed that the occurrence of hemorrhage results from the degradation of the vascular basement membrane of capillaries. Immunofluorescence confocal microscopy, immunochemical and proteomic analyses of tissue, and exudate in vivo have revealed a distinct pattern of P-I and P-III SVMP distribution in tissue. Observations from SVMPs labeled with Alexa Fluor 647 have found that P-III SVMP co-localized with capillary collagen IV, especially in those of microvesicles. P-I SVMPs applied to whole tissues appear to function primarily in the degradation of basement membrane components [56]. Hemorrhagic P-I and P-III SVMPs show a preference for type IV collagen in targeted degradation. J.M. Gutiérrez et al. provided a two-step hypothesis for SVMP mechanism of hemorrhage [56]. First, SVMPs hydrolyze type IV collagen and perlecan at the basement membrane components of capillaries and surrounding endothelial cells, resulting in a weakening of the mechanical stability of the basement membrane and microvessel wall. The second step occurs when the biophysical hemodynamic forces operating in microcirculation induce a distention in the wall, causing capillaries to disrupt, followed by consequent extravasation.

SVMP hemorrhage disrupts capillary networks, facilitating toxin dispersion. In 2016, reviews by Sanhajariya and colleagues investigated snake venom pharmacokinetics using an ELISA time course, varying venom concentrations mixed with the plasma of laboratory animals (rat, rabbit, and sheep) and humans [57]. In laboratory animals, two phases were observed in the metabolism of snake venom by intravenous injection of the venoms or toxins: the first phase consisting of rapid distribution with half-lives of 5–48 min and a second a slow elimination phase with half-lives of 0.8–28 h. Half-lives of the second phase did not show a significant difference among the species (*Bothrops alternatus*, *Vipera aspis*, and *Naja* sp.) explored under intravenous injection, but *Naja* sp. did show a twofold shorter phase time than *Vipera aspis* 32 hours after intermuscular injection. For humans, venom concentrations in plasma were examined from 24 pharmacokinetic studies in humans that used similar ELISA criteria. Venom concentrations of the patients bitten by vipers were typically higher than those of by elapids. Eventually, total 218 timed concentration data of 145 patients bitten by snakes of Viperidae and Elapid were used for the computational analysis within a nonlinear mixed-effects modeling framework with NONMEM. The result provided an estimated venom elimination half-life of 9.71 ± 1.29 h. Interestingly, these data also show that there is no big difference between Viperid and Elapid. It is very important to understand the certain pharmacokinetic of venom for post-treatment of inhibitor to neutralize toxicity of venoms.

3. Toxin resistance in venomous snakes

Given the toxic and proteolytic nature of venom, it is of the utmost importance that venomous snakes are protected against the activity of their own venom. This is an interesting area of research because venoms, especially viper venoms, have high concentrations of proteases that must be stored in an inactive state in the venom gland to prevent degradation of both the snake's own tissue and other proteins present in the venom. These proteases must then be readily activated when delivered into prey, requiring a finely tuned on/off switch. Here, we briefly summarize how these toxins are regulated in snake venom glands, with a focus on endogenous inhibitors, especially SVMP inhibitors, as SVMPs are one of the major venom compounds in Viperid snake venoms.

3.1 Mechanisms of toxin resistance

Three toxin resistance mechanisms have been proposed for venomous snakes: (1) target receptor mutations, (2) venom gland physiological conditions, and (3) inhibitors present in the venom gland or blood circulation. For the first mechanism, limited mutations on target receptors in snakes prevent the binding of their own toxins [58–60]. An example of this has been described by Takacs et al., where resistance against conspecific α-neurotoxins, major lethal components of Elapidae venoms, has been shown to be mediated by a unique N-glycosylation of the nicotinic acetylcholine receptor ligand binding domain of Elapidae snakes [58]. This observation has only been made for a few Elapidae species, but there is currently a limited amount of research in this area. The second mechanism involves the physiological conditions within the venom gland and those required for enzymatic toxins to be active. A high concentration of citrate is present in venom, and this results in a low pH environment. It is estimated that 25% of dried crude venom (30–150 mM) from *Crotalus* sp., *Agkistrodon* sp., *Bothrops* sp. *Dendroaspis* sp., *Sistrurus miliarius barbouri*, *Bitis gabonica gabonica*, *Vipera russellii russellii*, and *Lachesis muta* is citrate. Citrate concentrations of 18 or 27 mM exogenously added to whole venom have been shown to inhibit protease activity in vitro [61]. Secreted whole venom of *Crotalus* sp. has been observed to be acidic (pH 5.25–5.75), suggestive of an acidic storage condition for venom enzymes, which then when delivered into prey or human tissue at a pH of 7.2–7.4, these enzymes become activated [62]. In addition to the acidic storage conditions of the venom gland, four tripeptide inhibitors of venom metalloproteinases, pEKW, pENW, pEQW, and pERW, have been documented in the venoms of *Protobothrops mucrosquamatus* [63, 64], *Bothrops asper* [65], *Echis ocellatus*, *Cerastes cerastes cerastes* [66], and some rattlesnakes [67] and are likely present in the venom gland lumen. These inhibitors have been found in relatively large amounts (approximate concentrations in *P. mucrosquamatus* venom were reported greater than 5.0 mM), but their inhibitory activity is not strong, with IC_{50} values between 0.15 and 0.95 mM for different SVMPs in vitro [63, 67]. The X-ray crystal structure of a SVMP complexed with a pExW inhibitor revealed the indole ring of Trp in the pExW inhibitor stacked against the imidazole in the first histidine residue of the SVMP Zn^{2+} binding site [64]. In 2007, Philippe and colleagues discovered the 2–3 kDa polyHis-polyGly peptides in venom of *Atheris squamigera* by mass spectrometry-based strategies, and it was identified as a new class of peptides with clusters of histidine and glycine residues [68]. Similar peptides were found coded in C-type natriuretic peptide (CNP) and bradykinin-potentiating peptide (BPP)–CNP transcript precursors and were isolated from *E. ocellatus* and *Atheris* sp. venoms. Interestingly, these pHpGs have shown stronger inhibitory effect against SVMP in vivo than tripeptides [66].

In addition to inhibitors present in the venom and venom gland, serum proteins in some venomous snakes have also been found to bind toxins with high affinity and neutralize toxin pathophysiological effects [69]. These serum proteins and those found in the venom/venom gland are referred to as "endogenous inhibitors," but kinds of their inhibitor are different. Serum inhibitors circulate in the blood to effectively bind and neutralize host toxins, but they are different than immune antibodies. The roles of these endogenous inhibitors and their classifications will be discussed in the next sections.

3.2 Endogenous inhibitor protein families

There are three main endogenous inhibitor classes; these are phospholipase A2 inhibitors (PLI) [70, 71], anti-hemorrhagic factors [72], and small serum proteins [73–76], which have predominately been found in the blood of vipers. All endogenous inhibitors are stable at high temperatures and in acidic conditions and have been purified by reverse-phase high-performance liquid chromatography (RP-HPLC).

3.2.1 Phospholipase A_2 inhibitors (PLIs)

Snake venom PLA_2s are ubiquitous to Viperidae and Elapidae venoms and one of the primary components in viper venoms. These toxins are versatile and can induced a variety of effects, including neurotoxicity, myotoxicity, cardiotoxicity, hemolysis, and anticoagulation [77]. Inhibitors of PLA_2s, PLIs, have been identified and characterized from the blood sera of both venomous and nonvenomous snakes. PLI genes have been found uniquely expressed in snake liver tissues [78]. This suggests that the secretion of PLIs into blood circulation could be to provide protection against accidental self-envenomation in venomous snakes.

PLIs are divided into three groups (PLIα, PLIβ, and PLIγ) based on structural characteristics. PLIαs are glycoproteins with molecular masses ranging from 75 to 120 kDa and more than three non-covalently associated subunits. Their structural features demonstrate sequence homology to the carbohydrate-recognition domain of Ca^{2+}-dependent lectins (C-type lectin-like domain), but they lack the carbohydrate-binding ability. A highly conserved region (residues 49–143) shares 80–90% sequence identity between PLIαs and appears to be responsible for PLA_2 binding [79]. PLIβs are 150–160 kDa glycoproteins composed of three non-covalently bonded subunits and have nine tandem leucine-rich repeats. A homology analysis by BLAST shows similarity to human leucine-rich α_2-glycoproteins, which structurally forms horseshoe-shaped molecules, as observed in Toll-like receptors [80]. PLIβs have been purified and characterized from only one venomous snake, *Gloydius brevicaudus* [81], whereas there are a couple examples of these proteins that have been found in nonvenomous colubrids (*Elaphe quadrivirgata* and *Elaphe climacophora*) [82, 83]. The presence of a PLIβ gene in *Lachesis muta* was discovered by Lima et al., but the exact function of this inhibitor has not been identified [84]. PLIβs from *G. brevicaudus* specifically inhibited only group-II basic PLA_2s, forming stable toxin-inhibitor complexes at a 1:1 molar ratio [80]. PLIγs are acidic glycoproteins consisting of oligomers with 20–30 kDa subunits, the primary structure of which consists of conserved patterns of cysteine residues to form two units of repeats known as three-finger motifs. Structurally related proteins belong to the urokinase activating plasminogen receptor (u-PAR)/ly-6 superfamily [85]. This gamma class inhibitor comprises the greatest number of endogenous PLIs and has been isolated from the sera of many snake species, including those from Elapidae, Viperidae, Hydrophidae, Boidae, and Colubridae families [70].

Numerous studies have described highly effective inhibition of PLA_2 toxicity in vitro and in vivo by PLIs purified as a highly soluble protein from snake serum. However, binding sites, as well as inhibitory mechanism, have not been fully elucidated for these proteins because each PLIs' group targets different PLA_2s.

Currently, there are two review articles that have attempted to determine the PLA_2 targets of PLI classes based on structural predictions [70, 71]. In 2015, Zhen and colleagues successfully established recombinant expression of PLIγ in *Escherichia coli*. After expression optimization, the amount of recombinant PLIγ achieved was 23 mg/l of culture, and the recombinant PLIγ demonstrated inhibitory activity against *Deinagkistrodon acutus* venom purified PLA_2s, and *D. acutus*, *Naja atra*, and *Agkistrodon halys* crude venoms in vitro and in vivo. This type of experimental work will make it possible in the future to determine the inhibitory mechanism by inhibitor mutant analysis and/or obtaining the three-dimensional structure of the inhibitor and PLA_2 complexes.

3.2.2 Anti-hemorrhagic factors

As previously detailed, hemorrhage, one of the main symptoms of viper envenomation, is induced by snake venom metalloproteinases (SVMPs). The first anti-hemorrhagic factor, habu serum factor (HSF), was identified from the serum of *Protobothrops flavoviridis* by Omori-Satoh et al. in 1972 [86]; in 1992, the complete amino acid sequence was determined for this protein [87]. To date, anti-hemorrhagic factors habu serum factor (HSF), BJ46a [88], and mamushi serum factor (MSF) [89] have been purified and characterized from the venomous snakes *P. flavoviridis* (habu), *Bothrops jararaca,* and *Gloydius blomhoffii*, respectively (**Table 3**). These anti-hemorrhagic factors belong to the fetuin family, part of the cystatin superfamily, consisting of two cystatin-like domains and a His-rich domain. These anti-hemorrhagic factors show high sequence identity and are all single-chain, acidic glycoproteins. They also all demonstrate strong anti-hemorrhagic activity in vivo against the crude venom of the snake species they are isolated from. HSF and MSF showed relatively broad range inhibitory activity against both nonhemorrhagic and hemorrhagic SVMPs, as well as both P-I and P-III SVMP classes, but preferentially inhibited P-III SVMPs. These observations were also exhibited in the differences in the degree and specificity of inhibition against individual SVMP [89, 90]. HSF strongly inhibited the proteolytic and hemorrhagic activities in vivo and in vitro of HR1 and HR2 (P-III SVMPs), the main toxins in *P. flavoviridis* venom. Similarly, BJ46a is a potent inhibitor of atrolysin C (P-I SVMP) and jararhagin (P-III SVMP) proteolytic activities and the overall hemorrhagic activity of *B. jararaca* venom [88]. HSF and MSF did appear to be specific to SVMPs and were found to not inhibit cysteine proteases, such as papain and cathepsin B, serine proteases trypsin and chymotrypsin, or thermolysin, a bacterial MP. Binding studies of these factors suggest that they are forming noncovalent complexes with the MD of SVMPs; this has been hypothesized because they interacted with P-I SVMPs, but did not bind to the C-terminal region of SVMP jararhagin-C. Interestingly, the molar ratios for complex formation vary between inhibitors; for HSF and brevilysin H6 (P-III SVMP), a 1:1 ratio is required, but complex formation between BJ46a and jararhagin (or atrolysin C) was found in a 1:2 ratio. The N-terminal region of HSF (residues 5–89) has been found to be responsible for anti-hemorrhagic activity [91], and sequence comparisons between HSF and a HSF-like protein (HLP), which does not show SVMP inhibition, identified a substitution difference in the first cystatin-like domain [92]. These results suggested that N-terminal region of HSF is potentially responsible for SVMP binding.

Recently, BaltMPI [93] was found as a hemorrhagic inhibitor in *Bothrops alternatus* serum. BaltMPI should also be of the fetuin family as the N-terminal region consists of 60 amino acid residues (determined by Edman degradation) that showed high homology (97%) with BJ46a. BaltMPI has potent anti-hemorrhagic activity and inhibited the proteolytic activity of Batroxase and BjussuMP-I but has

Inhibitor name	Species	pI		Molecular Weight	Target MP	Family	Reference	Database accession numbers of sequence
venomous snake 1 (neutralized own toxin)		calculated*	observed	by SDS-PAGE** (kDa)				
Habu serum factor; HSF	*Protobothrops flavoviridis*	5.9	4	55	(Crude venom) Protobothrops flavoviridis (SVMPs from Protobothrops flavoviridis) HR1A (P-III), HR1B (P-III), HR2a (P-III), HR2b (P-III), H2 proteinase (P-I) (SVMP from *Gloydius blomhoffi brevicaudus*) Brevilysins H3, Brevilysins H4, Brevilysins H6, Brevilysins L4.	Cystatin super family (Fetuin family)	[87, 109]	AB058635
BJ46a	*Bothrops Jararaca*	5.7	5.2	55.4	(Crude venom) *B. jararaca* (SVMP) jararhagin (P-III from B. jararaca) atrolysin C (P-I from *Crotalus atrox*)		[88]	AF294836.1
Mamushi serum factor; jMSF (Japanese MSF)	*Gloydius blomhoffii blomhoffii*	5.6	N.D	48	(Crude venom) *Gloydius blomhoffi brevicaudus* (SVMP from *Gloydius blomhoffi brevicaudus*) brevilysin H2, brevilysin H3, brevilysin H4, brevilysin H6 (P-III SVMP from *Protobothrops flavoviridis*) HR2a (weak)		[89]	AB200169
cMSF (Chainese MSF)	*Gloydius blomhoffi brevicaudus*	5.6	N.D	48	(Crude venom) *Gloydius blomhoffi brevicaudus* (SVMP from *Gloydius blomhoffi brevicaudus*) brevilysin H3, brevilysin H4, brevilysin H6 (P-III SVMP from *Protobothrops flavoviridis*) HR1A, HR1B		[89]	Q5KQS4.1
BaSAH	*Bothrops asper*	N.D	5.2	66	(Crude venom) *Bothrops asper* (10 microgram) (SVMP) BaH1 (*Bothrops asper*, 0.18 microgram)	N.D	[98]	N.D
XX	*Agkistrodon contortrix mokasen*	N.D	4.6	64–68	(Crude venom) *Agkistrodon c. mokassen Agkistrodon piscivorus conanti*	N.D	[99]	N.D
XX	*Crotalus atrox*	N.D	N.D	65–80	(Crude venom) *Crotales atrox* (SVMP) hemorrhagic toxin-e (from *Crotales atrox*)	N.D	[100]	N.D
XX	*Vipera palaestinae*	N.D	4.7	80	(Crude venom) *Vipera palaestinae Echis colorata Cerastes cerastes.*	N.D	[101]	N.D

TMI	*Protobothrops mucrosquamatus*	N.D	N.D	47	(Crude venom) *P. mucrosquamatus P. flavoviridis P. stejnegeri* (SVMP from *P. mucrosquamatus*) TM-1, TM-2, TM-3	N.D	[102]	N.D
venomous snake 2 (neutralized toxin from other species)								
BaltMPI	*Bothrops alternatus*	N.D	5.27	60.5 and 42.4	(SVMP) Batroxase (P-I MP from *B. atrox*) BjussuMP-I (P-III MP from *B.jararacussu*)	N.D	[93]	N.D
Non-venomous								
NtAH (serum)	*Natrix tessellata*	N.D	N.D	880, 70, 100, 150	(Crude venom) *Bothrops asper* (SVMP from *Bothrops asper*) BaH1	N.D	[104]	N.D
XX	*Dinodon semicarinatu*	N.D	N.D	59 and 52	(Crude venom) *Trimeremrus flavovlridis*	N.D	[105]	N.D
XXX	*Drymarchon couperi*	N.D	N.D	Whole serum	(Crude venom) *Agkistrodon contortrix*	N.D	[106]	N.D

N.D; not determined, XX; not named or not determined,
[*]Theoretical Isoelectric point (pI) were calculated on the ProtParam of ExPASy server (https://web.expasy.org/protparam/),
[**]sodium dodecyl sulfate–polyacrylamide gel electrophoresis (SDS-PAGE) under reducing condition

Table 3.
Antihemorrhagic proteins from snake sera (or plasma).

yet to be investigated against the crude venom *Bothrops alternatus*, the snake species it originates from.

3.2.3 Small serum proteins (SSPs)

Since 2007, a new class of endogenous inhibitors, named small serum proteins (SSP-1 to SSP-5), has been characterized from Japanese vipers, *P. flavoviridis* (habu) and *G. b. blomhoffii*, that have been found to effectively neutralize various snake toxins [73, 75]. SSP-1, SSP-2, and SSP-5 consist of two domains of approximately 90 amino acid residues, while SSP-3 and SSP-4 have only a 60 residue N-terminal domain. All serum proteins have conserved cysteine residues and belong to the prostatic secretory protein of 94 amino acid (PSP94) family, despite only limited sequence identity to any mammalian PSP94 [94]. These inhibitors target different toxins; SSP-2 and SSP-5 have high affinity for CRISP family toxins [73, 95], while SSP-1, SSP-4, and SSP-3 inhibit distinct SVMPs. These results suggested SSP-1 to SSP-5 contributes to a snake's natural resistance against toxins. SSP-1 and SSP-4 complex with HSF, inhibiting apoptosis induced by HV1, a P-III SVMP from *P. flavoviridis* venom [74]. Each SSP alone could bind to target SVMPs, but SSP-1 and SSP-4 inhibit HV1 through a ternary complex involving HSF, SSPs, and HV1 (SSP-4, data has not published). In contrast, SSP-3 alone inhibits flavorase, a P-III SVMP from *P. flavoviridis* [76], and is not dependent on other proteins. These results suggested that the inhibition mechanisms of the SSP group are different, but they are noncompetitive. Recently, the crystal structure of complex SSP-2 and triflin, an ion channel-blocking CRISP toxin, was determined [96]. The interface between these two proteins consists of the two short β-strands of SSP-2 binding to the concave region centrally located in the N-terminal domain of triflin. Interestingly, the key β-strand on the N-terminal of SSPs is a hypervariable region, which might correspond to the ability to bind and target different venom toxins. This is in agreement with the molecular evolution of SSP genes, where the number of non-synonymous nucleotide substitutions is significantly greater than those of synonymous substitutions in N-terminal regions. Additionally, these mutational hotspots are found on the molecular surface, specifically located on the toxin interaction interface, while the protein scaffold structure is highly conserved [97].

4. Undetermined proteinous inhibitors

Isolated proteins from the serum of *Bothrops asper* [98], *Agkistrodon contortrix* [99], *Crotalus atrox* [100], and *Vipera palaestinae* [101] have shown effective neutralization of hemorrhagic activity in vivo from crude venom corresponding to each species or species-specific toxins (**Table 3**). The SVMP inhibitor isolated from *Protobothrops mucrosquamatus* serum, named TMI, demonstrated a 1000-fold stronger in vitro inhibitory activity than endogenous tripeptides (IC_{50} = 0.2–1.0 μM) and additionally inhibited venom proteolytic activity from other species [102]. Despite in vivo and in vitro experimental evidence, the sequence of these inhibitors has not yet been determined. A novel group of endogenous inhibitors may be responsible for this activity, as the molecule sizes of these proteins are different than what has been previously reported for other characterized inhibitors.

Venom resistant has been discovered in some species in mammals, birds, and reptiles, which are either predators or prey of venomous snakes. Natural inhibitors isolated from resistant animals are detailed in reviews by Domont et al. [69, 103] and Bastos et al. [72], which summarized toxin resistance corresponding to several snake species from the plasma, serum, and muscle of mammals. There are a few reports of natural inhibitors isolated from nonvenomous snakes, such as NtAH from *Natrix tessellate* [104] and a 59 kDa protein from *Dinodon semicarinatus* [105]. Recently, the whole serum of *Drymarchon couperi* [106] has also shown anti-hemorrhagic activity to venom, but the protein responsible for this activity has yet to be determined. These natural inhibitors in nonvenomous snakes are potentially protective for a diet that consists of venomous snakes, while resistance to SVMPs may be relatively widespread among snake species.

Endogenous inhibitor genes are expressed in the liver of venomous snakes, and these genes appear to be evolving by gene duplication and rapid diversification. This facilitates the neutralization of various toxins within venoms, which also are evolving under similar mechanism [97, 107]. Thus, a detailed characterization of inhibitors against species-specific toxins may help to decipher the evolution of endogenous natural resistance in venomous snakes. Unfortunately, the structural features that govern the inhibitor interaction are still unknown. Recently, there are reports that making a computational analysis predicted three-dimensional structure available [81], and one paper demonstrated that recombinantly expressed BJ46 was able to produce using the expression system of the methylotrophic yeast *Pichia pastoris* [108]. The ability to recombinantly produce these inhibitors will provide material for future work deciphering complex formations between inhibitors and toxins from mutation and structural analyses, providing insight into the molecular mechanisms behind toxin activity inhibition. With current technologies, it is not difficult to comprehensively evaluate venomous snake sera components or the sera from resistant animals. However, we have to be informed from structure-function studies to correlate amino acid sequence to the physiological activity of an inhibitor. It is possible that different inhibitors are operating under different mechanisms, even if they show high similarity, as has been the case for various venomous snake toxins. Thus, understanding in depth how toxin inhibitors function may aid in identifying novel inhibitors and new strategies for snakebite treatment.

5. Conclusions and remaining challenges

There are still many current challenges in the field of toxin inhibitors. Systemic effects of envenomation in humans by snakebite are often mitigated by antivenom therapy, the medically accepted treatment to date. Inhibitors have yet to gain acceptance in clinical use. However, local tissue damage is not neutralized by antivenom and results in permanent morbidity and disability in patients [109]. Local tissue damage is incurred by enzymatic toxins and thus is one of the reasons that Viperidae species occupy just over 60% of venomous snakes listed as Category 1 of highest importance to human health (**Tables 1** and **2**). Endogenous inhibitors isolated from almost all Viperidae show potent inhibition against their own venom and have also demonstrated to be selective toward highly lethal enzymes within these venoms. The serum inhibitor genes of venomous snakes might have evolved by gene duplication and rapid diversification to facilitate the neutralization of various venom toxins. These serum inhibitors are very stable (resistant to acidic, alkaline, and high temperature environments), selective in inhibitory activity against snake toxins, and are nontoxic, given they exist in blood serum and consist of amino acids (**Table 3**). However, the molecule mechanism of toxin neutralization involving endogenous inhibitors remains unclear due to a lack of three-dimensional structures detailing toxin and inhibitor complexes. By exploring molecular mechanisms responsible for natural toxin resistance in snakes, we may begin to understand the specificity and selectivity of endogenous inhibitors and use these insights in the design of better therapeutic agents for the treatment of snakebite victims.

Conflict of interest

The authors declare no conflict of interest.

Author details

Narumi Aoki-Shioi[1*] and Cassandra M. Modahl[2]

1 Department of Chemistry, Faculty of Science, Fukuoka University, Fukuoka, Japan

2 Department of Biological Sciences, National University of Singapore, Singapore

*Address all correspondence to: anarumi@fukuoka-u.ac.jp

References

[1] Fifty-ninth report/WHO Expert Committee on Biological Standardization. WHO Technical Report Series; No. 964. ISSN: 0512-3054, ISBN: 978 92 4 120964 6

[2] Hargreaves AD, Mulley JF. Assessing the utility of the Oxford Nanopore MinION for snake venom gland cDNA sequencing. PeerJ. 2015;**3**:e1441

[3] Calvete JJ. Next-generation snake venomics: Protein-locus resolution through venom proteome decomplexation. Expert Review of Proteomics. 2014;**11**:315-329

[4] Xu N, Zhao H-Y, Yin Y, et al. Combined venomics, antivenomics and venom gland transcriptome analysis of the monocoled cobra (*Naja kaouthia*) from China. Journal of Proteomics. 2017;**159**:19-31

[5] Tan KY, Tan CH, Chanhome L, et al. Comparative venom gland transcriptomics of Naja kaouthia (monocled cobra) from Malaysia and Thailand: elucidating geographical venom variation and insights into sequence novelty. PeerJ. 2017;**5**:e3142

[6] Ainsworth S, Petras D, Engmark M, et al. The medical threat of mamba envenoming in sub-Saharan Africa revealed by genus-wide analysis of venom composition, toxicity and antivenomics profiling of available antivenoms. Journal of Proteomics. 2018;**172**:173-189

[7] Reeks T, Lavergne V, Sunagar K, et al. Deep venomics of the Pseudonaja genus reveals inter- and intra-specific variation. Journal of Proteomics. 2016; **133**:20-32

[8] Jiang Y, Li Y, Lee W, et al. Venom gland transcriptomes of two elapid snakes (*Bungarus multicinctus* and *Naja atra*) and evolution of toxin genes. BMC Genomics. 2011;**12**:1

[9] Francischetti IMB, My-Pham V, Harrison J, et al. Bitis gabonica (*Gaboon viper*) snake venom gland: toward a catalog for the full-length transcripts (cDNA) and proteins. Gene. 2004;**337**: 55-69

[10] Cardoso KC, Da Silva MJ, Costa GG, et al. A transcriptomic analysis of gene expression in the venom gland of the snake *Bothrops alternatus* (urutu). BMC Genomics. 2010;**11**:605

[11] Durban J, Juárez P, Angulo Y, et al. Profiling the venom gland transcriptomes of Costa Rican snakes by 454 pyrosequencing. BMC Genomics. 2011;**12**:259

[12] Amazonas DR, Portes-Junior JA, Nishiyama MY Jr, et al. Molecular mechanisms underlying intraspecific variation in snake venom. Journal of Proteomics. 2018;**181**:60-72

[13] Junqueira-de-Azevedo ILM, Bastos CMV, Ho PL, et al. Venom-related transcripts from *Bothrops jararaca* tissues provide novel molecular insights into the production and evolution of snake venom. Molecular Biology and Evolution. 2015;**32**:754-766

[14] Neiva M, Arraes FBM, de Souza JV, et al. Transcriptome analysis of the Amazonian viper Bothrops atrox venom gland using expressed sequence tags (ESTs). Toxicon. 2009;**53**:427-436

[15] Cidade DAP, Simão TA, Dávila AMR, et al. Bothrops jararaca venom gland transcriptome: Analysis of the gene expression pattern. Toxicon. 2006; **48**:437-461

[16] Zelanis A, Andrade-Silva D, Rocha MM, et al. A transcriptomic view of the proteome variability of newborn and adult *Bothrops jararaca* snake venoms. PLoS Neglected Tropical Diseases. 2012; **6**:e1554

[17] Gonçalves-Machado L, Pla D, Sanz L, et al. Combined venomics, venom gland transcriptomics, bioactivities, and antivenomics of two *Bothrops jararaca* populations from geographic isolated regions within the Brazilian Atlantic rainforest. Journal of Proteomics. 2016; **135**:73-89

[18] Kashima S, Roberto PG, Soares AM, et al. Analysis of *Bothrops jararacussu* venomous gland transcriptome focusing on structural and functional aspects11All sequence data reported in this paper will appear in the GenBank database under the following accession numbers: BOJU-I (AY 185200), BOJU-II (AY 185206), BOJU-III (AY 145836), BOJUMET-I (AY 55005), BOJUMET-II (AY 25584), BOJUMET-III (AY 258153), C-type lectin (AY 251283), serine-proteases (AY 251282).: I—gene expression profile of highly expressed phospholipases A2. Biochimie. 2004;**86**:211-219

[19] Rokyta DR, Wray KP, Lemmon AR, et al. A high-throughput venom-gland transcriptome for the Eastern Diamondback Rattlesnake (*Crotalus adamanteus*) and evidence for pervasive positive selection across toxin classes. Toxicon. 2011;**57**:657-671

[20] Rokyta DR, Lemmon AR, Margres MJ, et al. The venom-gland transcriptome of the eastern diamondback rattlesnake (*Crotalus adamanteus*). BMC Genomics. 2012;**13**:312

[21] Amorim FG, Morandi-Filho R, Fujimura PT, et al. New findings from the first transcriptome of the *Bothrops moojeni* snake venom gland. Toxicon. 2017;**140**:105-117

[22] Nicolau CA, Carvalho PC, Junqueira-de-Azevedo ILM, et al. An in-depth snake venom proteopeptidome characterization: Benchmarking *Bothrops jararaca*. Journal of Proteomics. 2017;**151**:214-231

[23] Rokyta DR, Margres MJ, Ward MJ, et al. The genetics of venom ontogeny in the eastern diamondback rattlesnake (*Crotalus adamanteus*). PeerJ. 2017;**5**:e3249

[24] Rokyta DR, Wray KP, Margres MJ. The genesis of an exceptionally lethal venom in the timber rattlesnake (*Crotalus horridus*) revealed through comparative venom-gland transcriptomics. BMC Genomics. 2013; **14**:394

[25] Boldrini-França J, Rodrigues RS, Fonseca FPP, et al. Crotalus durissus collilineatus venom gland transcriptome: Analysis of gene expression profile. Biochimie. 2009;**91**: 586-595

[26] Strickland J, Mason A, Rokyta D, et al. Phenotypic variation in mojave rattlesnake (*Crotalus scutulatus*) venom is driven by four toxin families. Toxins. 2018;**10**:135

[27] Durban J, Pérez A, Sanz L, et al. Integrated "omics" profiling indicates that miRNAs are modulators of the ontogenetic venom composition shift in the Central American rattlesnake, *Crotalus simus simus*. BMC Genomics. 2013;**14**:234

[28] Durban J, Sanz L, Trevisan-Silva D, et al. Integrated venomics and venom gland transcriptome analysis of juvenile and adult mexican rattlesnakes *Crotalus simus*, *C. tzabcan*, and *C. culminatus* revealed miRNA-modulated ontogenetic shifts. Journal of Proteome Research. 2017;**16**:3370-3390

[29] Casewell NR, Harrison RA, Wüster W, et al. Comparative venom gland transcriptome surveys of the saw-scaled vipers (Viperidae: Echis) reveal substantial intra-family gene diversity and novel venom transcripts. BMC Genomics. 2009;**10**:564

[30] Aird SD, Watanabe Y, Villar-Briones A, et al. Quantitative high-throughput profiling of snake venom gland transcriptomes and proteomes

(*Ovophis okinavensis* and *Protobothrops flavoviridis*). BMC Genomics. 2013;**14**: 790

[31] Wagstaff SC, Harrison RA. Venom gland EST analysis of the saw-scaled viper, Echis ocellatus, reveals novel α9β1 integrin-binding motifs in venom metalloproteinases and a new group of putative toxins, renin-like aspartic proteases. Gene. 2006;**377**:21-32

[32] Junqueira-de-Azevedo ILM, Ching ATC, Carvalho E, et al. *Lachesis muta* (Viperidae) cDNAs Reveal Diverging Pit Viper Molecules and Scaffolds Typical of Cobra (Elapidae) Venoms: Implications for Snake Toxin Repertoire Evolution. Genetics. 2006;**173**:877-889

[33] Yin W, Wang Z, Li Q, et al. Evolutionary trajectories of snake genes and genomes revealed by comparative analyses of five-pacer viper. Nature Communications. 2016;**7**:13107

[34] Aird SD, Arora J, Barua A, et al. Population genomic analysis of a pitviper reveals microevolutionary forces underlying venom chemistry. Genome Biology and Evolution. 2017;**9**: 2640-2649

[35] Shibata H, Chijiwa T, Oda-Ueda N, et al. The habu genome reveals accelerated evolution of venom protein genes. Scientific Reports. 2018;**8**:11300

[36] Ullate-Agote A, Milinkovitch MC, Tzika AC. The genome sequence of the corn snake (*Pantherophis guttatus*), a valuable resource for EvoDevo studies in squamates. The International Journal of Developmental Biology. 2014;**58**: 881-888

[37] Li J-T, Gao Y-D, Xie L, et al. Comparative genomic investigation of high-elevation adaptation in ectothermic snakes. Proceedings of the National Academy of Sciences of the United States of America. 2018;**115**: 8406-8411

[38] Schield DR, Card DC, Hales NR, et al. The origins and evolution of chromosomes, dosage compensation, and mechanisms underlying venom regulation in snakes. Genome Research. 2019;**29**:590-601

[39] Tasoulis T, Isbister G. A review and database of Snake venom proteomes. Toxins. 2017;**9**:290

[40] Kini R, Sidhu S, Laustsen A. Biosynthetic Oligoclonal Antivenom (BOA) for snakebite and next-generation treatments for snakebite victims. Toxins. 2018;**10**:534

[41] Laustsen AH, Karatt-Vellatt A, Masters EW, et al. In vivo neutralization of dendrotoxin-mediated neurotoxicity of black mamba venom by oligoclonal human IgG antibodies. Nature Communications. 2018;**9**:3928

[42] Ainsworth S, Slagboom J, Alomran N, et al. The paraspecific neutralisation of snake venom induced coagulopathy by antivenoms. Communications Biology. 2018;**1**:34

[43] Lewin M, Gilliam L, Gilliam J, et al. Delayed LY333013 (Oral) and LY315920 (intravenous) reverse severe neurotoxicity and rescue juvenile pigs from lethal doses of *Micrurus fulvius* (eastern coral Snake) venom. Toxins. 2018;**10**:479

[44] Rawlings ND, Barrett AJ, Bateman A. MEROPS: The peptidase database. Nucleic Acids Research. 2010; **38**:D227-D233

[45] Herrera C, Escalante T, Rucavado A, et al. Metalloproteinases in disease: Identification of biomarkers of tissue damage through proteomics. Expert Review of Proteomics. 2018;**15**:967-982

[46] Bjarnason JB, Fox JW. Snake venom metalloendopeptidases: Reprolysins. Methods in Enzymology. 1995;**248**: 345-368

[47] Bahudhanapati H, Bhattacharya S, Wei S. Evolution of vertebrate Adam genes; duplication of testicular Adams from ancient Adam9/9-like loci. PLoS One. 2015;**10**:e0136281

[48] Jia L-G, Shimokawa K-I, Bjarnason JB, et al. Snake venom metalloproteinases: Structure, function and relationship to the ADAMs family of proteins. Toxicon. 1996;**34**: 1269-1276

[49] Sanz L, Calvete J. Insights into the evolution of a snake venom multi-gene family from the genomic organization of *Echis ocellatus* SVMP genes. Toxins. 2016;**8**:216

[50] Calvete JJ, Juárez P, Sanz L. Snake venomics. Strategy and applications. Journal of Mass Spectrometry. 2007;**42**: 1405-1414

[51] Fox JW, Serrano SMT. Exploring snake venom proteomes: Multifaceted analyses for complex toxin mixtures. Proteomics. 2008;**8**: 909-920

[52] Rucavado A, Nicolau C, Escalante T, et al. Viperid envenomation wound exudate contributes to increased vascular permeability via a DAMPs/TLR-4 mediated pathway. Toxins. 2016; **8**:349

[53] Kini RM, Koh CY. Metalloproteases affecting blood coagulation, fibrinolysis and platelet aggregation from snake venoms: Definition and nomenclature of interaction sites. Toxins (Basel). 2016;**8**. DOI: 10.3390/toxins8100284

[54] Escalante T, Rucavado A, Fox JW, et al. Key events in microvascular damage induced by snake venom hemorrhagic metalloproteinases. Journal of Proteomics. 2011;**74**:1781-1794

[55] Gutiérrez JM, Rucavado A, Escalante T, et al. Hemorrhage induced by snake venom metalloproteinases: Biochemical and biophysical mechanisms involved in microvessel damage. Toxicon. 2005;**45**:997-1011

[56] Baldo C, Jamora C, Yamanouye N, et al. Mechanisms of vascular damage by hemorrhagic snake venom metalloproteinases: Tissue distribution and in situ hydrolysis. PLoS Neglected Tropical Diseases. 2010;**4**:e727

[57] Sanhajariya S, Duffull S, Isbister G. Pharmacokinetics of snake venom. Toxins. 2018;**10**:73

[58] Takacs Z, Wilhelmsen KC, Sorota S. Cobra (*Naja* spp.) nicotinic acetylcholine receptor exhibits resistance to Erabu Sea Snake (*Laticauda semifasciata*) short-chain a-neurotoxin. Journal of Molecular Evolution. 2004;**58**:516-526

[59] Takacs Z, Wilhelmsen KC, Sorota S. Snake α-neurotoxin binding site on the Egyptian cobra (*Naja haje*) nicotinic acetylcholine receptor is conserved. Molecular Biology and Evolution. 2001; **18**:1800-1809

[60] 冀宪红, 张尚斐, 高斌, et al. 受体的多样性驱动蛇毒的进化. Zoological Research. 2018;**39**:431-436

[61] Odell GV, Ferry PC, Vick LM, et al. Citrate inhibition of snake venom proteases. Toxicon. 1998;**36**: 1801-1806

[62] Mackessy SP, Baxter LM. Bioweapons synthesis and storage: The venom gland of front-fanged snakes. Zoologischer Anzeiger—A Journal of Comparative Zoology. 2006;**245**: 147-159

[63] Huang K-F, Hung C-C, Wu S-H, et al. Characterization of three endogenous peptide inhibitors for multiple metalloproteinases with fibrinogenolytic activity from the venom of Taiwan Habu (*Trimeresurus mucrosquamatus*). Biochemical and

Biophysical Research Communications. 1998;**248**:562-568

[64] Huang K-F, Chiou S-H, Ko T-P, et al. Determinants of the inhibition of a Taiwan habu venom metalloproteinase by its endogenous inhibitors revealed by X-ray crystallography and synthetic inhibitor analogues: Inhibition of a SVMP by its endogenous inhibitors. European Journal of Biochemistry. 2002;**269**:3047-3056

[65] Francis B, Kaiser II. Inhibition of metalloproteinases in Bothrops asper venom by endogenous peptides. Toxicon. 1993;**31**:889-899

[66] Wagstaff SC, Favreau P, Cheneval O, et al. Molecular characterisation of endogenous snake venom metalloproteinase inhibitors. Biochemical and Biophysical Research Communications. 2008;**365**:650-656

[67] Munekiyo SM, Mackessy SP. Presence of peptide inhibitors in rattlesnake venoms and their effects on endogenous metalloproteases. Toxicon. 2005;**45**:255-263

[68] Favreau P, Cheneval O, Menin L, et al. The venom of the snake genus Atheris contains a new class of peptides with clusters of histidine and glycine residues. Rapid Communications in Mass Spectrometry. 2007;**21**:406-412

[69] Perales J, Neves-Ferreira AGC, Valente RH, et al. Natural inhibitors of snake venom hemorrhagic metalloproteinases. Toxicon. 2005;**45**: 1013-1020

[70] Campos PC, de Melo LA, Dias GLF, et al. Endogenous phospholipase A2 inhibitors in snakes: A brief overview. Journal of Venomous Animals and Toxins including Tropical Diseases. 2016;**22**:37

[71] Dunn RD, Broady KW. Snake inhibitors of phospholipase A2 enzymes. Biochimica et Biophysica Acta (BBA)—Molecular and Cell Biology of Lipids. 2001;**1533**:29-37

[72] Bastos V, Gomes-Neto F, Perales J, et al. Natural inhibitors of snake venom metalloendopeptidases: History and current challenges. Toxins. 2016;**8**:250

[73] Aoki N, Sakiyama A, Deshimaru M, et al. Identification of novel serum proteins in a Japanese viper: Homologs of mammalian PSP94. Biochemical and Biophysical Research Communications. 2007;**359**:330-334

[74] Shioi N, Ogawa E, Mizukami Y, et al. Small serum protein-1 changes the susceptibility of an apoptosis-inducing metalloproteinase HV1 to a metalloproteinase inhibitor in habu snake (*Trimeresurus flavoviridis*). Journal of Biochemistry. 2013;**153**:121-129

[75] Shioi N, Deshimaru M, Terada S. Structural analysis and characterization of new small serum proteins from the serum of a venomous snake (*Gloydius blomhoffii*). Bioscience, Biotechnology, and Biochemistry. 2014;**78**:410-419

[76] Shioi N, Nishijima A, Terada S. Flavorase, a novel non-haemorrhagic metalloproteinase in Protobothrops flavoviridis venom, is a target molecule of small serum protein-3. Journal of Biochemistry. 2015;**158**:37-48

[77] Manjunatha KR. Excitement ahead: Structure, function and mechanism of snake venom phospholipase A2 enzymes. Toxicon. 2003;**42**:827-840

[78] Kinkawa K, Shirai R, Watanabe S, et al. Up-regulation of the expressions of phospholipase A2 inhibitors in the liver of a venomous snake by its own venom phospholipase A2. Biochemical and Biophysical Research Communications. 2010;**395**:377-381

[79] Hains PG, Broady KW. Purification and inhibitory profile of phospholipase

A2 inhibitors from Australian elapid sera. The Biochemical Journal. 2000; **346**(Pt 1):139-146

[80] Okumura K, Ohkura N, Inoue S, et al. A novel phospholipase a $_2$ inhibitor with leucine-RICH repeats from the blood plasma of *Agkistrodon blomhoffii siniticus*: Sequence homologies with human leucine-rich α_2-glycoprotein. The Journal of Biological Chemistry. 1998;**273**:19469-19475

[81] Ohkura N, Okuhara H, Inoue S, et al. Purification and characterization of three distinct types of phospholipase A2 inhibitors from the blood plasma of the Chinese mamushi, *Agkistrodon blomhoffii siniticus*. The Biochemical Journal. 1997;**325**:527-531

[82] Okumura K, Inoue S, Ikeda K, et al. Identification of β-type phospholipase A2 inhibitor in a nonvenomous snake, *Elaphe quadrivirgata*. Archives of Biochemistry and Biophysics. 2002;**408**: 124-130

[83] Shirai R, Toriba M, Hayashi K, et al. Identification and characterization of phospholipase A2 inhibitors from the serum of the Japanese rat snake, *Elaphe climacophora*. Toxicon. 2009;**53**:685-692

[84] Lima RM, Estevão-Costa MI, Junqueira-de-Azevedo ILM, et al. Phospholipase A2 inhibitors (βPLIs) are encoded in the venom glands of *Lachesis muta* (Crotalinae, Viperidae) snakes. Toxicon. 2011;**57**:172-175

[85] Ohkura N, Inoue S, Ikeda K, et al. The two subunits of a phospholipase A2 inhibitor from the plasma of Thailand cobra having structural similarity to Urokinase-type plasminogen activator receptor and Ly-6 related proteins. Biochemical and Biophysical Research Communications. 1994;**204**: 1212-1218

[86] Omori-Satoh T, Sadahiro S, Ohsaka A, et al. Purification and characterization of an antihemorrhagic factor in the serum of Trimeresurus flavoviridis, a crotalid. Biochimica et Biophysica Acta (BBA)—Protein Structure. 1972;**285**:414-426

[87] Yamakawa Y, Omori-Satoh T. Primary structure of the Antihemorrhagic factor in serum of the Japanese Habu: A snake venom metalloproteinase inhibitor with a double-headed cystatin domain. The Journal of Biochemistry. 1992;**112**: 583-589

[88] Valente RH, Dragulev B, Perales J, et al. BJ46a, a snake venom metalloproteinase inhibitor: Isolation, characterization, cloning and insights into its mechanism of action. European Journal of Biochemistry. 2001;**268**: 3042-3052

[89] Aoki N, Tsutsumi K, Deshimaru M, et al. Properties and cDNA cloning of antihemorrhagic factors in sera of Chinese and Japanese mamushi (*Gloydius blomhoffi*). Toxicon. 2008;**51**: 251-261

[90] Deshimaru M, Tanaka C, Fujino K, et al. Properties and cDNA cloning of an antihemorrhagic factor (HSF) purified from the serum of *Trimeresurus flavoviridis*. Toxicon. 2005;**46**:937-945

[91] Aoki N, Deshimaru M, Terada S. Active fragments of the antihemorrhagic protein HSF from serum of habu (*Trimeresurus flavoviridis*). Toxicon. 2007;**49**:653-662

[92] Aoki N, Deshimaru M, Kihara K, et al. Snake fetuin: Isolation and structural analysis of new fetuin family proteins from the sera of venomous snakes. Toxicon. 2009;**54**:481-490

[93] Palacio TZ, Santos-Filho NA, Rosa JC, et al. Isolation and characterization of a novel metalloprotease inhibitor from *Bothrops alternatus* snake serum. International

Journal of Biological Macromolecules. 2017;**98**:436-446

[94] Aoki N, Matsuo H, Deshimaru M, et al. Accelerated evolution of small serum proteins (SSPs)—The PSP94 family proteins in a Japanese viper. Gene. 2008;**426**:7-14

[95] Aoki N, Sakiyama A, Kuroki K, et al. Serotriflin, a CRISP family protein with binding affinity for small serum protein-2 in snake serum. Biochimica et Biophysica Acta (BBA)—Proteins and Proteomics. 2008;**1784**:621-628

[96] Shioi N, Tadokoro T, Shioi S, et al. Crystal structure of the complex between venom toxin and serum inhibitor from Viperidae snake. The Journal of Biological Chemistry. 2019; **294**:1250-1256

[97] Tanaka Y, Oyama S, Hori S, et al. Accelerated evolution of Fetuin family proteins in *Protobothrops flavoviridis* (Habu Snake) serum and the discovery of an L1-like genomic element in the Intronic sequence of a Fetuin-encoding gene. Bioscience, Biotechnology, and Biochemistry. 2013;**77**:582-590

[98] Borkow G, Gutierrez JM, Ovadia M. Isolation, characterization and mode of neutralization of a potent antihemorrhagic factor from the serum of the snake *Bothrops asper*. Biochimica et Biophysica Acta (BBA)—General Subjects. 1995;**1245**:232-238

[99] Weinstein SA, Lafaye PJ, Smith LA. Observations on a venom neutralizing fraction isolated from serum of the northern copperhead. Agkistrodon contortrix mokasen. Copeia. 1991;**1991**: 777

[100] Weissenberg S, Ovadia M, Kochva E. Inhibition of the proteolytic activity of hemorrhagin-e from *Crotalus atrox* venom by antihemorrhagins from homologous serum. Toxicon. 1992;**30**: 591-597

[101] Ovadia M. Purification and characterization of an antihemorrhagic factor from the serum of the snake *Vipera palaestinae*. Toxicon. 1978;**16**: 661-672

[102] Huang K-F, Chow L-P, Chiou S-H. Isolation and characterization of a novel proteinase inhibitor from the Snake serum of Taiwan Habu (*Trimeresurus mucrosquamatus*). Biochemical and Biophysical Research Communications. 1999;**263**:610-616

[103] Domont GB, Perales J, Moussatché H. Natural anti-snake venom proteins. Toxicon. 1991;**29**: 1183-1194

[104] Borkow G, Gutierrez JM, Ovadia M. A potent antihemorrhagin in the serum of the non-poisonous water snake *Natrix tessellata*: Isolation, characterization and mechanism of neutralization. Biochimica et Biophysica Acta (BBA)—General Subjects. 1994; **1201**:482-490

[105] Goetz SM, Piccolomini S, Hoffman M, et al. Serum-based inhibition of pit viper venom by eastern indigo snakes (*Drymarchon couperi*). Biology Open. 2019;**8**:bio040964

[106] Tomihara Y, Yonaha K, Nozaki M, et al. Purification of an antihemorrhagic factor from the serum of the non-venomous snake *Dinodon semicarinatus*. Toxicon. 1988;**26**:420-423

[107] Chijiwa T, Inamaru K, Takeuchi A, et al. Unique structure (construction and configuration) and evolution of the array of small serum protein genes of *Protobothrops flavoviridis* snake. Bioscience Reports. 2019;**39**: BSR20190560

[108] Shi Y, Ji M-K, Xu J-W, et al. High-level expression, purification, characterization and structural prediction of a snake venom

metalloproteinase inhibitor in *Pichia pastoris*. The Protein Journal. 2012;**31**: 212-221

[109] Gutiérrez JM, Calvete JJ, Habib AG, et al. Snakebite envenoming. Nature Reviews. Disease Primers. 2017; **3**:17063

Chapter 4

The Effects of Snake Venom (*Bitis arietans*) on Embryonic Development

Charlotte Peters, Vladimir Petrilla, Lenka Luptakova and Eva Petrovova

Abstract

Venomous snake bites in pregnant women can lead to poor survival rates in both the foetus and mother; early bites can precipitate teratogenesis, miscarriages, preterm delivery, foetal death and antepartum haemorrhage. The chicken embryo poses as a valuable research model for venom research due to its advantages such as ease of availability, economic feasibility and its non-invasiveness. This study evaluates the embryotoxic effects of Puff adder venom (*Bitis arietans*) from Namibia, Kenya, South Africa and non-specified region of Africa at varying concentrations. The venoms were applied to chicken embryos on the fourth day of incubation and assessed on a ninth day, focusing on body weight, heart weight, liver weight and mortality rate. Nile blue staining was also performed to observe the occurrence of apoptosis amongst the venoms at the strongest concentrations. The information provided from our results suggested that there was a regional variation in venom toxicity, with the Kenyan venom producing the largest weight changes, whereas the non-specified African venom proved the most lethal across the concentrations. Further studies to assess venom protein concentrations in comparison with regional diet disparities are required.

Keywords: *Bitis arietans*, chicken embryo, development, embryotoxicity, snake venom

1. Chicken embryo as an animal model for biomedicine

The chick embryo has established itself within biomedical science as a crucial research model due to its similarity on a cellular and anatomical level to human embryos along with its rapid development, easy visibility and manipulation [1]. The cardiovascular system in the avian develops rapidly with the added benefit of the embryo remaining transparent during morphological development of primary organs, allowing visibility of vasculature formation using simple microscopy techniques [2].

1.1 Transgenic chicken egg as a bioreactor

The use of a chick egg as a bioreactor has been promoted over the use of standard large-scale fermenters due to its ability to produce large quantities of complex proteins and cheaper running costs [3]. A 2002 study placed a retroviral vector based on avian leucosis virus into the chicken genome and noted that biologically active enzymes were secreted into the serum and egg white of four generations of chickens. The levels of enzyme expression remained steady through each successive generation and remained constant for over 16 months in the magnum of hens indicating the expression of this enzyme was stable. This supports the possibility of chicken eggs in the role of a bioreactor for the production of biologically active proteins for therapeutic interest [4]. Human interferon a2b and β1a along with human granulocyte-colony stimulating factor have been successfully harvested from this method [5]. The egg is an ideal model for the recovery of these proteins as the content is sterile and provides a long half-life [6]. Production of human proteins in hens could become the method of choice for proteins that are toxic to mammals, an example of this is human erythropoietin which is damaging to the mammary gland of rabbits but remains inactive in chickens [7].

1.2 Chicken egg used for drug screening and production

The avian chorioallantoic membrane (CAM) refers to the outermost membrane that is highly vascularised for gas exchange and calcium transportation between the embryo and its environment [8]. It has been widely used to discover targets and measure the in vivo angiogenic effects of factors such as vascular endothelial growth [9] and P13 kinase [5]. The chorioallantoic membrane provides advantageous exposure to the embryo with minimal invasiveness [5]. The chicken egg is a reliable candidate in assessing angiogenic responses to drugs as well as being cost and time-effective [10]. In 1984, inactivated rabies vaccine for human use was developed which had been adapted to proliferate in primary chick egg cultures [11]. This vaccine provided similar antigenicity to the human diploid cell strain with the advantages of cheaper and faster production. This purified chick embryo cell culture vaccine has now been licenced in over 60 countries worldwide for 30 years [12]. The influenza vaccine has been developed in the embryonated chicken eggs since the 1940s, the egg provides high titre capabilities and large-scale production opportunity which has led to the streamlined process of today which provides vaccination for millions worldwide [13].

1.3 Chicken egg used in retinal development

The chicken embryo is advantageous in studying retinal development due to its significant similarity to the human embryo at a molecular, cellular and anatomical level and its rapid development [1]. It is an important model in regenerative research as the neural retina can regenerate from the pigmented epithelium as late as stage 24 [14]. The regeneration can occur from the cup margin or patches of pigmented epithelium far from the margin. The lens does not have to be present for the regeneration, and the regenerating tissue develops faster than normal [14]. The chicken model is used in the vision research community to study human retinogenesis and develop new ways to battle human blindness and eye disease by allowing scientists an insight into the complex regulatory network of neurons and glial cells [15]. In America, diabetic retinopathy is the leading cause of blindness amongst over 40-year-olds [16] with all type 1 diabetes developing DR and more than 60% with type 2 [17]. Chickens, like humans, are diurnal with complex colour vision and as their retina is cone-dominant it makes them an ideal model for photoreceptor-degenerative blindness [18]. In a 2014 study, chicken embryos were injected with either streptozotocin or high concentration of glucose at day 11; in both groups, cataracts occurred in varying degrees making them a promising animal model for diabetes research [19].

1.4 Chicken embryo as an animal model for research in Alzheimer's disease

Studies by Murphy and LeVine [20] and Carrodeguas et al. [21] revealed that the chick embryo has an active process for the formulation and degeneration of the amyloid-beta peptide deposits associated with Alzheimer's disease. The distribution of the peptide sequence in chick embryos is similar to humans, predominating in the nervous system. This study also discovered that the chick embryo produces neprilysin (ADAM-17), a protease that degrades the peptide [21]. Due to the easy access of chick embryos, it's an ideal candidate for developing a potential system for drug regulation and regression for this neurodegenerative disease [22]. In a 2003 study, the chick embryo was a model for supporting the use of *Ginkgo biloba* extract as Alzheimer's therapy. The embryo was exposed to cyanide, with and without therapeutic use of the extract. Results show an increase function in cultured neurons from the telencephalon and a reduction in apoptotic damage caused by serum deprivation after 24 hours [23].

1.5 The role of the chicken embryo in oncology research

The chick embryo allows the unique research of oncology in vivo. Along with being highly accessible and easy to manipulate, the CAM is naturally immune-deficient which can support engraftment of both normal and cancerous tissue up until developmental day 18 [24]. The CAM has also been used for research into carcinogenesis [25] and tumour angiogenesis [26]. In 1911, by inoculating the Rouse Sarcoma virus into chick embryos, it was suggested for the first time that viruses could cause cancer [27]. It is now estimated that 15–20% of human cancers worldwide involve tumour inducing viruses, such as T-cell leukaemia virus type 1 and hepatitis C [28]. In 2002, Zijlstra et al. [29] developed a highly sensitive assay to monitor metastatic dissemination of human cancer cells in the chick embryo by using the CAM as an established biological platform. In 2014, Mu et al. concluded that chicken embryo extract may promote the reversion of metastatic phenotypes of osteosarcoma cells, which could lead to tumour reversion through epigenetics [30].

1.6 Role of the chicken embryo in stem cell research

In 1996, Pain et al. displayed that early chicken blastoderm cells or avian embryonic stem cells can be maintained in vitro for long term culture. These cells model traits of murine stem cells in morphology, reactivity to antibodies and high telomerase activity along with the high capability to differentiate into various cell types [31]. When blastoderm embryonic stem cells are grafted onto the CAM, they organise into complex structures such as embryoid bodies and derivatives of the three primary germ layers. These cells can provide an in vitro model of cell differentiation and maturation along with means of targeted genome control [32]. Germline stem cell research is associated with the manufacture of transgenic animals using male spermatogonial stem cells [33] for the production of pharmaceutical proteins [34]. Recently direct reprogramming has been created to convert differentiated somatic cells into pluripotent embryo stem-like cells; this is an advantageous medical method avoiding ethical issues surrounding human egg use [33]. Amniotic stem cells isolated from the amniotic cavity can create clonal cell lines and due to their ease of isolation, are considered a potential source for regenerative medicine application [35].

1.7 Chick embryotoxicity screening test

Developed by Jelinek in 1977 the chick embryotoxicity screening test (CHEST) is a standardised technique to allow administration of small amounts of test compounds and the quantitative measurement of results. This method is advantageous as it requires limited materials. Fertilised eggs, micropipettes for administration, incubator and a dissection kit are all that is needed. The CHEST test allows the use of a chick embryo to study experimental teratogenicity. The number of dead, malformed, and growth-retarded foetuses (weight <650 mg and with no malformation) are totalled for each concentration and stage of the embryo at the time of exposure. The proportion of affected embryos is plotted against the concentration of test compound, and the embryo-stage of administration. The proportion of effects on particular organs in surviving embryos is considered separately to establish a profile of effects for each compound [36]. The screening test has been used to determine the toxicity of many substances, establishing parameters of dose–response and stage-response [37].

2. Snake venom

2.1 The role of snake venom

Venom is defined as 'a secretion, produced in a specialised gland in one animal and delivered to a target animal through the infliction of a wound, which contains molecules that disrupt normal physiological or biochemical processes to facilitate feeding or defence' [38].

Venom is composed of proteins and polypeptides, it has two primary functions—to paralyse their prey and start the digestive process with hydrolysing proteins leading to tissue necrosis and blood clotting [39]. These venom components can be grouped according to the mode of action:

1. Binding to cholinergic receptors, often leading to respiratory muscle paralysis.

2. Inhibition or increase release of acetylcholine, causing muscle cells to not react to nerve stimulus, leading to spasms, damage of the skin and disruption connective tissues.

3. Cytotoxic and cardiotoxic, which harm cell membranes and disrupt the transport of substances across the membranes [39].

In broad terms, snake venoms are classified as inflammatory, cytotoxic, neurotoxic or haemotoxic [40].

2.2 The venom delivery system

Many snakes use fangs, specialised dentition associated with the venom gland (Duvernoy gland) to introduce venom into prey. Fangs can either be posteriorly (grass snake) or anteriorly (vipers) positioned within the upper jaw [41].

Many poisonous snakes possess different types of dentition; vipers and atractaspidids have a shortened maxilla which rotates allowing the fangs to move; whereas elapids fangs are fixed at the front of the maxilla. Colubrids can possess an enlarged rear positioned fang or no fang at all. The venom gland, also known as the Duvernoy gland in posteriorly positioned fanged species, is innervated by the maxillary branch of the trigeminal nerve, facial nerve and supplied by the internal carotid artery [42]. The Duvernoy gland is positioned posteriorly to the eye, encased in a thin layer of connective tissue and consists mainly of serous cells; a single duct extends from the gland to the base of the fang; whereas the venom gland is encased in a fibrous sheath varying in position depending on species. The viperid gland is large, isosceles with the longest side along the upper lip directed dorsally; the gland is divided into lobules by the outer sheath with the lumen becoming a primary duct which passes through a mucous accessory duct into a secondary duct extending the length of the fang [43]. In contrast, the elapid venom gland is oval made from many branching tubules, its lumen is narrow and therefore most of the venom is stored in the surrounding cells [44]. The atractaspidid species possess a cylindrical gland extending posteriorly beyond the head, its lumen has a characteristic pattern of unbranched tubules radiating outwards [45].

2.3 Snakebite classification

Bites can be classified as cytotoxic bites characterised by a painful swelling with watery blood leaking from the wound followed by shock, blistering and discolouration. Venomous snake bites in pregnant women can lead to poor survival rates in both the foetus and mother; early bites can precipitate teratogenesis, miscarriages, preterm delivery, foetal death and antepartum haemorrhage [46]. The bite will cause severe pain to the limb affected. Species associated with this bite include the puff adder, Gaboon adder and spitting cobras. Black and green mambas along with non-spitting cobras produce a neurotoxic bite in victims which leads to moderate swelling, cold and clammy extremities, dilated pupils and drooping of the eyelids. Patients suffering these bites will develop swollen lymph glands, vomiting, ptyalism and breathing difficulties. Haemotoxic bites associated with boomslang and vine snakes cause bleeding from the gums, nose, corner of eyes and old wounds and scratches. Certain snake species can produce more than one type of bites such as the *Bitis arietans* that produces a haemotoxic and cytotoxic bite [47].

2.4 Composition of snake venom

Medically significant venomous snakes are all front-fanged and are classified into three families: Atractaspididae, Elapidae and Viperidae; the glands of these snakes are homologous [48], with current evidence suggesting these evolved from non-front fanged venomous snakes [49]. These glands contain the snake venom, made from a combination of different protein families, each containing a variety of toxin isoforms along with carbohydrates, lipids, nucleosides and metals. Although homologous, the venom proteome is not due to the influence of genetic mutations and natural selection [50]. In a 2017 review, 59 protein families were identified in these three species, with four dominant proteins: phospholipase A2s, metalloproteases, serine proteases and three-finger toxins; six secondary families: cysteine-rich secretory proteins, L-amino acid oxidases, Kunitz peptides, c-type lectins, disintegrins and natriuretic peptides; nine minor proteins and 36 rare. Results revealed that elapid venom contained a less diverse range of protein families than the others, mostly consisting of phospholipases and three-finger toxins. Viper venom showed to scarcely contain three-finger toxin [51].

2.4.1 Phospholipase A_2

These enzymes play an important role in the regulation of phospholipid turnover, membrane permeability, cell maintenance and growth, apoptosis and the production of leukotrienes and prostaglandins [50]. Of the four types of PLAs, only type one and two are found in snake venom with several isoforms. These PLAs target the motor nerve terminal and the terminal part of the motor axon, by initiating hydrolysis of the lipids of the outer leaf of the plasma membrane of the nerve terminal resulting in its depolarization. Synaptic vesicles are also destroyed by the PLA and the products of lipid hydrolysis [52]. Exposure of skeletal muscle to venom PLAs causes a severe inflammatory degenerative response, with the first clinical signs apparent less than 1 hour after inoculation, with affected fibres rapidly depolarising [50].

2.4.2 Metalloprotease

Haemorrhaging is a common clinical sign associated with viper and crotaline snake bites and has been associated with the proteolytic activity of metalloprotease [53]. The proteases induce direct damage of the microvessels [54]. Snake venom metalloproteases are classified into four main groups based on their domain structure: PI—possesses a metalloprotease domain only, PII—consists of both metalloprotease and disintegrin-like domains, PIII—compromised of metalloprotease, disintegrin-like and high-cysteine domains, PIV—in addition to metalloprotease, disintegrin and cysteine also possesses a lectin-like polypeptide [53]. The disintegrin-like domain inhibits platelet aggregation by binding to the fibrinogen receptor in platelet plasma membranes and although the role of the other domains is not clear, venoms with cysteine and disintegrin domains are more active at inducing haemorrhage than enzymes with only metalloprotease domains [55]. Investigations suggest pathogenesis is associated with a per rhexis mechanism whereby endothelial cells of capillary blood vessels rapidly thin and detach from surrounding basal lamina, progressive degeneration of these vessels leads to breaks in the endothelial lining, allowing blood to enter interstitial space [56].

2.4.3 Serine protease

Serine proteases are major components of snake venom, mostly identified in snakes of the Viperidae family and certain Elapidae, Colubridae and Hydrophiidae families [57]. These venom enzymes affect the haemostatic system by acting on the coagulation cascade and possess strong pro-coagulant effects through the activation of platelets, production of thrombin-like enzymes which clot fibrinogen and the creation anti-coagulant enzymes such as protein C [58], these serine protease produced thrombins are not susceptible to hirudin or heparin, other proteases possess kininogenase activity which releases hypotensive bradykinin [59].

2.4.4 Three-finger toxin (3FTs)

This family of non-enzymatic polypeptides exhibit potent toxic effects. Based on their biological properties, they can be classified as postsynaptic neurotoxins targeting the nicotinic and muscarinic acetylcholinesterase receptors; fasciculins targeting acetylcholinesterase; calciseptins and FS2 toxins targeting L-type calcium channels; anticoagulants; β-blockers targeting β_1 and β_2 adrenergic receptors; dendroaspin targeting specific glycoproteins; cardiotoxin A5 targeting integrins and antagonists of α_1A and α_2A adrenergic receptors [60]. A large number of 3FTs are neurotoxic, interfering with cholinergic transmission at post-synaptic sites in the peripheral and central nervous system; mipartoxin-I, a 3FT, is the most abundant protein found in coral snake venom from northern South America and possesses a lethal effect in mice and a clear neuromuscular blockade in avian and mice subjects with an affinity for the cholinergic nicotinic receptor [61]. A group of cardiotoxic 3FTs found only in cobra venom is the second-largest group, at low concentrations they elevate heart rates and at high concentrations, cause death by cardiac arrest [62].

2.5 The use of *Bitis arietans* snake venom in biopharmaceutical research

Biscetin, a platelet adhesion inducer, isolated from the venom of *Bitis arietans* has been shown to activate the binding of the Von Willebrand factor to glycoprotein without altering the binding site; this factor plays a key role in haemostatic response to vascular injury [63]. In a 2015 study, bitistatin a disintegrin isolated from the Puff adder was demonstrated to have an affinity for the integrin receptor avβ3, a marker used for tumour angiogenesis. This can be radiolabeled, injected and then detected on imaging. The ability to detect these receptors via diagnostic imaging has been used to successfully diagnose thrombosis in a canine model [64]. Studies researching strategies to enhance immunological responses against venoms observed the cross-immunoreactivity of antivenoms of the *Echis* and *Bitis* species, supporting the hypothesis that immunising horses with a mixture of *Echis ocellatus*, *Bitis arietans* and *Naja nigricollis* generates enough antibodies that can recognise all medically relevant viper venoms in sub-Saharan Africa [65].

2.6 The Puff adder (*Bitis arietans*)

The Puff adder (*Bitis arietans*) is venomous snake from the Viperidae family found in the Middle East, North and sub-Saharan Africa. The species has a broad, flattened, lanceolate shaped head covered with small keeled scales attached to a narrow neck. Puff adders along with Russell's vipers can make a loud hissing sound by expelling air through their large nostrils. These snakes are distinguishable by their distinctive repeated U or V dorsal pattern [66]. *Bitis arietans* feed on a variety of small animals including hares, hedgehogs, rodents, lizards and birds; they can actively forage by visiting birds' nests to feed on eggs, nestling or the adult birds themselves. This species can also deploy ambush tactics by camouflaging themselves in areas where bird encounters are common, such as water pools [67].

2.7 The occurrence of snake bites

A global review by White in 2000 estimated that between 1.25 and 5.5 million snakebites occur annually [68]. These primarily occur in developing countries where there is a dense population of humans, an abundance of snakes and a lack of medical treatment facilities. In 1987 in South Africa, pregnant women accounted for 0–4% of cases admitted to hospital, in India, they accounted for 1% of admissions [46]. Venomous snakebites may lead to poor foetal development and adversely affect the mother's health; previous studies determined that foetal death occurred in 38–43% of snakebite cases, whereas maternal death accounted for 10% [69]. The African puff adder, along with the carpet viper, is the two most common species responsible for fatalities following bites in Africa. These adder venoms possess cardiotoxic and haemorrhagic effects which can lead to hypovolemic shock, necrosis, systemic haemorrhage and arrhythmias [70].

2.8 The geographical variations in snake venom

Variation in venom composition occurs between species of snake as well as within a species. These variations can have a significant impact on venom toxicity and medical management. Different toxin-encoding genes in the genome attribute to these variations [28], however the mechanisms by which these gene expressions are controlled are poorly understood [71]. Results from Barlow et al. [72] provides evidence for the theory of diet affecting venom composition, by observing *Echis* snake species diet and the LD50 by which to incapacitate their natural scorpion prey; their study findings suggested that variations in composition are derived from adaptive evolution, driven by natural selection, for different diets. It has more recently been hypothesised by other literature that variation in venom composition is the result of adaption to dietary selection [28]. In a 2015 study, the intraspecific variations of venom activities of *E. ocellatus* snakes from Nigeria and Cameroon were observed; the Nigerian venom showed higher lethality and coagulation in comparison to the Cameroonian venom. The antivenoms produced by both snakes were similarly effective in neutralising the venom, however, the coagulant activity was better neutralised by the Nigerian antivenom than the Cameroonian venom [73]. Further studies in geographical variations involving envenomation by *N. naja* revealed that the median lethal dose in mice differed between northern (0.55 mg/kg), central (0.66), western (0.68), southern (0.62) and Sabaragamuwa (0.7) regions respectively. Histopathological changes of these regional venoms, however, showed a higher affinity for certain bodily systems, with northern venom observing a significantly higher infiltration of inflammatory and necrotic cells into skeletal muscle and central venom demonstrating high cardiotoxic effects, these results confirm venom disparity [74]. Geographical location showed a remarkable degree of variation amongst *Bitis arietans* species originating from the same geographical origin, most evident by the venom components metalloproteinases [71]. These metalloproteinases are responsible for inducing haemorrhaging, myonecrosis and degradation of extracellular matrix components which in turn affects local inflammatory response to a bite [53].

3. Materials and methods

3.1 Ethics and morality of research

In accordance with the European Union Directive 2010/63/EU section nine, embryos were not developed beyond the first two-thirds of development. This also corresponds with mandates of The Institutional Animal Care and Use Committee, Association of New England Medical Centre (Tufts) and the National Institute of Health, USA which dictate that a chick embryo that has not reached the 14th day of its gestation period will not experience pain and therefore can be used for experimentation without ethical restrictions.

3.2 CHEST II

For this research, the chick embryotoxicity screening test was used. This standardised technique allows for the administration of small amounts of test compounds into the fertilised egg on 4th embryonic day (ED4) and the measurement of a quantitative endpoint on ED9.

3.2.1 Materials

1. Fertilised eggs: alive and morphologically normal (breed Lohmann Brown, Hatchery Farm Párovské Háje, Nitra, Slovakia).

2. Incubator (ART 549/A).

3. Dissection kit: including tissue forceps, dissecting scissors and blunt scissors.

4. Micropipette with disposable tips.

5. Stereomicroscope (Olympus SZ 61 with digital camera ARTCAM-300MI).

6. Observing dish with fixing pins.

7. Distilled water: to aid observation.

3.3 Application of snake venom: CHEST II

Eggs were placed in an incubator on day 0 at 37–38°C with a 50–60% relative humidity and rotated periodically until (ED4). Then eggs were removed and blunt end of eggs was cleaned with 70% alcohol and covered by a transparent adhesive tape. Subsequently, using serrated scissors (FST 14071-12), an opening was cut for application of the respective doses of snake venom (100 μl). The tested concentration was applied directly over the embryo on the top of inner shell membrane (*membrana papyracea*). Controls received the same volume of sterile distilled water—100 μl (**Figure 1**). The ranges of concentration as well as the total number of embryos and the days of application are listed in **Tables 1** and **2**. A small hole was then covered by micro-tape and labelled, before being returned to the incubator without rotation. On ED9 the eggs were removed from the incubator, the tape was removed and the survived chicken embryos were removed from the eggs using a crook, weighed and examined under a dissecting microscope. Hearts and livers were dissected from the chicken embryos and they were weighted separately (**Figure 1**).

3.4 Preparation of snake venom concentrations

Venoms from *Bitis arietans* (*B.A.*) of different regions were extracted in the breeding garden Pata near Hlohovec (Slovakia), which had been designed for reptiles' conservation of the gene pool under the veterinary certificate No. CHEZ-TT-01. We used the snake venom of *Bitis arietans* from three different regions (Kenya, South Africa, Namibia). Also, we used one more snake venom sample without specific region determination (B.A. nonspecific). The breeding garden also serves as a quarantine station for imported animals and is an official importer of exotic animals from around the world, having the permission of the State Nature Protection of the Slovak Republic under the No. 03418/06, the trade with endangered species of wild fauna and flora and on amendments to certain laws under Law No. 237/2002.

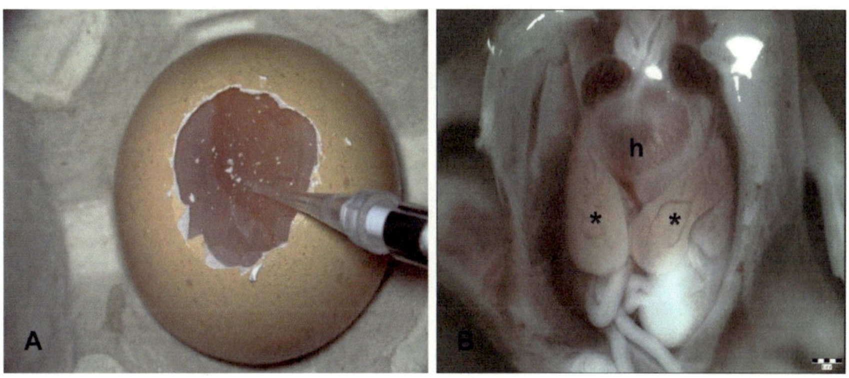

Figure 1.
Graphical illustration of snake venom administration on ED4 (A) and visualisation of developing heart and liver on ED9 (B); asterisk—lobes of liver, h—heart.

Snake venom	**Concentrations (mg/ml)**			
	E-1	**E-2**	**E-3**	**E-4**
Control (sterile distilled water)				
B.A. nonspecific region	100.00	10.00	1.00	0.10
B.A. Kenya	100.00	10.00	1.00	0.10
B.A. Namibia	100.00	10.00	1.00	0.10
B.A. South Africa	100.00	10.00	1.00	0.10

Table 1.
Concentrations of snake venom used for each venom.

Snake venom	**Dose (mg/ml)**	***N***	**Dead embryos**	**Mortality (%)**	**Mean body weight (g)**	**Mean heart weight (mg)**	**Mean liver weight (mg)**
Bitis arietans— nonspecific region	0	10	1	10	1.73	22.9	31.6
	100	10	7	70	1.42	16.3	20.7
	10	10	3	30	1.66	**18.3**	**20.9**
	1	10	2	20	1.59	17.0	**19.9**
	0.1	10	1	10	1.66	**18.8**	**22.2**
Bitis arietans— Kenya	0	10	1	10	1,53	18.7	28.5
	100	10	2	20	**1.16**	**13.5**	**15.5**
	10	10	4	40	**1.19**	**13.3**	**14.8**
	1	10	1	10	**1.19**	**15.6**	**14.2**
	0.1	10	3	30	1.57	18.3	**20.4**
Bitis arietans— South Africa	0	10	1	10	1.62	18.0	28.8
	100	10	2	20	1.67	18.5	**19.3**
	10	10	2	20	1.62	19.9	**19.6**
	1	10	2	20	1.66	19.9	26.8
	0.1	10	0	0	1.43	**15.4**	**20.7**
Bitis arietans— Namibia	0	10	1	10	1.70	21.0	31.2
	100	10	2	20	1.47	17.3	**20.8**
	10	11	3	27	1.72	20.6	35.3
	1	11	1	9	1.60	20.1	31.4
	0.1	11	2	18	1.54	20.1	30.1
Total		**203**	**41**				

N, number of chicken embryos; numbers in bold represent statistically significant results ($P \leq 0.05$).

Table 2.
Embryotoxic effect of Bitis arietans *venom from different regions of Africa.*

A sterile plastic cup was used for venom extraction with plastic food wrap, and rubber bands fixed the plastic wrap. For the application, we used snake venoms immediately after their extracting. Before use, it was ensured the venoms were continuously kept in cold storage to ensure that they retained their full toxicological potential. The venoms were diluted with sterile distilled water to give equal concentrations (based on molecular weights) of E-1, E-2, E-3 and E-4 when required (**Table 1**). The composition of tested snake venoms used in our study has been already described and determined in previous studies [75, 76].

3.5 Nile blue staining

For this staining method, embryos with the highest concentration of snake venom (10-1) were used. The blue stain was applied on ED4. The embryos were then dissected on day ED6 and incubated in a 1/8000 solution of Nile Blue A (Sigma) and PBS for 15 minutes at 37°C in an incubator. Following this, embryos were transferred to cold PBS (4 °C) and washed for 4 hours. Embryos were then photographed with a stereomicroscope Olympus SZ 61 with digital camera ARTCAM-300MI and Quick Photo 2.3 software. These embryos were lastly compared with control embryos (sterile distilled water applied only) dissected on ED6.

3.6 Evaluation

The number of dead or growth-retarded embryos (those <650 mg) were totalled for each concentration. The proportion of effects on heart and liver in surviving embryos were considered separately to establish a profile of each concentration. The result of the CHEST was rank venom in order of their teratogenic potency in chickens; these ranges can be compared for an assessment of human risk. For statistical analysis, the programme GraphPad Prism 6.0 was utilised (one-way ANOVA, with a P-value of 0.05).

4. Results

The following results were analysed—body weight, heart weight and liver weight. These results were compared between control samples and the venom of *Bitis arietans* from four different regions of Africa (Namibia, Kenya, South Africa and non-specified region).

4.1 Body weight

All living embryos were weighed on ED 9 in grams. **Figure 2** presents the following concentrations E1 (10-1), E2 (10-2), E3 (10-3) and E4 (10-4).

4.1.1 Kenya

The average body weight of the control embryos was 1.73 g, whereas embryos infused with venom concentration 10-1 (E1), 10-2 (E2) and 10-3 (E3) were significantly reduced ($P < 0.05$) in comparison. E1 averaged at 1.15 g in body weight, E2 was slightly increased at 1.18 g and E3 at 1.19 g. There was a large increase between E3 and 10-4 (E4) body weight, with E4 averaging at 1.5 g.

4.1.2 Namibia

The embryos injected with venoms of the Namibian snake showed no statistically significant changes in body weight in comparison with the control embryos. E1 body weight averaged at 1.4 g in comparison with the 1.72 g of control embryos. E2 average body weight was 1.7 g whereas E3 averaged at 1.6 g. E4 embryos body weight was less than E2 and E3 at 1.54 g.

4.1.3 South Africa

None of the embryos impregnated with South African Puff adder venom showed a statistically significant change in body weight compared to the control group. E1, E2 and E3 body weights were all similar, averaging at 1.67, 1.62 and 1.66 g respectively. E4 averaged the smallest body weight at 1.43 g.

4.1.4 Non-specific region

None of the embryos infused with the non-specific venom showed significant differences in body weight compared to the control group. E1 averaged the smallest body weight at 1.42 g, E2 averaged at 1.66 g, E3 at 1.58 g and E4 at 1.66 g.

4.2 Heart weight

Hearts were cut from surviving embryos at the level of the aorta and weighed in milligrams (**Figure 3**).

4.2.1 Kenya

The control heart mean weighed 23 mg; the embryo hearts infused with venom were significantly smaller in E1, E2 and E3. E1 and E2 weighed in at 13 mg, E3 had a slight increase in weight at 15 mg. There was a large increase between E3 and E4 with the latter averaging 18 mg.

4.2.2 Namibia

None of the concentrations had a significant effect on heart weight in comparison to the control group. E1 mean heart weight came in at 17 mg. E2 was the largest weights at 21 mg, E3 and E4 averaged 20 mg.

4.2.3 South Africa

The largest average heart weight was seen in E3 and E2 at 19.8 mg. E1 averaged at 18.5 mg. E4 had the lowest body weight of 15 mg; this result was statistically significant.

4.2.4 Non-specified region

E1 and E3 results were both deemed statistically significant. E1 averaged the lowest heart weight of 16 mg. E2 averaged 18 mg whereas E3 mean was lower than E2 at 17 mg. E4 weighed in with the largest heart weight of 18 mg.

4.3 Liver weight

Livers were cut at the level of the portal vein, cut from surviving embryos and weighed in milligrams (**Figure 4**).

4.3.1 Kenya

All four concentrations of snake venom s were proven statistically significant. The mean control group liver weighed 31.6 mg, larger than all four test groups. E1

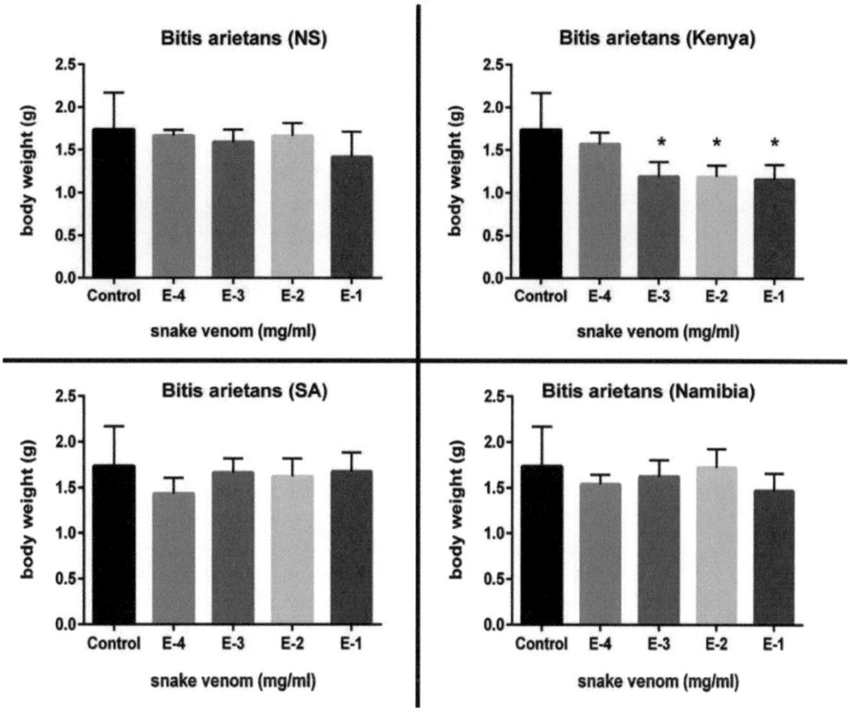

Figure 2.
Graphs depicting body weights of the Bitis arietans *venoms of Kenya, non-specified (NS), South Africa (SA) and Namibia, (*): statistically significant (P ≤ 0.05).*

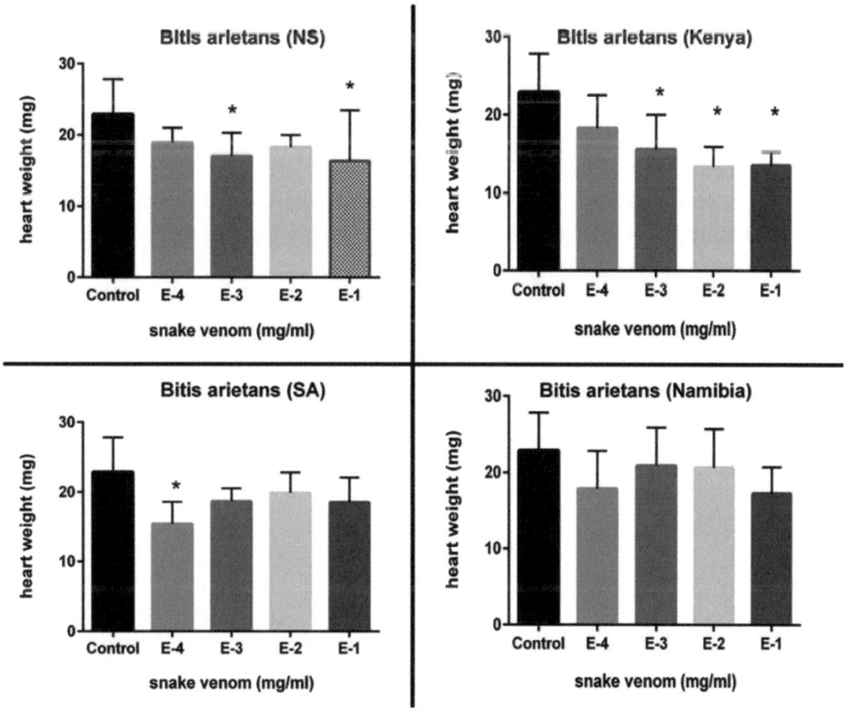

Figure 3.
Graphs depicting heart weights of the Bitis arietans *venoms of Kenya, non-specified (NS), South Africa (SA) and Namibia, (*): Statistically significant (P ≤ 0.05).*

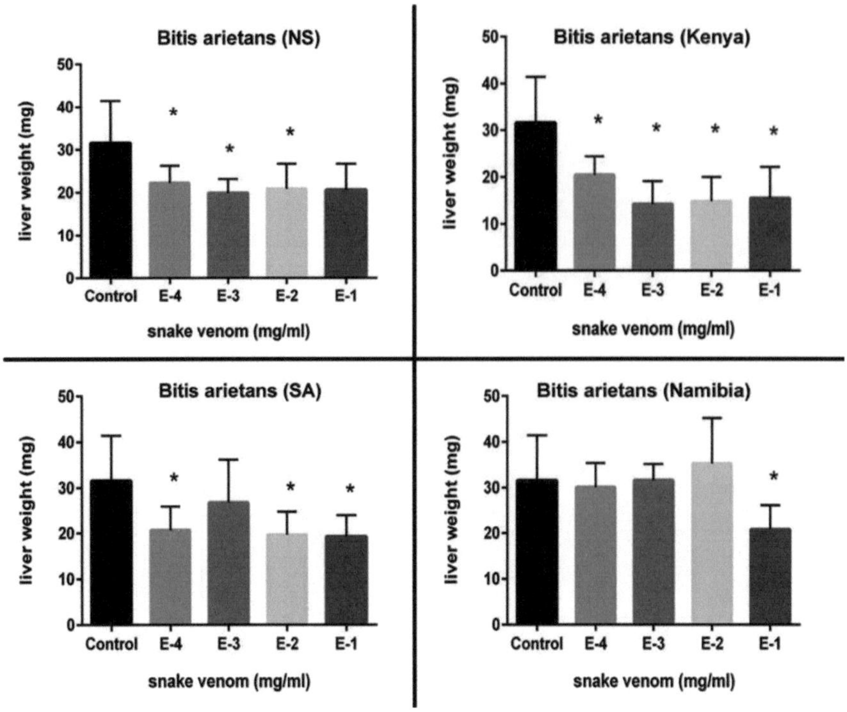

Figure 4.
Graphs depicting liver weights of the Bitis arietans *venoms of Kenya, non-specified (NS), South Africa (SA) and Namibia, (*): Statistically significant ($P \leq 0.05$).*

liver weight mean was recorded as 15.5 mg, E2 weighed in at 14.8 mg; E3 was the lowest average liver weight of 14 mg. E4 average liver weight was the largest at 20 mg.

4.3.2 Namibia

Venom concentration E1 was the only statistically significant result in this test group, with its average weight calculated at 20 mg. E2 liver weight averaged heavier than the control group (31.6 mg) with 35 mg. E3 mean weight was similar to the control at 31.4 mg and E4 averaged 30 mg.

4.3.3 South Africa

E1, E2 and E4 concentrations were proven statistically significant; whereas E3, with the largest liver weight of 26 mg, was not. E1 had the lowest average liver weight of 19.2 mg; E2 was marginally heavier at 19.8 mg. E4 liver weight averaged at 20.7 mg.

4.3.4 Non-specified region

Three of the four concentrations of non-specified venom had a statistically significant effect on the liver weight (E2, E3 and E4). E1 mean result weighed in at 20 mg; E2 was faintly heavier at 20.9 mg. E3 weighed the least with 19.9 mg. E4 had the heaviest weight within the test group at 22.2 mg.

4.4 Mortality rates

The highest mortality rate was seen in the highest concentration, in this maximum venom concentration (E1) the non-specific venom samples had a 70% death occurrence (embryos not surviving to day 9); the Kenyan, Namibian and South African E1 all had a 20% mortality rate. All groups at each concentration had a fatality, except the South African E4 group.

The non-specified venom produced the highest overall amount of fatalities, with the Kenyan being second, Namibian third and South African venom being the least lethal. The 10 mg/ml (E2) concentration saw the highest mortality rates overall, with the Kenyan test group showing a 40% mortality, the Namibian and non-specific test group perceiving 30% mortality and the South African group a 20% mortality. E3 showed 20% fatality in the South African and non-specific test groups, in Namibia and Kenyan groups only 10% fatality rate was recorded. In the lowest concentration (E4) the highest mortality rate was recorded in the Kenyan group with 30%. No fatalities were recorded in the South African group. The Namibian test group showing a 20% mortality and the non-specific test group a 10% mortality (**Figure 5**, **Table 2**).

4.5 Nile blue staining

The embryos were stained on ED4 and removed from their eggs on ED6; all were envenomed with the strongest concentrations of venom (10-1; **Figure 6**).

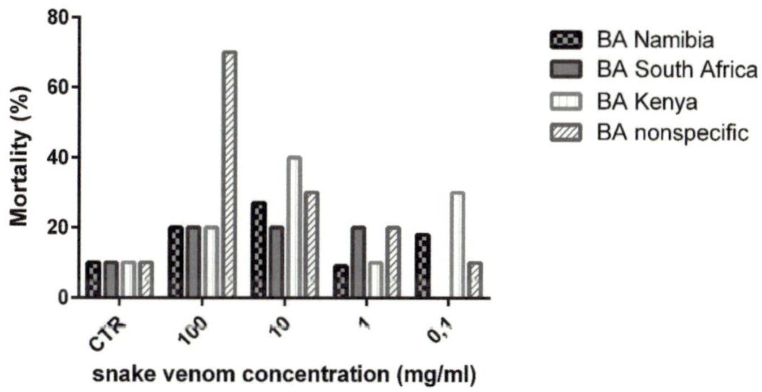

Figure 5.
Mortality rates of chicken embryos against snake venom.

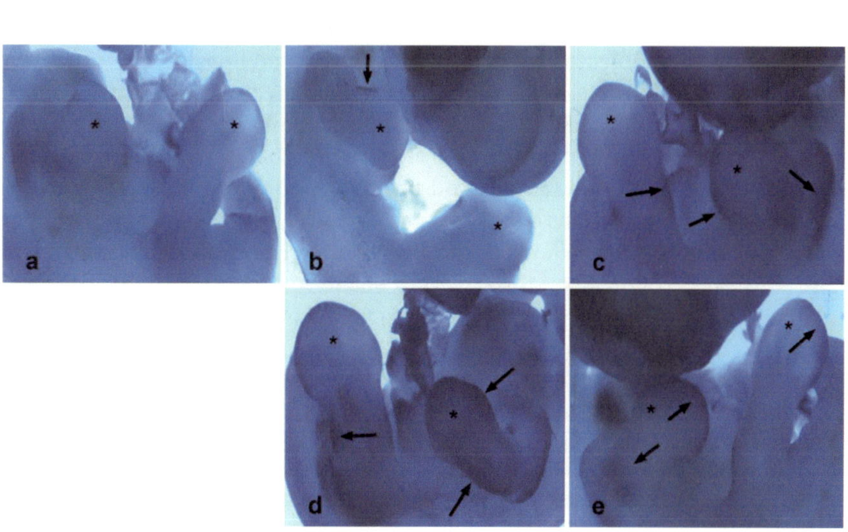

Figure 6.
Nile blue staining results. (a) Control, (b) B.A. nonspecific region, (c) B.A. South Africa, (d) B.A. Kenya, (e) B.A. Namibia; asterisk—wing and leg buds on ED9, arrows—dark coloured areas with apoptotic response.

The arrows on the above images highlight the darkened areas of apoptotic cells. These images show that initial cell death is initiated on the wing buds. The control embryo (a), infused with distilled sterile water only, demonstrates no apoptosis. The nonspecific venom (b) indicates a small amount of apoptosis located on the wing buds. Embryos envenomed with South African (c) and Kenyan (d) B.A. showed significant apoptosis along with the entire wing buds, with the Kenyan spreading to the extremities. The Namibian embryo showed less severe cell apoptosis than (c) and (d) along with the wing buds.

5. Discussion

5.1 Bodyweight

Although the body weights varied amongst regional snakes and concentrations, they all presented similarly which was anticipated as they are the same species of snake. Generalised haemorrhaging was present across all four venom groups, which was expected due to the haemotoxic nature of *Bitis arietans* [47]. The Kenyan test group was the only one to have statistically significant changes in body weight with envenomation (E1, E2 and E3); the average weights for this group were also notably smaller than the rest, suggesting a larger detrimental effect than the other venom groups. The South African, Namibian and non-specific groups had similar mean weights across all four concentrations, which could propose a similar toxicity level across these regions. Further research into regional diet variations could strengthen the hypothesis that venom composition is derived from a natural dietary selection [28].

5.2 Heart weight

All heart weights of embryos envenomed with *Bitis arietans* were reduced, with the Kenyan group showing the highest rate of statistical significance, with E1, E2 and E3 all being significant; this group also presented the lowest mean weights at 13–15 mg. These findings support the proposal that the Kenyan venom has a stronger effect than the other regions. A histopathological study observed that *Vipera raddei*, from the family Viperidae, venom caused cardiomyocyte disruption, fibrosis and blood vessel congestion in post mortem specimens [77]. Another study found *Naja nigricollis* venom injected into pregnant mice caused hepatic and myocardial damage as well as pulmonary vascular congestion and accumulation of blood in the intestinal lumen of the foetus [78]. One of the venom components of *Bitis arietans* is a serine protease, a bioactive protein, which plays a role in the regulation of the blood coagulation cascade and affects the circulatory haemostasis [59]. Disturbances by these proteins could lead to adverse effects on embryonic organ development, which may account for the reduction in heart weights; however, to date, no studies are focusing on the effects of snake venom on the heart function.

5.3 Liver weight

All groups had a minimum of one statistically significant concentration, suggesting the liver was the most affected parameter (in comparison with heart and body weight). In furtherance with the proposal that the Kenyan venom has the highest potency, E1, E2 and E3 all proved statistically significant as well as being of the lowest median body weights of the groups surveyed. All livers exhibited a decrease in mean weight, varying yellow colour change along with increased susceptibility to disintegration on removal; this substantiates the results from a previous study on the effects of *Echis coloratus* venom on sheep liver, where biochemical and histological alterations were observed. The study reported an elevation in glucose, aspartate aminotransferase, alanine transferase, triglyceride and total bilirubin whilst cholesterol levels were reduced. Histologically, pyknosis, karyorrhexis, cytoplasmic vacuolation, necrosis, fatty changes and hepatocyte atrophy were observed [79].

5.4 Mortality

The highest incidence of mortality was observed in E1 by the non-specified test group, with a 70% mortality; whereas Kenya, Namibia and South Africa observed a 40–10% death rate. This evidence proposes that although the Kenyan venom has the most significant impact on development, the non-specific venom has the strongest potency. Furthers study with a larger specimen pool is needed to confirm these findings.

5.5 Apoptotic cell appearance (Nile blue staining)

A 1993 study observed that haemorrhagic snake venom (*Bitis arietans*) induced apoptosis of vascular endothelial cells whereas neurotoxic venom did not induce programmed cell death; instead it caused necrosis at much higher doses of venom [80]. This corroborates with the findings of the Nile blue staining of this study which revealed varying levels of cell death along with the wing buds and limb extremities of *Bitis arietans* envenomed embryos. The development of limb vasculature may explain why apoptosis was seen the distal limbs, clustered away from the tips of the extremities. Interestingly, apoptosis was primarily seen on the wing buds, which develop later than the legs [81]. Previous studies may have explained the affinity for wing bud cells over leg bud cells due to the principle of non-equivalence meaning that cells in different areas of the body have different intrinsic characters and positional information [82]; however it has more recently been proven that these cells are interchangeable and not restricted in their development [83].

6. Conclusions

In conclusion, it was seen that the test group envenomed by *Bitis arietans* from Kenya exhibited the highest incidence of detrimental effects. Concentration 100, 10 and 1 mg/ml of venom all showed statistically significant changes to the body, heart and liver weight. This venom also produced the smallest average weights in comparison to the other test groups. The highest mortality rate, however, was observed in the non-specific venom, with the strongest concentration resulting in 70% fatalities. This suggests that the most fatal of the four venoms observed was the non-specific African *Bitis arietans*. The induced cell death was observed in all four venom specimens, which correlates to *Bitis arietans* previously documented haemotoxic potential. The results showed that the Kenyan venom, along with having the most significant effect on organ weights of the embryo, also initiated the strongest apoptosis.

These results suggest a geographical variation in potency of *Bitis arietans* venom, however further study is required to determine the cause of this variation. Current hypotheses suggest a natural dietary evolution influencing the venom composition; future studies examining if there is a regional difference in the diet of these snakes along with an analysis of their venom enzymes could aid in confirming this hypothesis.

Acknowledgements

This work was realized within the framework of the project of the Ministry of Education VEGA No. 1/0050/19 and APVV-17-0017.

Author details

Charlotte Peters[1], Vladimir Petrilla[2], Lenka Luptakova[3] and Eva Petrovova[1*]

1 Institute of Anatomy, University of Veterinary Medicine and Pharmacy in Kosice, Kosice, Slovakia

2 Institute of Physiology, University of Veterinary Medicine and Pharmacy in Kosice, Kosice, Slovakia

3 Institute of Biology, Zoology and Radiobiology, University of Veterinary Medicine and Pharmacy in Kosice, Kosice, Slovakia

*Address all correspondence to: eva.petrovova@uvlf.sk

References

[1] Vergara MN, Canto-Soler MV. Rediscovering the chick embryo as a model to study retinal development. Neural Development. 2012;**7**:22. DOI: 10.1186/1749-8104-7-22

[2] Bressan M, Mikawa T. Avian as a model system of vascular development. Methods in Molecular Biology. 2015;**1214**:225-242. DOI: 10.1007/978-1-4939-1462-3_14

[3] Lillico SG, McGrew MJ, Sherman A, Sang HM. Transgenic chickens as bioreactors for protein-based drugs. Drug Discovery Today. 2005;**10**:191-196. DOI: 10.1016/S1359-6446(04)03317-3

[4] Harvey AJ, Speksnijder G, Baugh LR, Morris JA, Ivarie R. Expression of exogenous protein in the egg white of transgenic chickens. Nature Biotechnology. 2002;**20**:396-399. DOI: 10.1038/nbt0402-396

[5] Rashidi H, Sottile V. The chick embryo: Hatching a model for contemporary biomedical research. BioEssays. 2009;**31**:459-465. DOI: 10.1002/bies.200800168

[6] Harvey AJ, Ivarie R. Validating the hen as a bioreactor for the production of exogenous proteins in egg white. Poultry Science. 2003;**82**:927-930. DOI: 10.1093/ps/82.6.927

[7] Steinlein P, Deiner E, Leutz A, Beug H. Recombinant murine erythropoietin receptor expressed in avian erythroid progenitors mediates terminal erythroid differentiation *in vitro*. Growth Factors. 1994;**10**:1-16

[8] Kue CS, Tan KY, Lam ML, Lee HB. Chick embryo chorioallantoic membrane (CAM): An alternative predictive model in acute toxicological studies for anti-cancer drugs. Experimental Animals. 2015;**64**: 129-138. DOI: 10.1538/expanim.14-0059

[9] Wilting J, Christ B, Bokeloh M, Weich HA. *In vivo* effects of vascular endothelial growth factor on the chicken chorioallantoic membrane. Cell and Tissue Research. 1993;**274**:163-172. DOI: 10.1007/bf00327997

[10] Nowak-Sliwinska P, Segura T, Iruela-Arispe ML. The chicken chorioallantoic membrane model in biology, medicine and bioengineering. Angiogenesis. 2014;**17**:779-804. DOI: 10.1007/s10456-014-9440-7

[11] Barth R, Gruschkau H, Jaeger O, Milcke L, Weinmann E. Purified chick embryo cell (PCEC) rabies vaccine for human use. Laboratory data. Behring Institute Mitteilungen. 1984;**76**:142-154

[12] Giesen A, Gniel D, Malerczyk C. 30 years of rabies vaccination with Rabipur: A summary of clinical data and global experience. Expert Review of Vaccines. 2015;**14**:351-367. DOI: 10.1586/14760584.2015.1011134

[13] Hegde NR. Cell culture-based influenza vaccines: A necessary and indispensable investment for the future. Human Vaccines and Immunotherapeutics. 2015;**11**:1223-1234. DOI: 10.1080/21645515.2015.1016666

[14] Coulombre JL, Coulombre AJ. Regeneration of neural retina from the pigmented epithelium in the chick embryo. Developmental Biology. 1965;**12**:79-92. DOI: 10.1016/0012-1606(65)90022-9

[15] Langouet-Astrie CJ, Meinsen AL, Grunwald ER, Turner SD, Enke RA. RNA sequencing analysis of the developing chicken retina. Scientific Data. 2016;**3**:160117. DOI: 10.1038/sdata.2016.117

[16] Ola M, Mawaz M, Siddiquei M, Al-Amro S, Abu El-Asrar A. Recent

advances in understanding the biochemical and molecular mechanism of diabetic retinopathy. Journal of Diabetes and Its Complications. 2012;**26**:56-64. DOI: 10.1016/j.jdiacomp.2011.11.004

[17] Fong DS, Aiello L, Gardner TW, King GL, Blankenship G, Cavallerano JD, et al. Retinopathy in diabetes. Diabetes Care. 2004;**27**(Suppl 1):84-87. DOI: 10.2337/diacare.27.2007.s84

[18] Valdez DJ, Nieto PS, Díaz NM, Garbarino-Pico E, Guido ME. Differential regulation of feeding rhythms through a multiple-photoreceptor system in an avian model of blindness. FASEB Journal. 2013;**27**:2702-2712. DOI: 10.1096/fj.12-222885

[19] Shi L, Ko ML, Huang CC, Park S, Hong M, Wu C, et al. Chicken embryos as a potential new model for early onset type I diabetes. Journal of Diabetes Research. 2014;**2014**:1-10. DOI: 10.1155/2014/354094

[20] Murphy MP, LeVine H 3rd. Alzheimer's disease and the amyloid-beta peptide. Journal of Alzheimer's Disease. 2010;**19**:311-323. DOI: 10.3233/JAD-2010-1221

[21] Carrodeguas JA, Rodolosse A, Garza MV, Sanz-Clemente A, Pérez-Pé R, Lacosta AM, et al. The chick embryo appears as a natural model for research in beta-amyloid precursor protein processing. Neuroscience. 2005;**134**:1285-1300. DOI: 10.1016/j.neuroscience.2005.05.020

[22] Sarasa M, Pesini P. Natural non-trasgenic animal models for research in Alzheimer's disease. Current Alzheimer Research. 2009;**6**:171-178

[23] Ahlemeyer B, Krieglstein J. Pharmacological studies supporting the therapeutic use of Ginkgo biloba extract for Alzheimer's disease. Pharmacopsychiatry. 2003;**36**:8-14. DOI: 10.1055/s-2003-40454

[24] Kain KH, Miller JWI, Jones-Paris CR, Thomason RT, Lewis JD, Bader DM, et al. The chick embryo as an expanding experimental model for cancer and cardiovascular research. Developmental Dynamics. 2014;**24**:216-228. DOI: 10.1002/dvdy.24093

[25] Bader AG, Kang S, Vogt PK. Cancer-specific mutations in PIK3CA are oncogenic *in vivo*. Proceedings of the National Academy of Sciences. 2006;**103**:1475-1479. DOI: 10.1073/pnas.0510857103

[26] Ribatti D. The chick embryo chorioallantoic membrane in the study of tumor angiogenesis. Romanian Journal of Morphology and Embryology. 2008;**49**:131-135

[27] Rous P. A sarcoma of the fowl transmissible by an agent separable from the tumor cells. The Journal of Experimental Medicine. 1911;**13**:397-411. DOI: 10.1084/jem.13.4.397

[28] Javier RT, Butel J. The history of tumour virology. Cancer Research. 2008;**68**:7693-7706. DOI: 10.1158/0008-5472.CAN-08-3301

[29] Zijlstra A, Mellor R, Panzarella G, Aimes RT, Hooper JD, Marchenko ND, et al. A quantitative analysis of rate-limiting steps in the metastatic cascade using human-specific real-time polymerase chain reaction. Cancer Research. 2002;**62**:7083-7092

[30] Mu X, Sultankulov B, Agarwal R, Mahjoub A, Schott T, Greco N, et al. Chick embryo extract demethylates tumor suppressor genes in osteosarcoma cells. Clinical Orthopaedics and Related Research. 2014;**472**:865-873. DOI: 10.1007/s11999-013-3104-6

[31] Pain B, Clark ME, Shen M, Nakazawa H, Sakurai M, Samarut J,

et al. Long-term in vitro culture and characterisation of avian embryonic stem cells with multiple morphogenetic potentialities. Development (Cambridge, England). 1996;**122**:2339-2348

[32] Petitte JN, Liu G, Yang Z. Avian pluripotent stem cells. Mechanisms of Development. 2004;**121**:1159-1168

[33] Intarapat S, Stern CD. Chick stem cells: Current progress and future prospects. Stem Cell Research. 2013;**11**:1378-1392. DOI: 10.1016/j.scr.2013.09.005

[34] Naito M. Development of avian embryo manipulation techniques and their application to germ cell manipulation. Animal Science Journal. 2003;**74**:157-168. DOI: 10.1046/j.1344-3941.2003.00101.x

[35] Bajada S, Mazakova I, Richardson JB, Ashammakhi N. Updates on stem cells and their applications in regenerative medicine. Journal of Tissue Engineering and Regenerative Medicine. 2008;**2**:169-183. DOI: 10.1002/term.83

[36] Davies WJ, Freeman SJ. Chick embryotoxicity screening test (CHEST I and II). Methods in Molecular Biology. 1995;**43**:307-310. DOI: 10.1385/0-89603-282-5:307

[37] Jelinek R, Peterka M, Rychter Z. Chick embryotoxicity screening test—130 substances tested. Indian Journal of Experimental Biology. 1985;**23**:588-595

[38] Casewell NR, Wüster W, Vonk FJ, Harrison RA, Fry BG. Complex cocktails: The evolutionary novelty of venoms. Trends in Ecology and Evolution. 2013;**28**:219-229. DOI: 10.1016/j.tree.2012.10.020

[39] Vyas VK, Brahmbhatt K, Bhatt H, Parmar U. Therapeutic potential of snake venom in cancer therapy: Current perspectives. Asian Pacific Journal of Tropical Biomedicine. 2013;**3**:156-162. DOI: 10.1016/S2221-1691(13)60042-8

[40] Langley RL. Snakebite during pregnancy: A literature review. Wilderness and Environmental Medicine. 2010;**21**:54-60. DOI: 10.1016/j.wem.2009.12.025

[41] Jackson K. The evolution of venom-conducting fangs: Insights from developmental biology. Toxicon. 2007;**49**:975-981. DOI: 10.1016/j.toxicon.2007.01.007

[42] Kochva E. The development of the venom gland in the Opisthoglyph snake *Telescopus fallax* with remarks on *Thamnophis sirtalis* (Colubridae, Reptilia). Copeia. 1965;**2**:147-154. DOI: 10.2307/1440716

[43] Kochva E, Gans C. The venom gland of Vipera palaestinae with comments on the glands of some other viperines. Cells, Tissues, Organs. 1965;**62**:365-401. DOI: 10.1159/000142760

[44] Rosenberg HI. Histology, histochemistry, and emptying mechanism of the venom glands of some elapid snakes. Journal of Morphology. 1967;**123**:133-155. DOI: 10.1002/jmor.1051230204

[45] Underwood G, Kochva E. On the affinities of the burrowing asps Atractaspis (Serpentes: Atractaspididae). Zoological Journal of the Linnean Society. 1993;**107**:3-64. DOI: 10.1006/zjls.1993.1002

[46] Adewole AA, Ugiagbe OA, Onile TG, Joseph GA, Kassim OD, Medupin PF, et al. Case reports in Women's Health Snake bite in third trimester of pregnancy with systemic envenomation and delivery of a live baby in a low resource setting : A case report. Case Reports in Women's Health. 2017;**16**:14-17. DOI: 10.1016/j.crwh.2017.10.001

[47] Chisale M. Snake and snakebites–Part 2. WHO Pharmaceuticals Newsletter. 2008;**5**:1-4

[48] Jackson TNW, Young B, Underwood G, McCarthy CJ, Kochva E, Vidal N, et al. Endless forms most beautiful: The evolution of ophidian oral glands, including the venom system, and the use of appropriate terminology for homologous structures. Zoomorphology. 2017;**136**:107-130. DOI: 10.1007/s00435-016-0332-9

[49] Vonk FJ, Admiraal JF, Jackson K, Reshef R, de Bakker MAG, Vanderschoot K, et al. Evolutionary origin and development of snake fangs. Nature. 2008;**454**:630-633. DOI: 10.1038/nature07178

[50] Harris JB, Scott-Davey T. Secreted phospholipases A2 of snake venoms: Effects on the peripheral neuromuscular system with comments on the role of phospholipases A2 in disorders of the CNS and their uses in industry. Toxins. 2013;**5**:2533-2571. DOI: 10.3390/toxins5122533

[51] Tasoulis T, Isbister G. A review and database of snake venom proteomes. Toxins. 2017;**9**:E290. DOI: 10.3390/toxins9090290

[52] Rigoni M, Caccin P, Gschmeissner S, Koster G, Postle AD, Rossetto O, et al. Equivalent effects of snake PLA2 neurotoxins and lysophospholipid—fatty acid mixtures. Science. 2005;**310**:1678-1680. DOI: 10.1126/science.1120640

[53] Gutiérrez JM, Rucavado A. Snake venom metalloproteinases: Their role in the pathogenesis of local tissue damage. Biochimie. 2000;**82**:841-850

[54] Baldo C, Jamora C, Yamanouye N, Zorn TM, Moura-da-Silva AM. Mechanisms of vascular damage by hemorrhagic snake venom metalloproteinases: Tissue distribution and *in Situ* hydrolysis. PLoS Neglected Tropical Diseases. 2010;**4**:E727. DOI: 10.1371/journal.pntd.0000727

[55] Bjarnason JB, Fox JW. Hemorrhagic metalloproteinases from snake venoms. Pharmacology & Therapeutics. 1994;**62**:325-372

[56] Moreira L, Borkow G, Ovadia M, Gutiérrez JM. Pathological changes induced by BaH1, a hemorrhagic proteinase isolated from *Bothrops asper* (Terciopelo) snake venom, on mouse capillary blood vessels. Toxicon. 1994;**32**:976-987

[57] Serrano SMT, Maroun RC. Snake venom serine proteinases: Sequence homology vs. substrate specificity, a paradox to be solved. Toxicon. 2005;**45**:1115-1132. DOI: 10.1016/j.toxicon.2005.02.020

[58] Markland FS. Review paper snake venoms and the hemostatic system. Toxicon. 1998;**36**:1749-1800

[59] Matsui T, Fujimura Y, Titani K. Snake venom proteases affecting hemostasis and thrombosis. Biochimica et Biophysica Acta. 2000;**1477**:146-156. DOI: 10.1016/s0167-4838(99)00268-x

[60] Girish VM, Kumar S, Joseph L, Jobichen C, Kini RM, Sivaraman J. Identification and structural characterization of a new three-finger toxin hemachatoxin from Hemachatus haemachatus venom. PLoS One. 2012;7:E48112. DOI: 10.1371/journal.pone.0048112

[61] Rey-Suárez P, Floriano RS, Rostelato-Ferreira S, Saldarriaga-Córdoba M, Núñez V, Rodrigues-Simioni L, et al. Mipartoxin-I, a novel three-finger toxin, is the major neurotoxic component in the venom of the redtail coral snake Micrurus mipartitus (Elapidae). Toxicon. 2012;**60**:851-863. DOI: 10.1016/j.toxicon.2012.05.023

[62] Dufton MJ, Hider RC. Structure and pharmacology of elapid cytotoxins. Pharmacology and Therapeutics. 1988;**36**:1-40

[63] Matsui T, Hamako J, Matsushita T, Nakayama T, Fujimura Y, Titani K. Binding site on human von Willebrand factor of bitiscetin, a snake venom-derived platelet aggregation inducer. Biochemistry. 2002;**41**:7939-7946. DOI: 10.1021/bi020004b

[64] Knight LC, Baidoo KE, Romano JE, Gabriel JL, Maurer AH. Imaging pulmonary emboli and deep venous thrombi with 99mTc-bitistatin, a platelet-binding polypeptide from viper venom. Journal of Nuclear Medicine. 2000;**41**:1056-1064

[65] Calvete JJ, Harrison RA, Casewell NR, Wagstaff SC, Bolton FMS, Sanz L, et al. Medically important differences in snake venom composition are dictated by distinct postgenomic mechanisms. Proceedings of the National Academy of Sciences. 2014;**111**:9205-9210. DOI: 10.1073/pnas.1405484111

[66] Warrell DA. Venomous and poisonous animals. In: Farrar J, Hotez PJ, Junghanss T, Kang G, Lalloo D, White NJ, editors. Manson's Tropical Diseases. 23rd ed. China: Elsevier; 2014. pp. 1096-1127. DOI: 10.1016/B978-0-7020-5101-2.00076-5

[67] Glaudas X, Graham A. Natural history notes: *Bitis arietans* (puff adder). Foraging behavior. Herpetelogical Review. 2014;**45**:139-140

[68] White J. Bites and stings from venomous animal: A global overview. Therapeutic Drug Monitoring. 2000;**22**:65-68

[69] Dunnihoo DR, Rush BM, Wise RB, Brooks GG, Otterson WN. Snake bite poisoning in pregnancy. A review of the literature. The Journal of Reproductive Medicine. 1992;**37**:653-658

[70] Pollach G. A 14-year-old boy from Malawi who has been bitten by a snake. In: Rothe C, editor. Clinical Cases in Tropical Medicine. 1st ed. China: Elsevier; 2014. pp. 126-129. DOI: 10.1016/C2012-0-03630-7

[71] Currier R. Investigating venom synthesis: Exploring the composition, variation and gene expression dynamics of *Bitis arietans* venom. [PhD thesis]. University of Liverpool. 320 p

[72] Barlow A, Pook CE, Harrison RA, Wüster W. Coevolution of diet and prey-specific venom activity supports the role of selection in snake venom evolution. Proceedings of the Royal Society B: Biological Sciences: The Royal Society. 2009;**276**:2443-2449. DOI: 10.1098/rspb.2009.0048

[73] Sánchez LV, Pla D, Herrera M, Chippaux JP, Calvete JJ, Gutiérrez JM. Evaluation of the preclinical efficacy of four antivenoms, distributed in sub-Saharan Africa, to neutralize the venom of the carpet viper, Echis ocellatus, from Mali, Cameroon, and Nigeria. Toxicon. 2015;**106**:97-107. DOI: 10.1016/j.toxicon.2015.09.027

[74] Dissanayake DSB, Thewarage LD, Waduge RN, Ranasinghe JGS, Kularatne SAM, Rajapakse RPVJ. The venom of spectacled cobra (Elapidae: *Naja naja*): *In Vitro* study from distinct geographical origins in Sri Lanka. Journal of Toxicology. 2018;**2018**:1-14. DOI: 10.1155/2018/7358472

[75] Fasoli E, Sanz L, Wagstaff S, Harrison RA, Righetti PG, Calvete JJ. Exploring the venom proteome of the African puff adder, Bitis arietans, using a combinatorial peptide ligand library approach at different pHs. Journal of Proteomics. 2010;**73**:932-942. DOI: 10.1016/j.prot.2009.12.006

[76] Mackessy SP. Handbook of Venoms and Toxins of Reptiles. Florida: CBC Press; 2010. 528 p. ISBN: 978-0-8493-9165-1

[77] Aznaurian AV, Amiryan SV. Histopathological changes induced

by the venom of the snake *Vipera raddei* (Armenian adder). Toxicon. 2006;**47**:141-143. DOI: 10.1016/j.toxicon.2004.11.012

[78] Mohamed AH, Nawar NN, Hanna MM. Some effects of *Naja nigricollis* envenomation on developing fetal tissue. Toxicon. 1974;**12**:477-480

[79] Jarrar BM. Histological alterations and biochemical changes in the liver of sheep following *Echis coloratus* envenomation. Saudi Journal of Biological Sciences. 2011;**18**:169-174. DOI: 10.1016/j.sjbs.2010.12.002

[80] Araki S, Ishida T, Yamamoto T, Kaji K, Hayashi H. Induction of apoptosis by hemorrhagic snake venom in vascular endothelial cells. Biochemical and Biophysical Research Communications. 1993;**190**:148-153. DOI: 10.1006/bbrc.1993.1023

[81] Hamburger V, Hamilton HL. A series of normal stages in the development of the chick embryo. Journal of Morphology. 1951;**88**:49-92

[82] Lewis JH, Wolpert L. The principle of non-equivalence in development. Journal of Theoretical Biology. 1976;**62**:479-490. DOI: 10.1016/0022-5193(76)90132-6

[83] Krabbenhoft KM, Fallon JF. The formation of leg or wing specific structures by leg bud cells grafted to the wing bud is influenced by proximity to the apical ridge. Developmental Biology. 1989;**131**:373-382. DOI: 10.1016/s0012-1606(89)80011-9

Chapter 5

Toxicosis of Snake, Scorpion, Honeybee, Spider, and Wasp Venoms: Part 1

Saganuwan Alhaji Saganuwan

Abstract

Toxicosis is a poisoning caused by venomous animals such as snake, scorpion, honeybee, spider, and wasp. Their poisons contain amino acids, peptides, proteins, enzymes, and metallic ions that are responsible for neurotoxicity, hemotoxicity, and myotoxicity. Because of in vivo therapeutic challenges posed by toxicosis, there is need for ideal therapeutic agents against envenomation caused by venomous animals. Findings have shown that toxicosis could be treated symptomatically. Snake and scorpion antivenins could be used for treatment of poisoning caused by snake, scorpion, honeybee, spider, and wasp. The amount of antivenin is dependent on the quantity of venom injected into the affected individuals. More so, symptomatic treatments are also done according to the systems affected. Hospitalization is necessary for assessment of therapeutic success.

Keywords: toxicosis, snake, scorpion, toxin, antivenin, lethality, hemotoxicity, neurotoxicity, myotoxicity, hospitalization

1. Introduction

Venomous animals such as snake, scorpion, honeybee, spider, and wasp constitute very significant health hazard in the world. The snake venom contains many toxic and non-toxic molecules [1]. Forty-seven out of 50 US States have venomous snakes. Southwestern US are mostly affected. About 4700 venomous snakes bite human and 150,000 primarily dogs and cats are bitten by venomous snakes every year in the US, with human mortality of 0.06% and that of dog is 1–30% [2]. Scorpionism is caused by many poisonous scorpions including Tityus species endemic to Panama, whereas *Centruroides* are endemic to Guatemala, Belize, El Salvador, Nicaragua, and Costa Rica. They are wildly toxic via unchannel active toxins. In Panama, the incidence was 52 cases per 100,000 in 2007 and 28 deaths were recorded between 1998 and 2006, respectively. *Tityus* species present in the Atlantic coast of Costa Rica is responsible for fatalities in Panama. *Tityus pachyurus* [3] and *Parabuthus granulatus* are of the most medical importance in the Western Cape of South Africa. *P. transvaalicus* venom is used for production of *P. granulatus* venom [4]. About 200,000 cases of scorpionism are reported in Mexico and cause 310 deaths every year and 20,000 out of 38,068 affected persons were successfully treated using equine antiserum (serotherapy) and no life was lost [5]. The first case of scorpionism was reported in Canada in a 36 year old man in 1962. The rate of scorpionism in Amazon region of Brazil is 8.14–273 cases per 100,000. Most species involved in envenomation belong to the genus of Tityus [6]. *M. gibbosus* is endemic to a small geographic area of Erbalj on terra rossa soil [7]. The incidence of scorpion sting in Iran was 61.2 per 100,000 populations [8], as against 1.2 million people with estimated 3250 death per year. The mean annual rate was 17.4 per woman population [9]. The highest rate of sting occurred in Iran among individuals of 25- to 34-year-old [8]. The global mortality rate was 10 per 1000 cases. Most of the stings were seen on lower limbs (58.6%) and upper limbs (34.3%) during the hot season [10]. The scorpion that had envenomated for the first time may have less toxic envenomation for the second time as reported in the case of sting from *Leiurus abdullahbayrami* [11]. In India, envenomation was more common in males than in females [12].

Honeybee (*Apis mellifera*) constitutes a significant nuisance and of medical importance in Africa, Europe and other parts of the world. Other subspecies are *A. mellifera carnica*, *A. mellifera ligustica*, and *A. mellifera scutellata* [13]. Honeybee stings reported in Ceara, Brazil showed 1307 cases affecting men between 20 and 29 years of age [14] translating to 19 cases per 100,000 in Campina Grade [15]. Bee envenomation is a problem in India, China, Latin America, Middle East, and North and South Africa [16]. About 200 stings from *Apis mellifera* could cause envenoming syndrome in children and elderly [17] as multiple stings, not increased venom potency or delivery cause serious reactions [18]. Bee venoms differ in weight and concentrations of phospholipase and melittin [19]. Unfortunately, no specific antivenom for bee envenomation; hence, proper removal of stings, first aid treatment and chemotherapy should be considered as medical emergency [20]. Administration of hydrocortisone, calcium, analgesic, and 0.9% sodium chloride and application of ice to the site of stung pregnant woman resulted in recovery from the pain and the fetus was stable and delivered 3 months after treatment without sequela [21]. There are 42,473 species of spiders grouped into 110 families (Platnick) [22]. *Hadronyche formidabilis* and *H. cerberea* have very high envenoming rates [23]. Black widow spider (*Latrodectus mactans*) and brown recluse spider (*Loxosceles reclusa*) are of most concern [24]. In view of the increased challenges and negligence of envenomation caused by venomous snake, scorpion, spider, wasp, and bee, there is need for thorough search for their therapeutic regimens with a view to having lasting solution against fatality.

2. Methodology

Literatures were searched on venomous snakes, scorpions, honeybees, spiders, and wasps with an intent to identifying their toxicity potentials, epidemiology of their toxicosis, signs of toxicity, treatment, and development of vaccines against their venoms. Sought also are information on medicinal plants, phytochemicals and other therapeutic agents, structures of some chemicals present in the venoms, and their medical applications and medicinal uses. Mathematical formulas were also derived for calculation of body weight, body surface area, packed cell volume, hemoglobin, total blood volume, lost blood volume, median lethal dose (LD_{50}), median effective dose (ED_{50}), number of bee stings, total dose of bee venom, and relationship between renotoxicity and hemotoxicity.

3. Results

Findings have shown that venoms from poisonous species of snakes, scorpions, honeybees, spiders and wasps are highly toxic and could cause various degrees of hemotoxicity, myotoxicity, and neurotoxicity including death (**Tables 1** and **2** and **Figures 1–77**).

System	Age (year)	Sting(s)	Sex	Signs	Treatment
Nervous	6,70 70	1 each 1	Female Male	Axonal polyneuropathy, seizure Brachial plexitis, Parkinsonism	Immunoglobulin I.V., anti-inflammatory, oxygen
Muscular	34	3	Male	Rhabdomyolysis, muscle pain, allergy	Analgesic, anti-inflammatory
Circulatory	35–42	Many	Male	Myocardial infarction, ischemic attack, cardiac arrest, Kounis syndrome, anaphylaxis	Angioplasty, steroids, antihistaminics
Renal	2	1	Male	Nephrotic syndrome, anasarca, acute renal failure	Corticosteriod
Ocular	21–50	1	Male Female	Cataract, glaucoma	Surgery, keratoplasty, antibiotics, corticosteroid
Miscellaneous	40	Multiple	Male	Intravascular coagulopathy, coma	Hydrocortisone, analgesic, pheniramine

Table 1.
Toxicity signs of honeybee sting in human.

Animal	Weight (kg)	Number of stings	Dose of stings (mg)	LD_{50} (mg/kg)	ED_{50} (mg/kg)	Lethal time (hour)
Child	10	94	28.2	1.41	11.2	2.10
Adult	60	1000	300	2.5	7.5	3.72

Table 2.
Calculated median lethal dose and effective dose 50 of honeybee venom and antivenom in human.

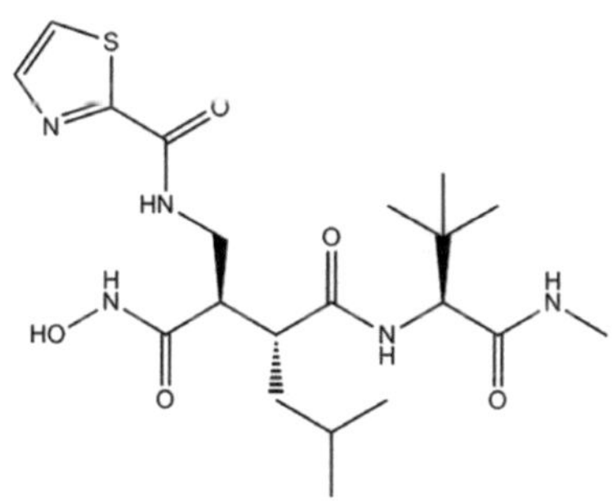

Figure 1.
Metalloproteinase of rattlesnake's venom.

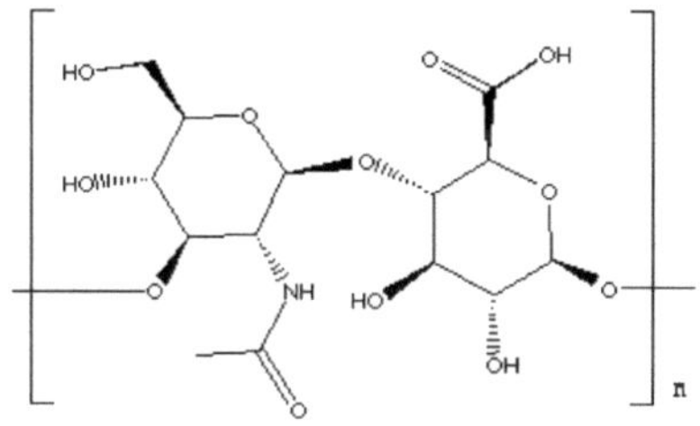

Figure 2.
Hyaluronidase of black mamba's venom enzyme.

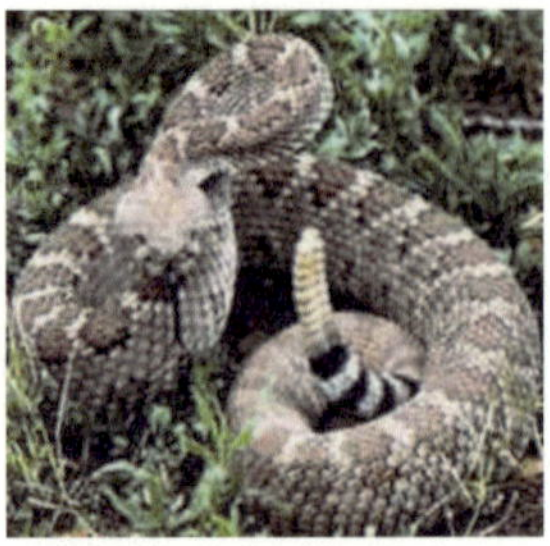

Figure 3.
Eastern diamondback rattlesnake (Crotalus adamanteus) *found in southeastern United States.*

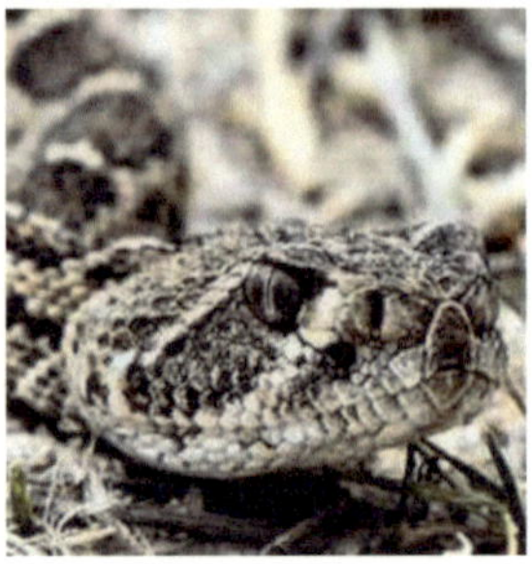

Figure 4.
Western diamondback rattlesnake (Crotalus atrox) *can be found, from California to West Texas, Oklahoma, the southern parts of New Mexico and Arizona and northern parts of Mexico. This species is also found in several islands in the Gulf of California.*

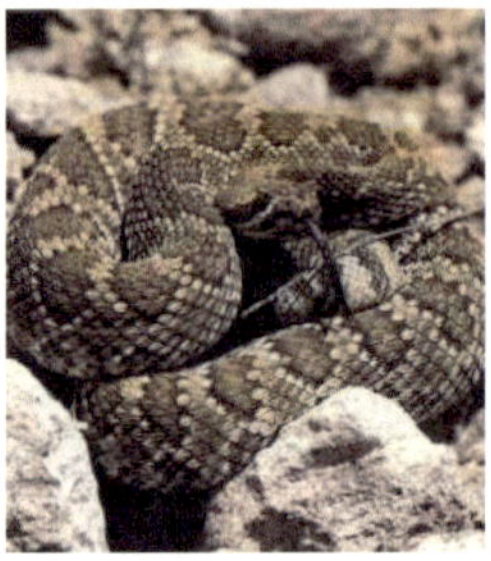

Figure 5.
Mojave rattlesnake (Crotalus scutulatus) *found in the deserts of the southwestern United States and central Mexico.*

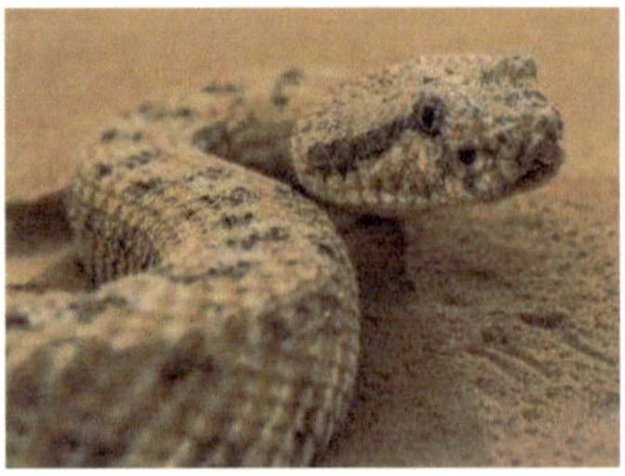

Figure 6.
Sidewinder (Crotalus cerastes) *found in the desert regions of the southwestern United States and northwestern Mexico.*

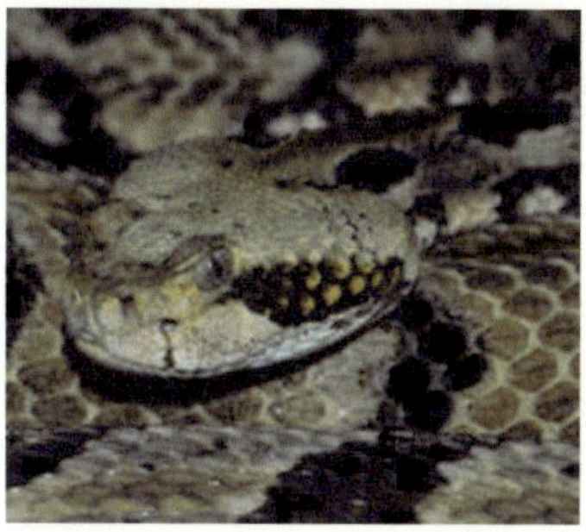

Figure 7.
Timber rattlesnake *(*Crotalus horridus*) also commonly known as canebrake rattlesnake or banded rattlesnake found in the eastern region of the United States.*

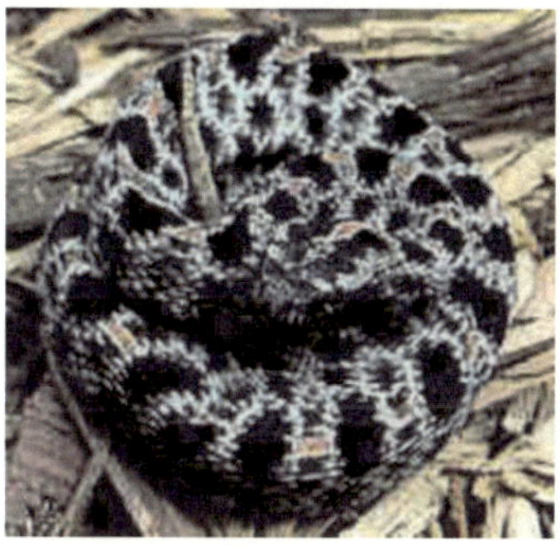

Figure 8.
Pigmy rattlesnake *(*Sistrurus miliarius*) found in the southeastern part of the United States.*

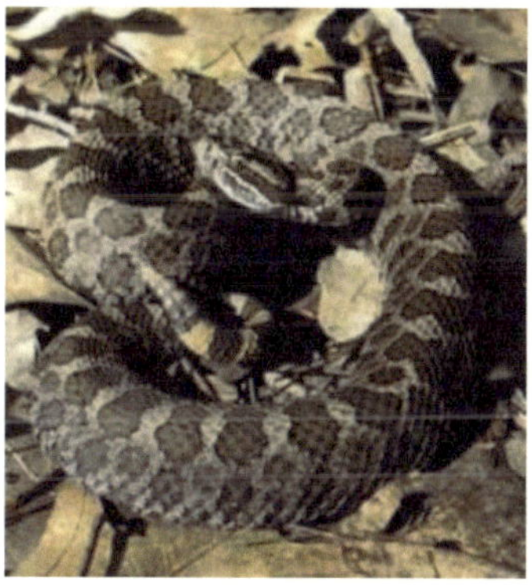

Figure 9.
Massasauga rattlesnake *(*Sistrurus catenatus*) found in several states of the United States, southern Ontario in Canada and in northern Mexico on the border with Texas.*

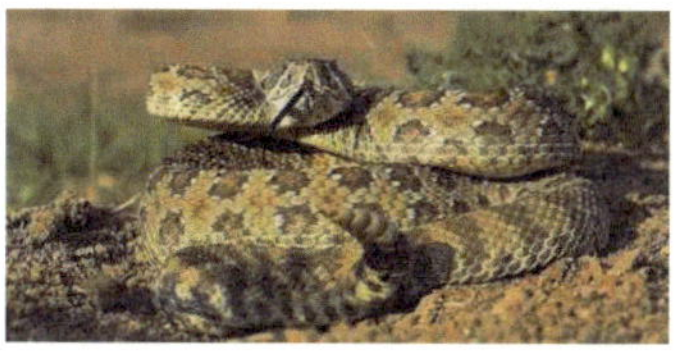

Figure 10.
Prairie rattlesnake *or* ***Great Plains rattlesnake*** *(*Crotalus viridis*) found in the western United States. They are also found in southwestern Canada and northern regions of Mexico.*

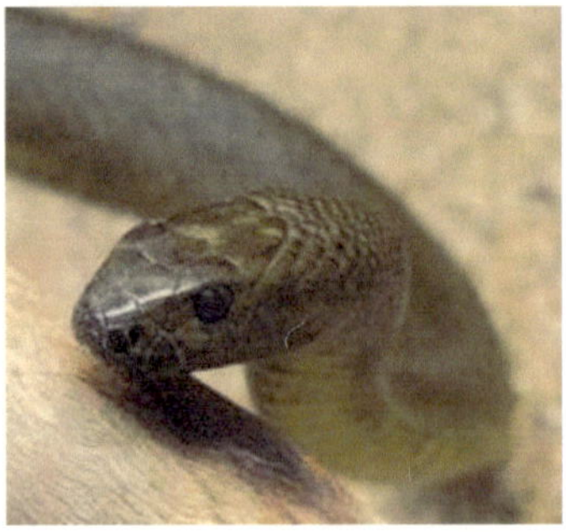

Figure 11.
Inland taipan *(*Oxyuranus microlepidotus*) found in semi-arid regions of central east Australia.*

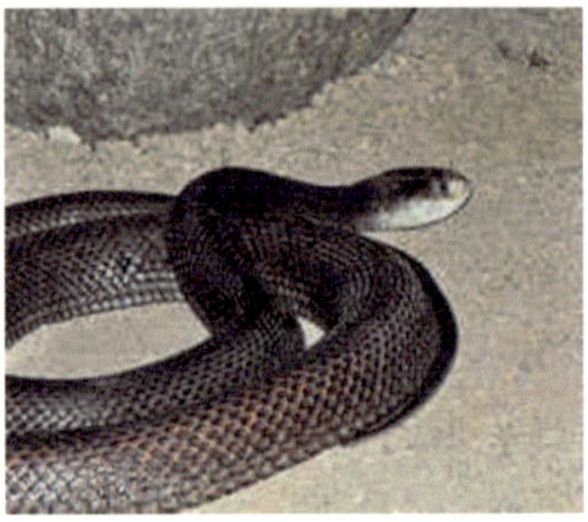

Figure 12.
Coastal taipan *also known as the common or eastern taipan (*Oxyuranus scutellatus*). It's found throughout the coastal regions of northern and eastern Australia and also on the island of New Guinea.*

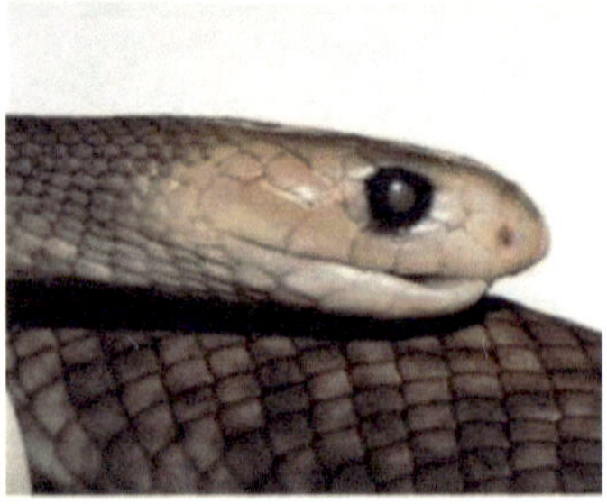

Figure 13.
Central Ranges taipan *(*Oxyuranus temporalis*).*

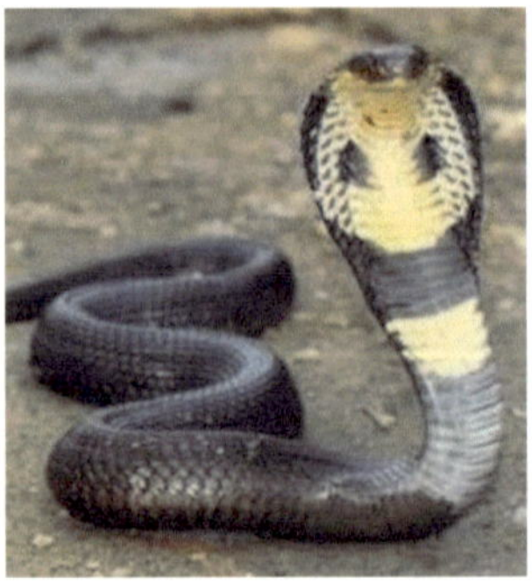

Figure 14.
King cobra *(*Ophiophagus hannah*). King cobras live in Southeast Asia mainly in the plains and rainforests of India where they are abundant and revered in some places, southern China, Malaysia, and the Philippines.*

DOI: http://dx.doi.org/10.5772/intechopen.92804

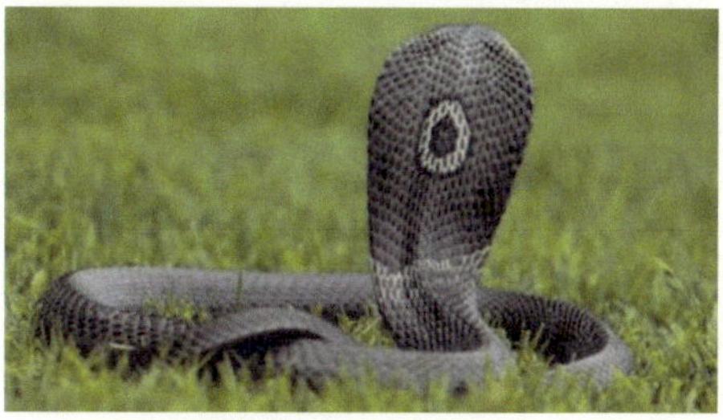

Figure 15.
Monocled cobra *(*Naja kaouthia*) can be found in China, India, Vietnam, Nepal, and Cambodia, but also Malaysia, Bangladesh, Bhutan, Laos, Myanmar, and Thailand.*

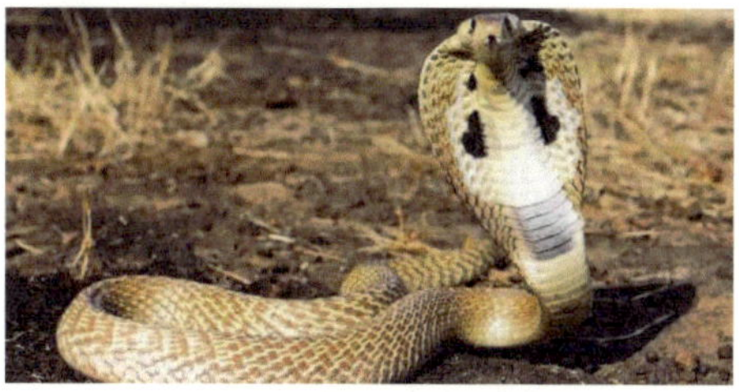

Figure 16.
Indian cobra *(*Naja naja*). They are found in several countries including India, Pakistan, Sri Lanka, Myanmar, southern Nepal, Bangladesh, Bhutan, and possibly in the extreme eastern Afghanistan in the Kabul River Valley.*

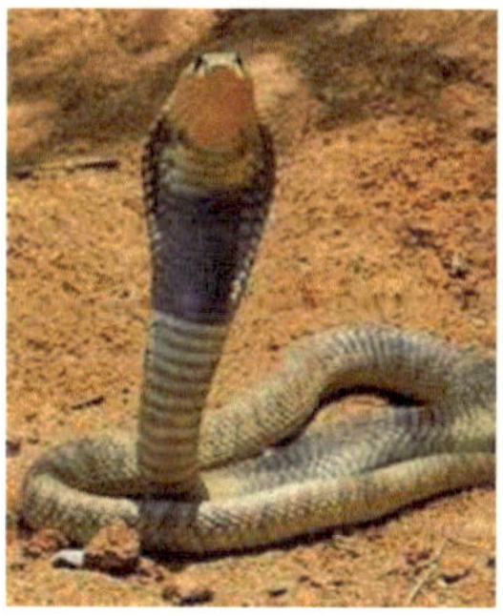

Figure 17.
Egyptian cobra *(*Naja haje*) is found throughout most of North Africa north of the* ***Sahara desert****, and also south of the Sahara through West Africa, in the Congo Basin, Kenya and Tanzania and the southern part of the Arabian Peninsula.*

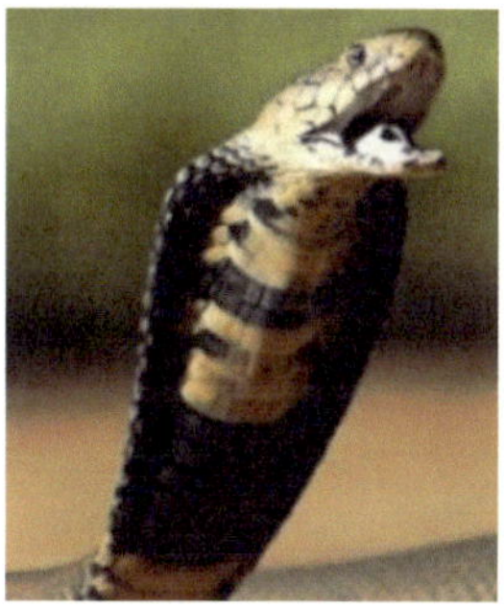

Figure 18.
Mozambique spitting cobra *(*Naja mossambica*)—eastern parts of southern Africa, most of Mozambique, Swaziland, Zimbabwe, southern Angola, Zambia, Malawi, northeastern Namibia, northern Botswana, and southern Tanzania including Pemba island.*

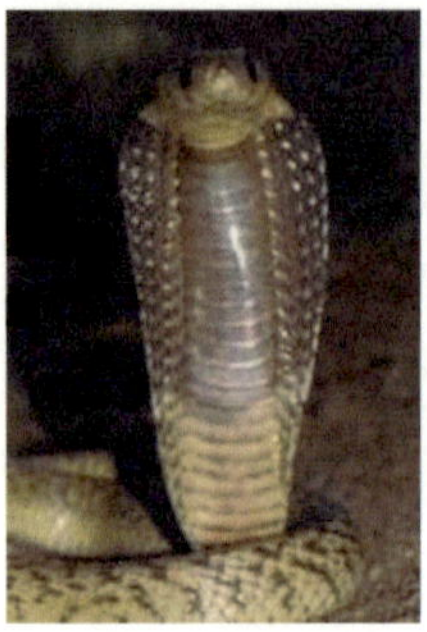

Figure 19.
Cape cobra (Naja nivea) *found in southern Africa, particularly in South Africa and in parts of Botswana and south part of Namibia.*

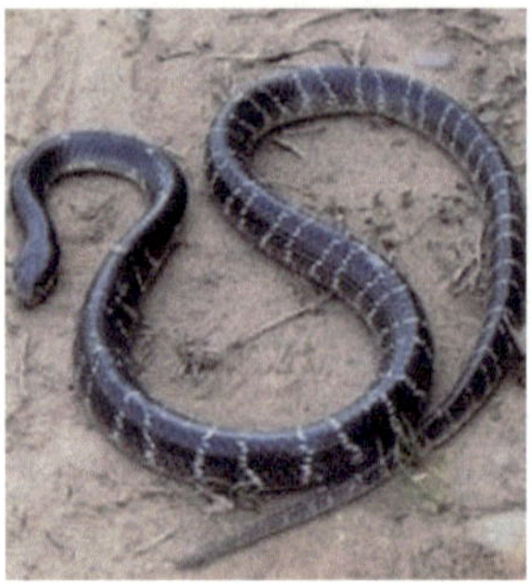

Figure 20.
Common krait (Bungarus caeruleus) *found in the Indian subcontinent. These snakes are found almost all over Peninsular India but not in the offshore Islands. They are also found in other neighboring countries such as Pakistan, Bangladesh, Nepal, and Sri Lanka.*

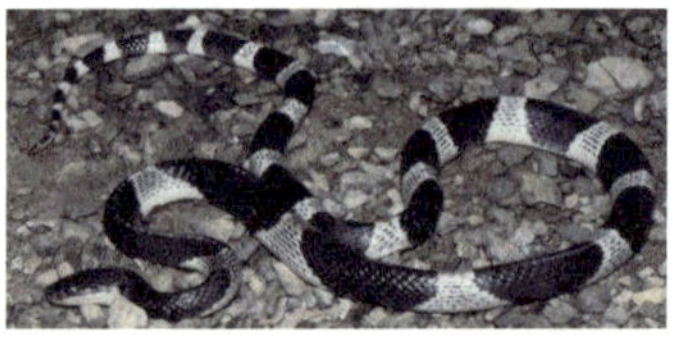

Figure 21.
Blue krait *is also known as the* ***Malayan krait*** (Bungarus candidus). *These snakes are found in Peninsular Malaysia, central Vietnam, Thailand, Bali, Lao People's Democratic Republic, Indonesia, Singapore, and Sumatra.*

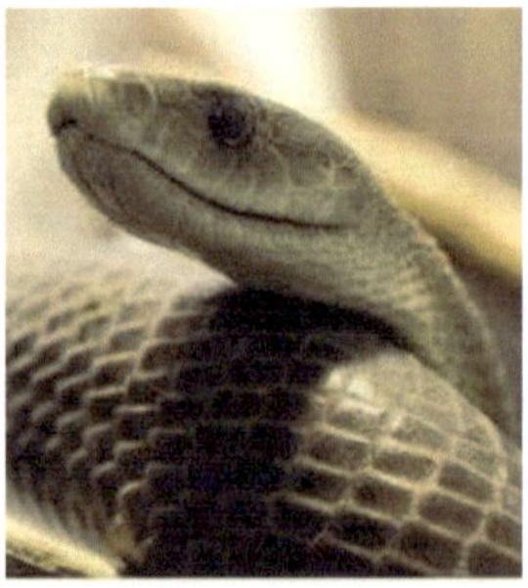

Figure 22.
Black mamba (Dendroaspis polylepis). *The black mamba lives in the savannas and rocky hills of southern and eastern Africa. Its fragmented range includes many African countries like the Democratic Republic of the Congo, Sudan, Ethiopia, Eritrea, Somalia, Kenya, Uganda, Tanzania, Burundi, Rwanda, Angola, Mozambique, Swaziland, Malawi, Zambia, Zimbabwe, Botswana, Namibia, and South Africa.*

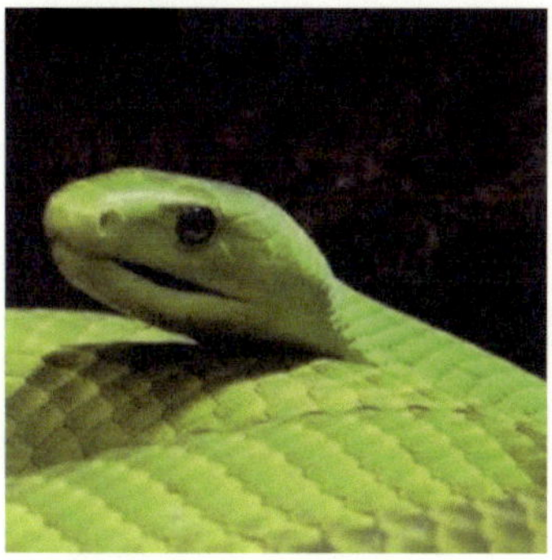

Figure 23.
Eastern green mamba *(*Dendroaspis angusticeps*). Their range stretches from the eastern Cape in South Africa through Kenya, Mozambique, Tanzania, eastern Zimbabwe, and southern Malawi.*

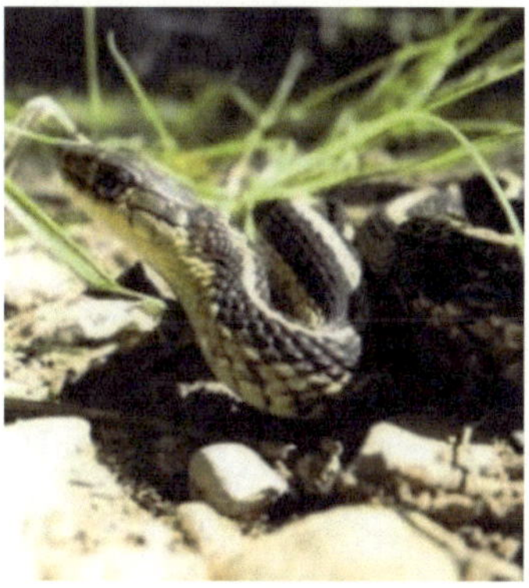

Figure 24.
Eastern gartersnake *or* ***Eastern garter snake***(Thamnophis sirtalis sirtalis)*. They have a wide range across eastern North America, extending as far north as southern Ontario and Quebec in Canada, to the Gulf of Mexico in the south, along the eastern shores of America to the Mississippi River.*

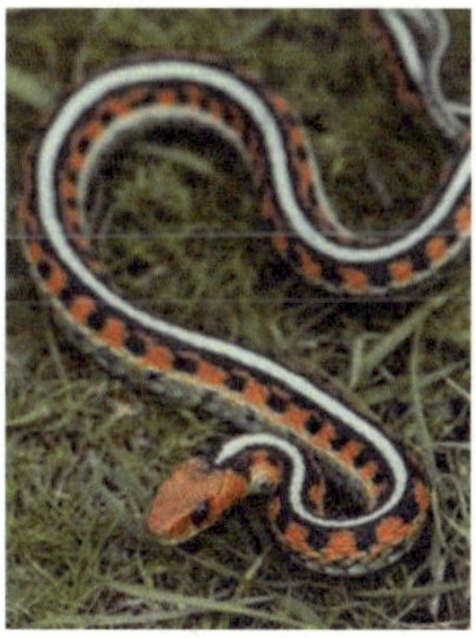

Figure 25.
California red-sided garter snake *(*Thamnophis sirtalis infernalis*) found in California.*

4. Discussion

4.1 Signs of ophidism

Difference between cobra and viper venom in terms of molecular weight, route of administration and nature of toxin could account for differences in their venoms

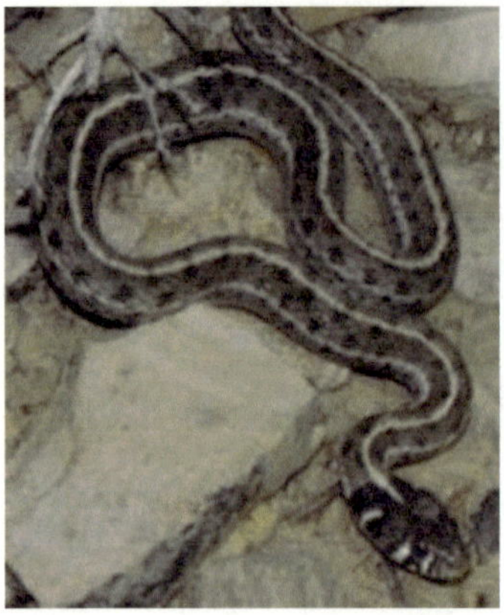

Figure 26.
Checkered garter snake *(*Thamnophis marcianus*) found in the southwestern United States southwards into Mexico and Central America as far south as Costa Rica.*

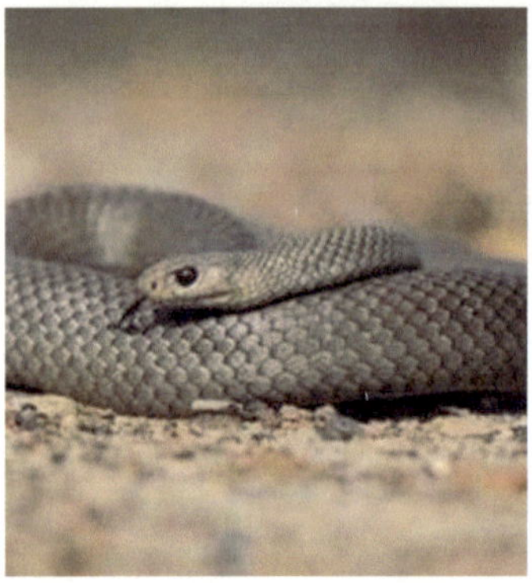

Figure 27.
Eastern brown snake *(*Pseudonaja textilis*) found in the eastern half of Australia, except in Tasmania.*

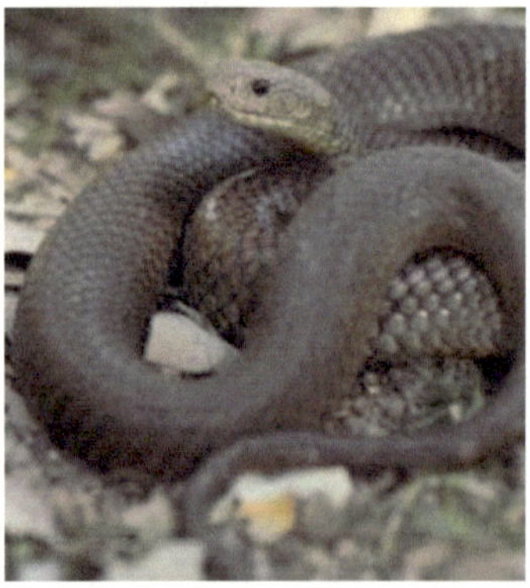

Figure 28.
King brown snake *or* ***mulga snake*** *(*Pseudechis australis*) found over most of mainland Australia, except for the extreme south and the southeast coastal regions.*

lethality. Venom of *Cerastes cerastes* is more toxic than that of *Bitis arietans* and *Macrovipera lebetina* and toxin of *Naja haje* is more toxic than that of *C. cerastes, M. lebetina* and *B. occitanus*. Vipers have toxins with high molecular weight [25]. Therefore, venom quality has to be standardized for development of efficient anti-venom, [26]. When the time of injected antivenom is shorter than fatal limit time,

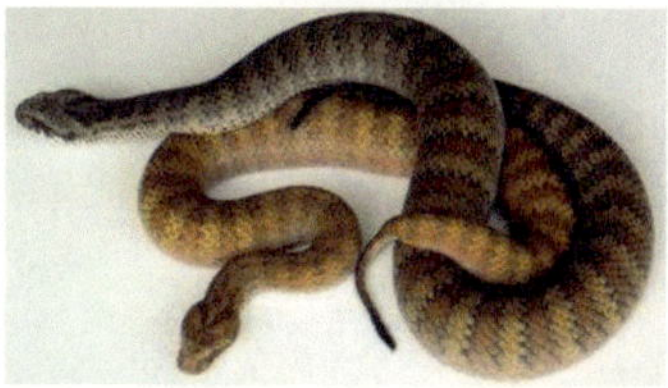

Figure 29.
Death adder *(genus* Acanthophis*) found in Australia, Indonesia, New Guinea and its nearby islands.*

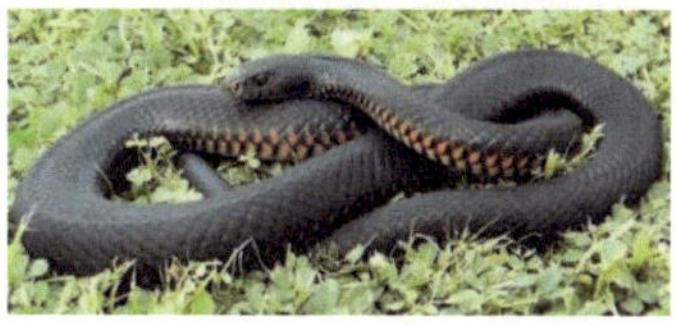

Figure 30.
Red-bellied black snake *(*Pseudechis porphyriacus*) native to eastern Australia. The red-bellied black snakes are found in a more or less continuous range from southeastern Queensland south through eastern New South Wales and Victoria.*

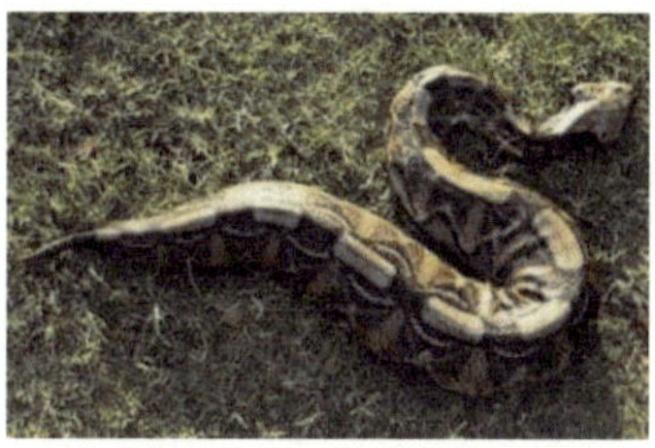

Figure 31.
Gaboon viper *(*Bitis gabonica*) found along the equatorial belt of Africa, East and Central Africa, and southeast Africa. In the African Portuguese-speaking countries, it can be found in Guinea-Bissau, Angola, and northern Mozambique.*

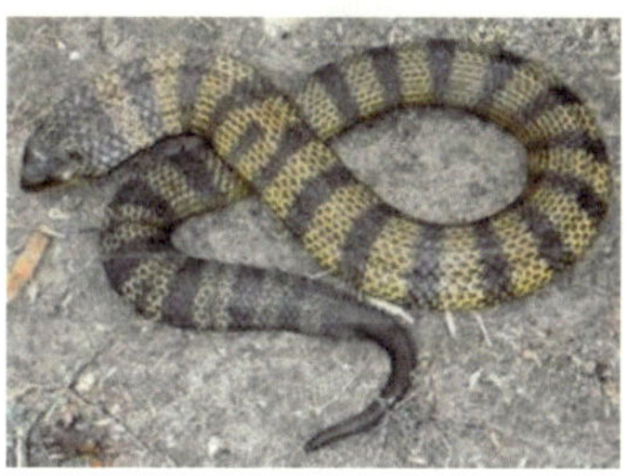

Figure 32.
Tiger snake *(*Notechis*) found in Australia.*

the envenomated may be protected by increasing the dose of antivenom. But when the antivenom is injected closer to the fatal limit time, the chance of death is one-half [27].

4.2 Treatment of snake envenomations

Rational dosage of snake antivenom requires larger randomized controlled trials and further strategies are required to reduce morbidity in children bitten by *Naja atra* [28]. Neurotoxic envenomations and complications thereafter correlate positively with snake antivenom dosage; hence higher doses are required which may

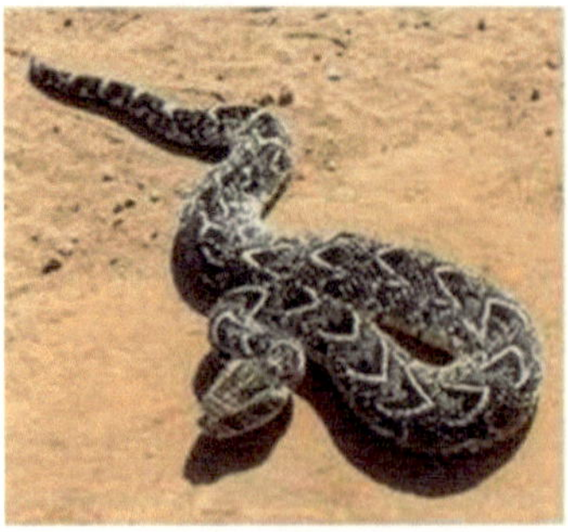

Figure 33.
Puff adder *(*Bitis arietans*) found in African savannah and grasslands.*

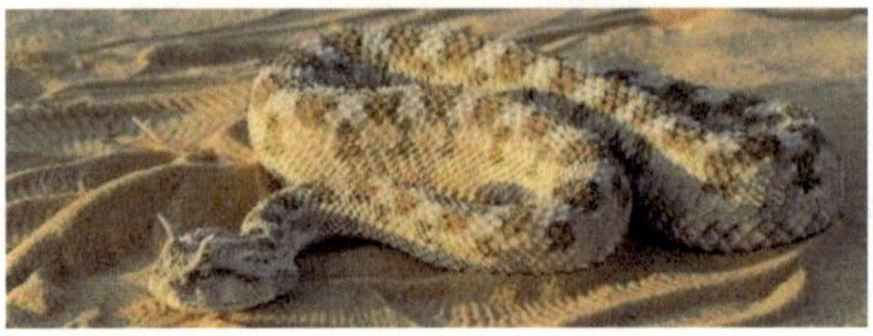

Figure 34.
Horned viper *(*Cerastes cerastes*). It is found in many north African countries like Morocco, Mauritania, Mali, eastward through Algeria, Niger, Tunisia, Libya and Egypt, Chad, Sudan, Ethiopia, Somalia, and northern Israel.*

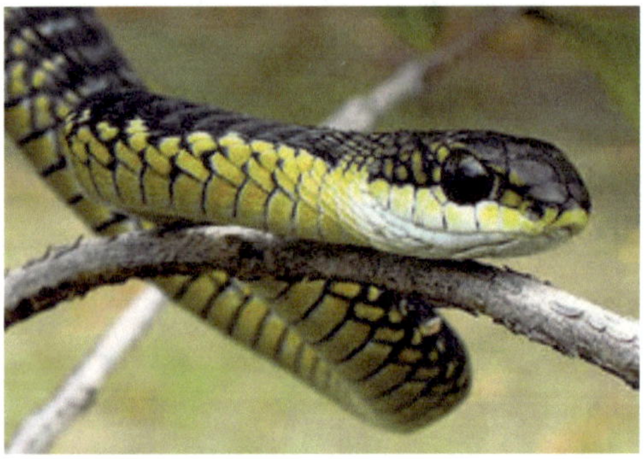

Figure 35.
Boomslang (Dispholidus typus*) found in sub-Saharan Africa in the central and southern regions of the continent. The boomslang is most abundant in Botswana, Swaziland, Namibia, Mozambique, and Zimbabwe, but the species has been reported as far north as southern Chad and Nigeria, and as far east as eastern Guinea.*

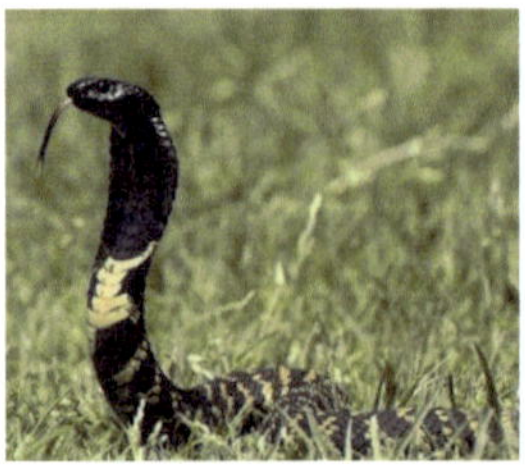

Figure 36.
Rinkhals *(*Hemachatus haemachatus*). The rinkhals is found in most provinces of South Africa, like western and eastern Cape along the south coast, Mpumalanga, Free State, southern Gauteng and Kwazulu Natal.*

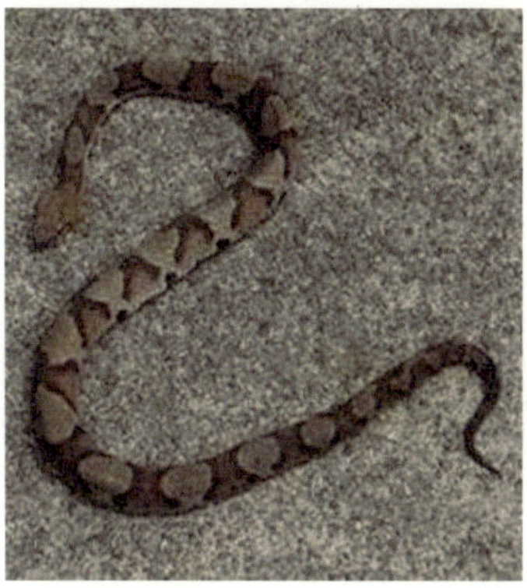

Figure 37.
***Copperhead** or **water moccasin** (*Agkistrodon contortrix*). These snakes are found in the United States and in northern Mexico. In the USA, they are found in the states of Alabama, Arkansas, Florida, Georgia, Illinois, Connecticut, Delaware, Indiana, Iowa, Kansas, Kentucky, Louisiana, Ohio, Mississippi, Missouri, Oklahoma, Maryland, Massachusetts, New Jersey, New York, North Carolina, Tennessee, Texas, Pennsylvania, South Carolina, Virginia, and West Virginia. In Mexico, it occurs in Coahuila and Chihuahua regions.*

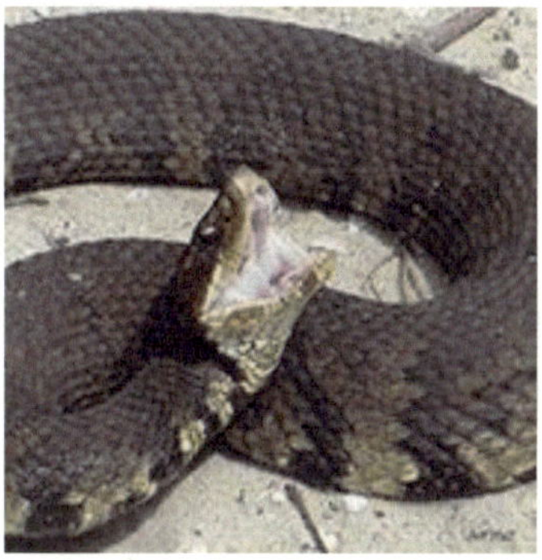

Figure 38.
***Cottonmouth** (*Agkistrodon piscivorus*) found in the southeastern United States.*

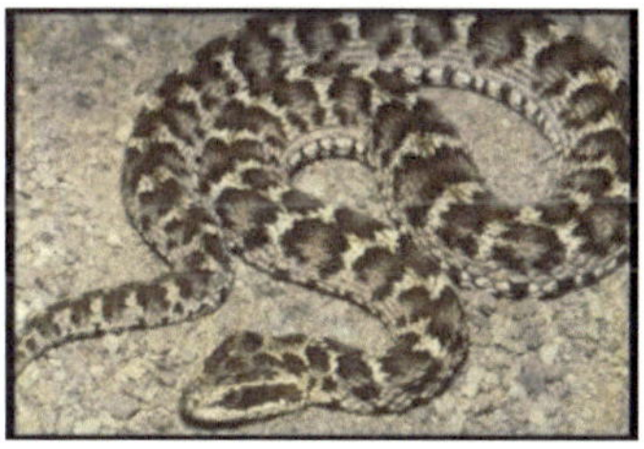

Figure 39.
***Mamushi** or **Japanese Mamushi** (*Gloydius blomhoffii*) found in Japan, China, and Korea.*

also cause adverse reactions [29]. Neutralization capacity of antivenom may be related to geographic proximity of snake species [30]. *Cerestes cerestes* antivenom and *Macrovipera mauritanica* antivenom cross react with *Bitis arietans* antivenom due to presence of antigens common to them [31]. Tenerplasminin-1 (TP_1), a plasmin inhibitor isolated from *Micrurus tener tener* venom was similar to Kunitz-type serine peptidase inhibitors [32]. *Rauwolfia serpentina* inhibits *Daboia russelii* venom [33].

The therapeutic dose of antivenom is relative to the quantity of venom [34]. Therefore, postmortem lesions are required to provide the cause of death [35].

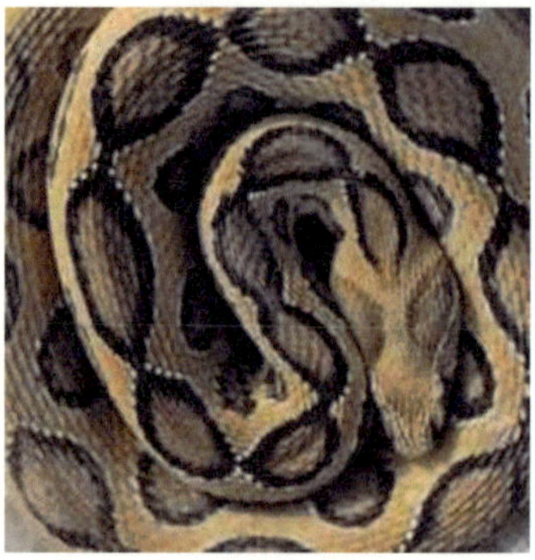

Figure 40.
Russell's viper *(*Daboia russelii*) is found throughout Asia, in the Indian subcontinent, much of Southeast Asia in southern parts of China and Taiwan. The species is found in many countries India, Pakistan, Sri Lanka, Myanmar, Bangladesh, Nepal, Thailand, Cambodia, China, Taiwan, and Indonesia.*

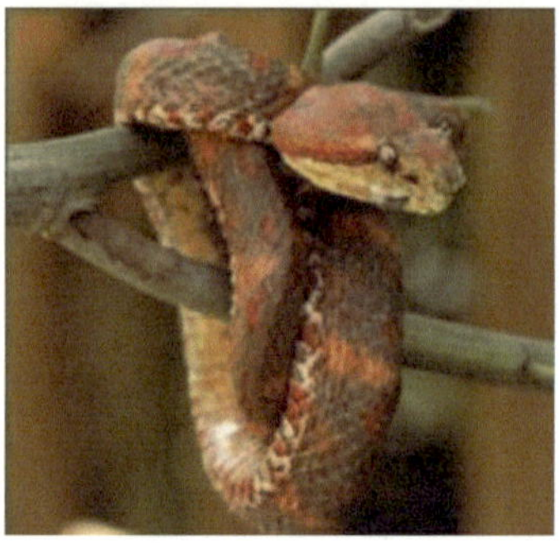

Figure 41.
Eyelash viper or eyelash palm-pit viper *(*Bothriechis schlegelii*) found in central America and northern South America.*

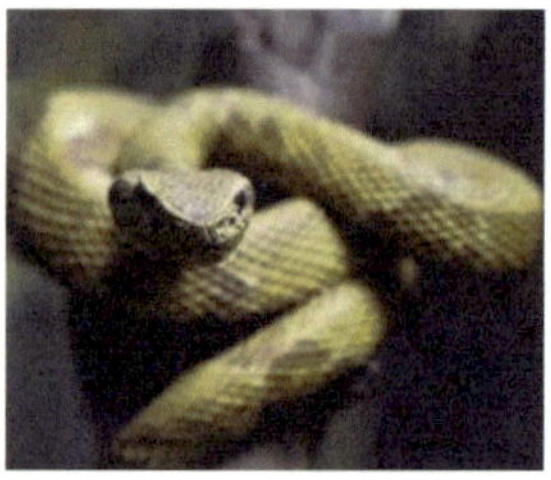

Figure 42.
Golden lancehead *(*Bothrops insularis*).*

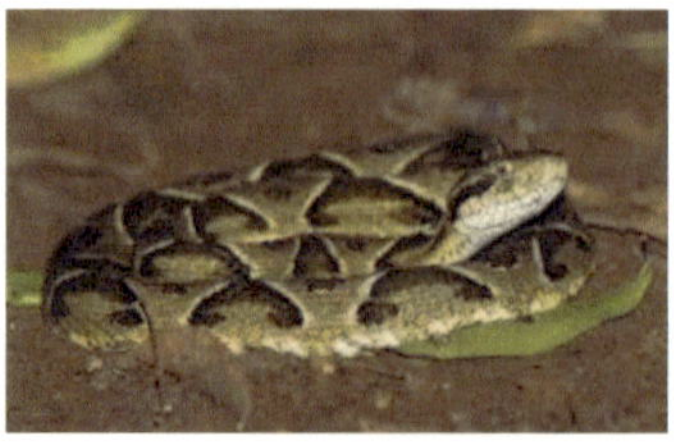

Figure 43.
Jararaca (Bothrops jararaca*). They are found in southern Brazil, northeastern Paraguay, and Misiones province in northern Argentina. It is also found in several islands off the coasts of Argentina and Paraguay, some as far as 35 km offshore.*

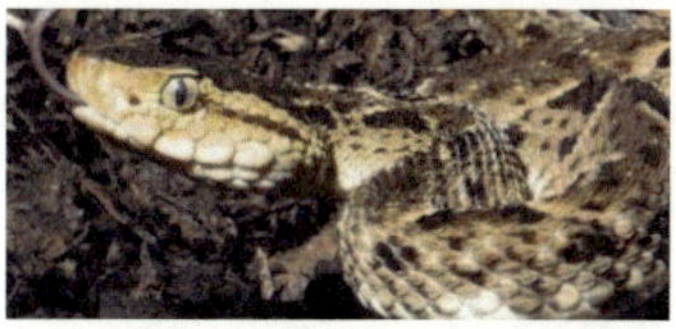

Figure 44.
***Fer-de-lance** or **terciopelo** (*Bothrops asper*) inhabits the region from southern Mexico to northern South America.*

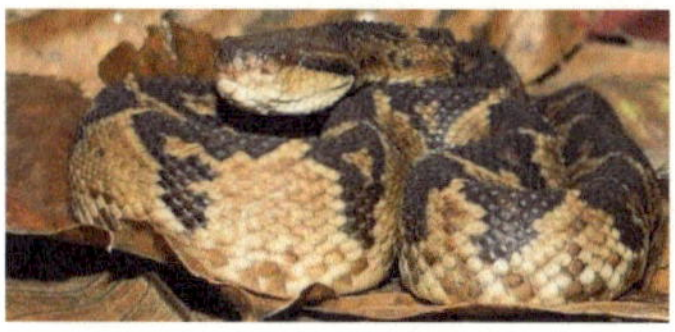

Figure 45.
***Bushmaster** (*Lachesis muta*) found in southern Central America and the northern half of South America including the island of Trinidad.*

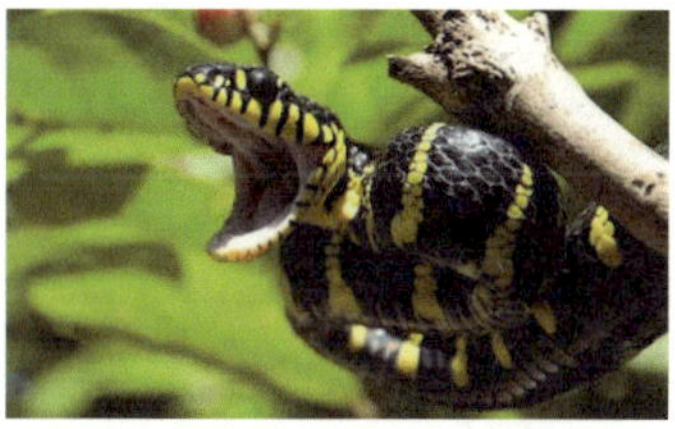

Figure 46.
***Mangrove snake** (*Boiga dendrophila*) found in Indonesia, Malaysia, Thailand, Singapore, Vietnam, Cambodia and Philippines.*

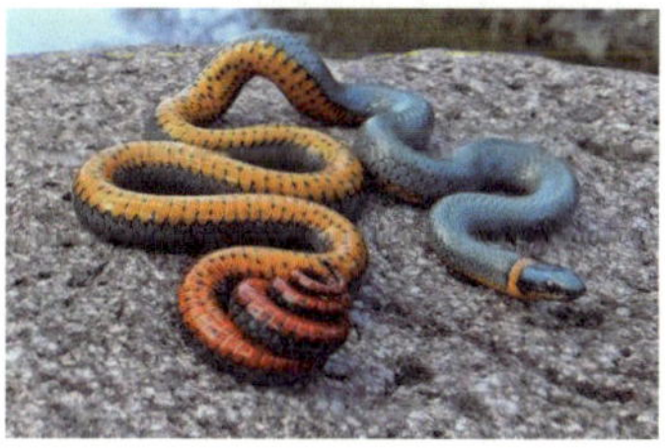

Figure 47.
***Ringneck snake** (*Diadophis punctatus*) found in southeastern Canada and throughout most of the United States southward into Central Mexico.*

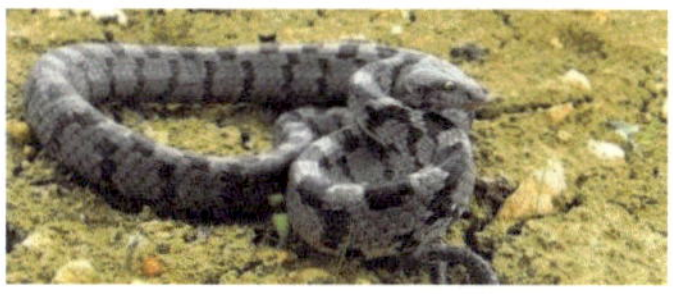

Figure 48.
***European cat snake** or **European Catsnake** (*Telescopus fallax*).*

Hence, neutralizing capacity of antivenins must be standardized [36] because of complex nature of venom composition [37]. Pro-coagulant is used to assess anti-venom activity and the results of antivenin test in rodents may not prove efficacious in human [37] which is considered very important [38]. Hence, changes in dosing

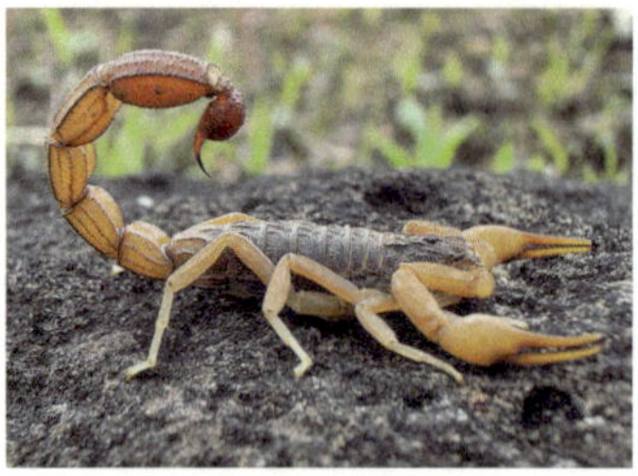

Figure 49.
Indian red scorpion *(*Hottentotta tamulus*) found throughout most of India, eastern Pakistan and the eastern lowlands of Nepal.*

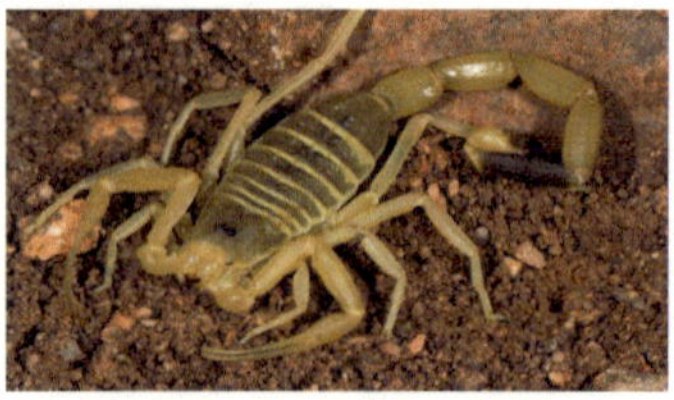

Figure 50.
Deathstalker scorpion (Leiurus quinquestriatus). *The deathstalker scorpion's range covers a wide sweep of territory in the Sahara, Arabian Desert, Thar Desert, and Central Asia, from Algeria and Mali in the west through to Egypt, Ethiopia, Asia Minor and the Arabian Peninsula, eastward to Kazakhstan, and western India.*

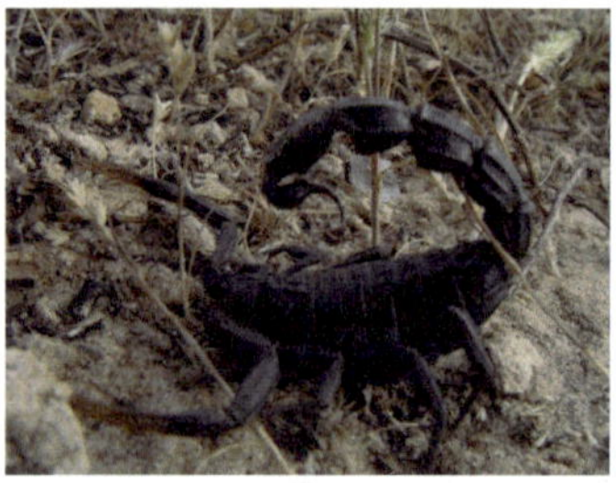

Figure 51.
Arabian fat-tailed scorpion *(*Androctonus crassicauda*) found mainly in the Palaearctic region. It is commonly found in Saudi Arabia, Kuwait, Qatar, Iraq, Iran, Turkey, and in north African nations.*

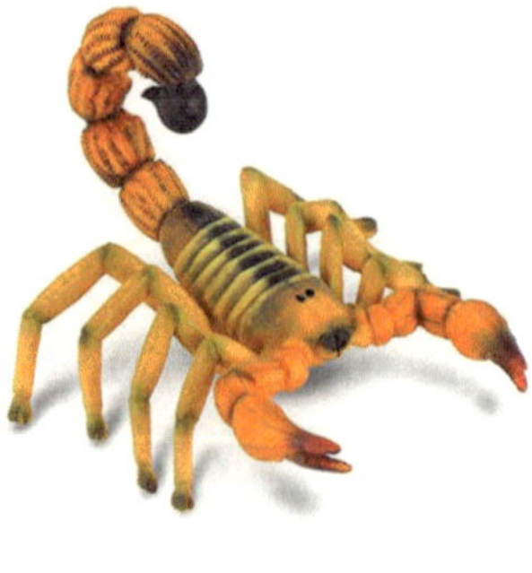

Figure 52.
Yellow fat-tailed scorpion (Androctonus australis). *The yellow fat-tailed scorpion is found in north and west Africa, the Middle East, and eastward to the Hindu Kush region. Countries where* Androctonus *species live include Armenia, Morocco, Algeria, Tunisia, Libya, Egypt, Togo, Palestine, Israel, India, Lebanon, Turkey, Jordan, Saudi Arabia, Yemen, Oman, United Arab Emirates, Qatar, Kuwait, Iraq, Iran, Afghanistan, Bahrain, and Pakistan.*

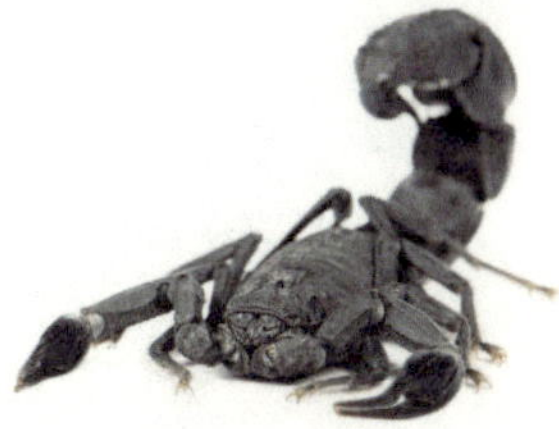

Figure 53.
Black spitting thick-tailed scorpion *(*Parabuthus transvaalicus*)—southern Africa.*

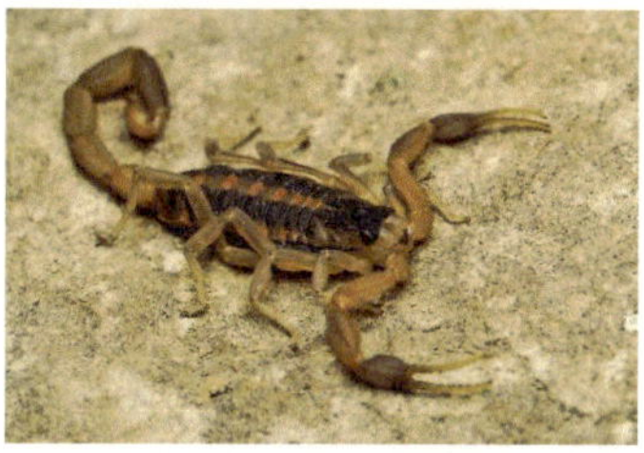

Figure 54.
Striped bark scorpion *(*Centruroides vittatus*) is distributed throughout the South-Central U.S. states and throughout northern Mexico. Beginning in the northern Mexico Border States, Chihuahua, Coahuila, Nuevo León, and Tamaulipas,* C. vittatus' *range extends upward longitudinally through Texas, Oklahoma, and Kansas, to reach as far north as Thayer County, Nebraska.*

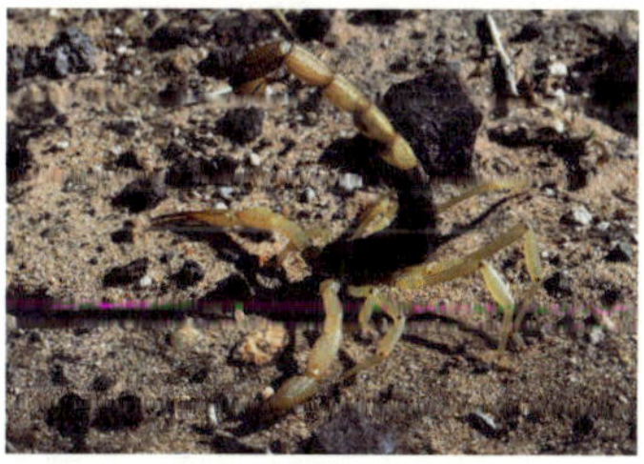

Figure 55.
Arizona bark scorpion *(*Centruroides exilicauda*) found in the deserts of Arizona, California and Utah.*

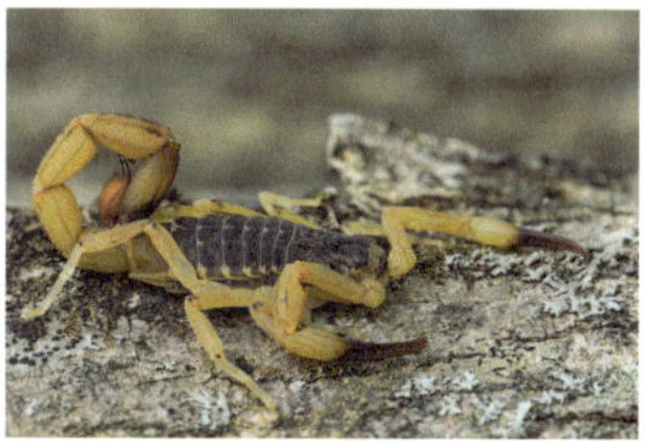

Figure 56.
Brazilian yellow scorpion *(*Tityus serrulatus*)—South America.*

and development of new antivenins have been recommended [39]. However, low effective dose can be used with beneficial results [40]. The most effective treatment for snake envenomation is the specific heterologous serum [41] and additional dose is unnecessary in brown snake envenomation [42]. Antivenom cause anaphylactic

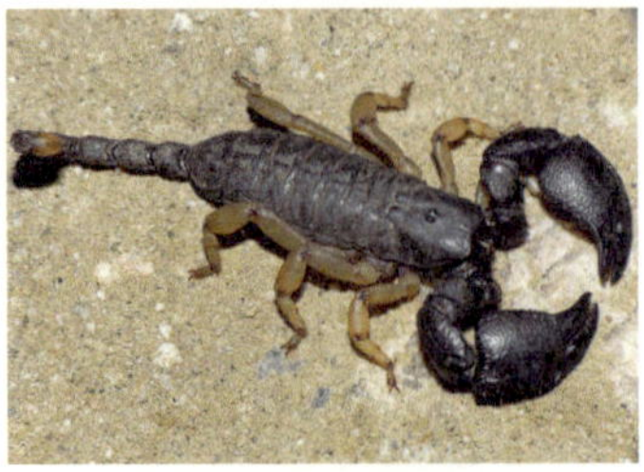

Figure 57.
Yellow-legged burrowing scorpion *(*Opistophthalmus glabrifrons*)—southern Africa.*

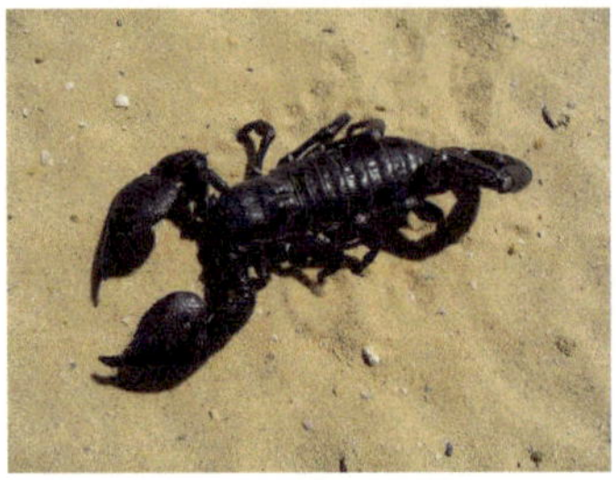

Figure 58.
Tanzanian red clawed scorpion *(***Pandinus cavimanus***)—Tanzanian, Africa.*

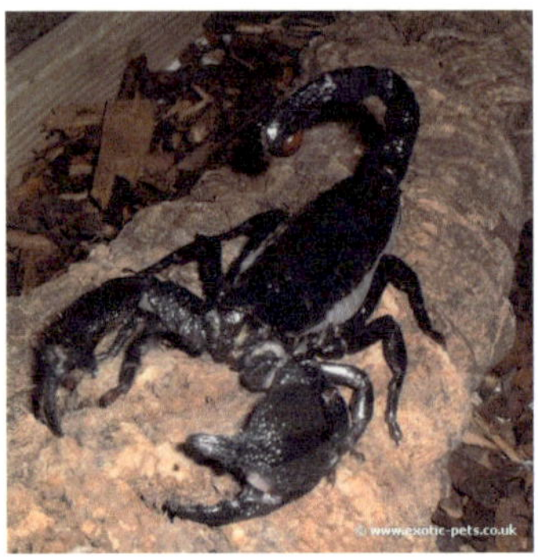

Figure 59.
Emperor scorpion *(***Pandinus imperator***) found living in the rain forest or wet savannah, throughout Africa from Mauritania to Zaire.*

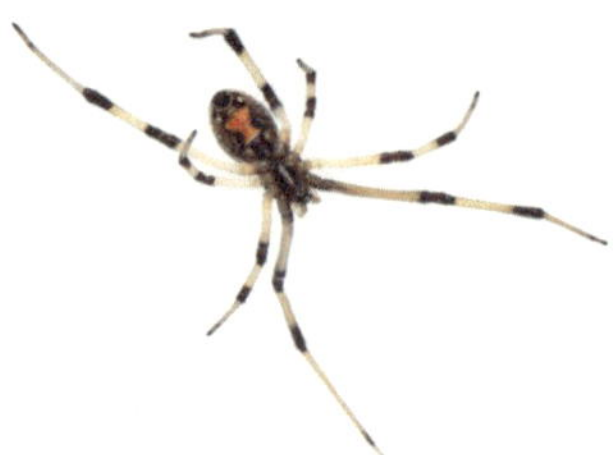

Figure 60.
Brown widow spider *(*Latrodectus geometricus*) found throughout the world, including Africa, the United States, Europe, Asia, the Middle East, and South America.*

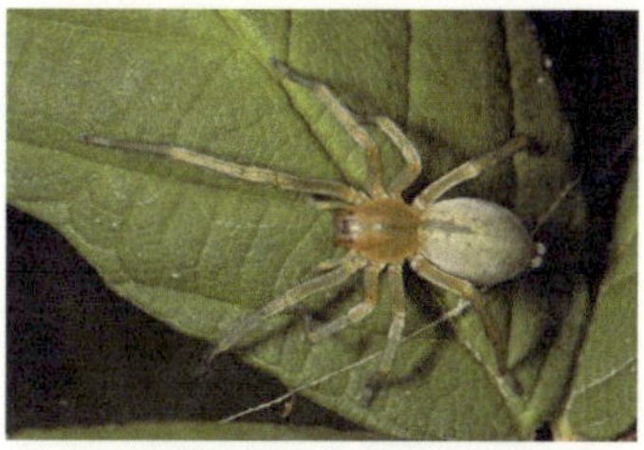

Figure 61.
Yellow sac spider (Cheiracanthium) *is a species endemic to the Americas.*

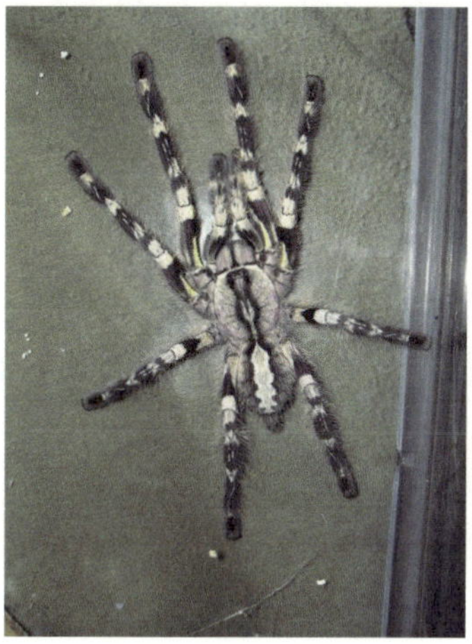

Figure 62.
Indian ornamental tarantula (Poecilotheria regalis) *is a species of spider found in South Asia, as well as southeastern India.*

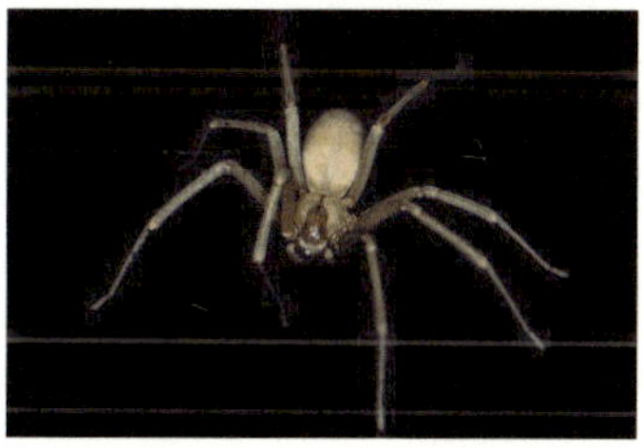

Figure 63.
Brown recluse (Loxosceles reclusa) *primarily found in North America (throughout the Midwest and Southern United States in particular).*

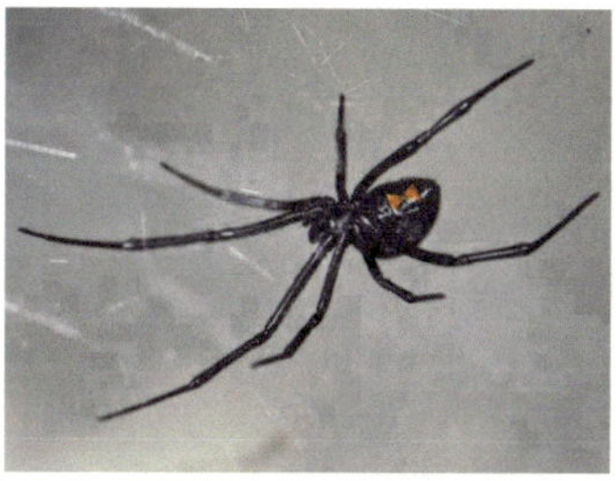

Figure 64.
Black widow spider (Latrodectus) *found on every continent of the world (with the exception of Antarctica).*

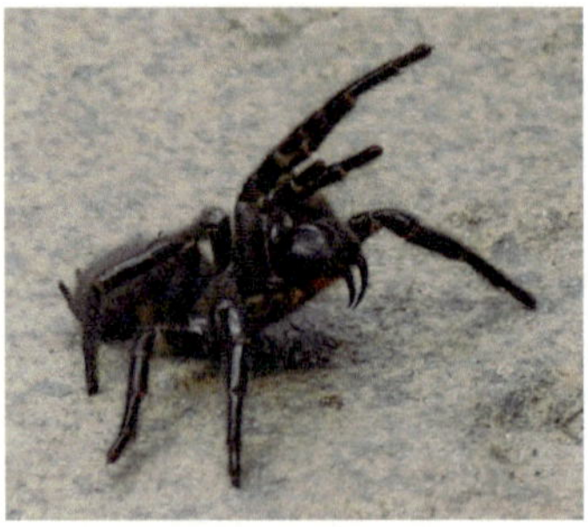

Figure 65.
Sydney funnel-web spider (Atrax robustus) *is native to eastern Australia.*

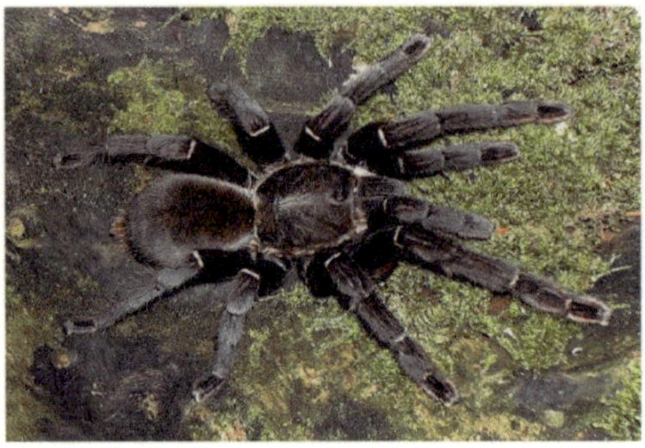

Figure 66.
Chinese bird spider (Cyriopagopus hainanus) *is found predominantly in China and Southeast Asia.*

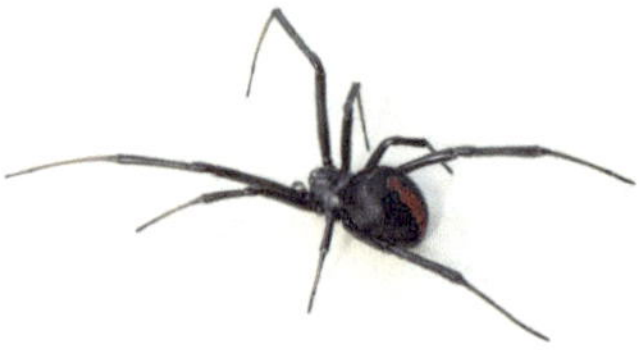

Figure 67.
Redback spider (Latrodectus hasseltii) *found predominantly in Australia, Southeast Asia, and New Zealand.*

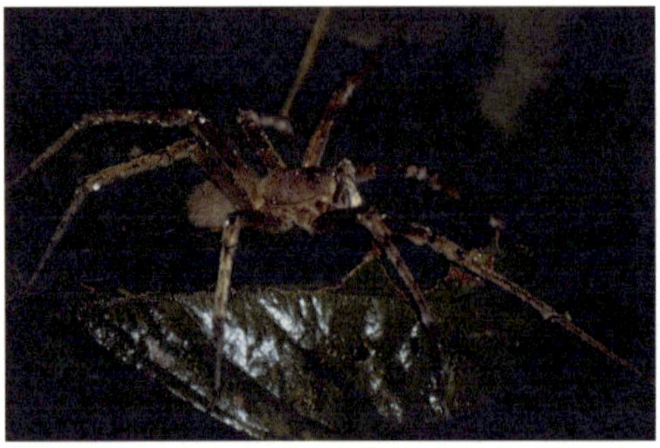

Figure 68.
Brazilian wandering spider (Phoneutria fera) *endemic to the tropical regions of South America.*

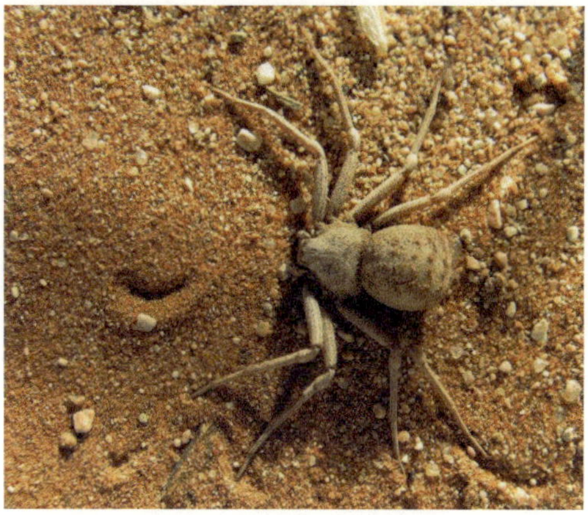

Figure 69.
Six-eyed sand spider *(*Hexophthalma*) is found predominantly in the deserts of southern Africa.*

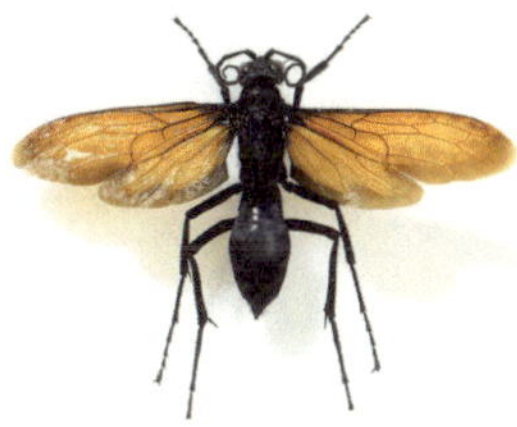

Figure 70.
Tarantula hawks *(*Pepsis *species) found across South and Central America and in the southern United States.*

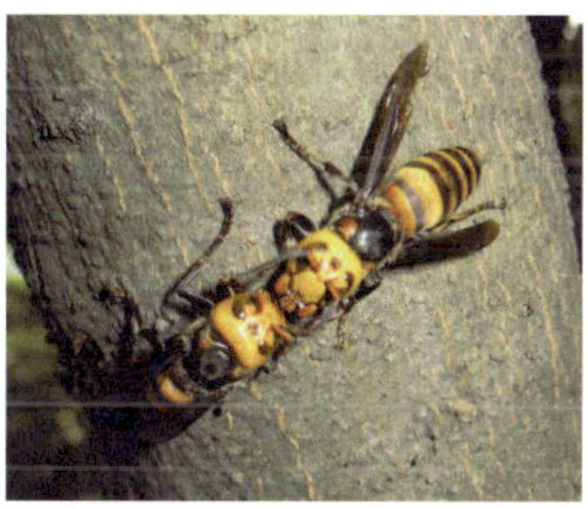

Figure 71.
Giant Japanese hornet*.*

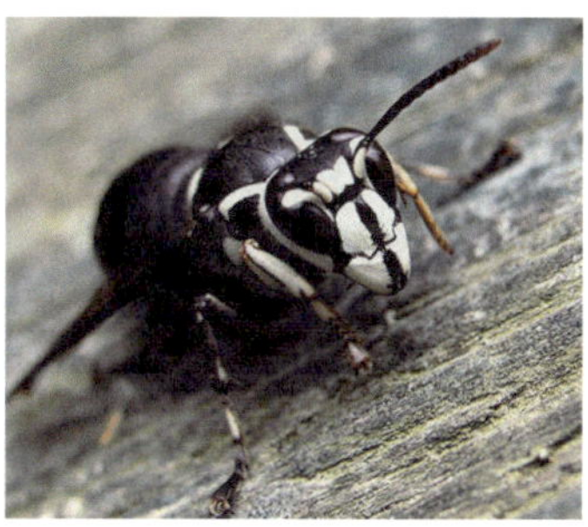

Figure 72.
Bald-faced hornet *(*Dolichovespula maculata*) is found throughout North America.*

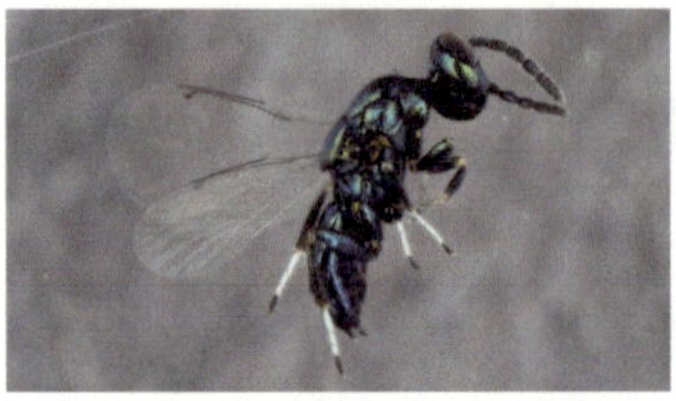

Figure 73.
Crypt-keeper wasp *(*Euderus*).*

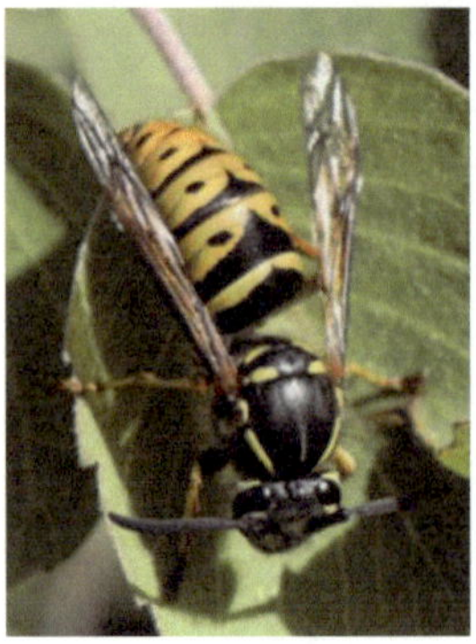

Figure 74.
German yellowjacket Paravespula germanica *(Linnaeus) found throughout North America.*

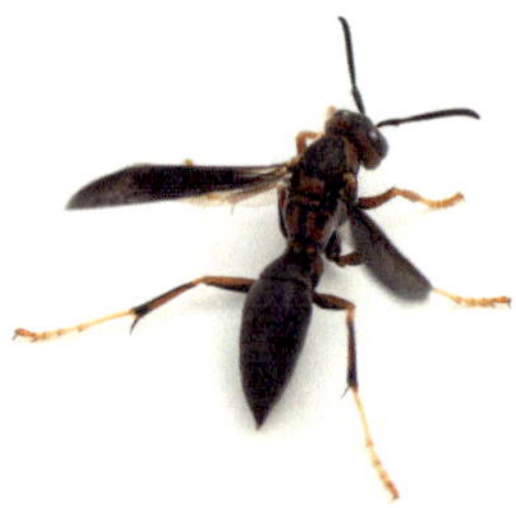

Figure 75.
Paper wasps (Polistes *species)—southern United States.*

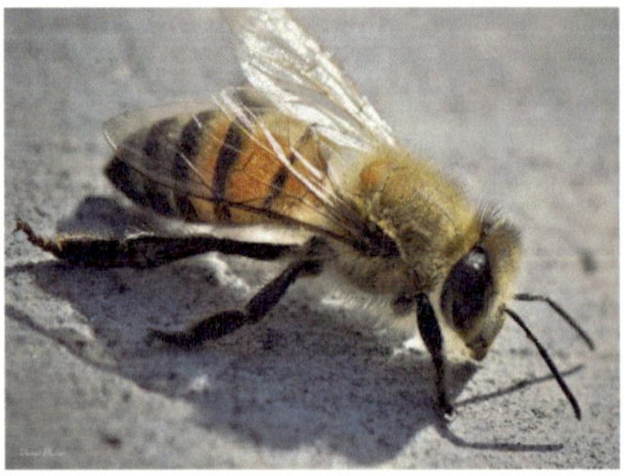

Figure 76.
Africanized honey bee *(*Apis mellifera scutellata *Lepeletier) occurs naturally in sub-Saharan Africa but has been introduced into the Americas.*

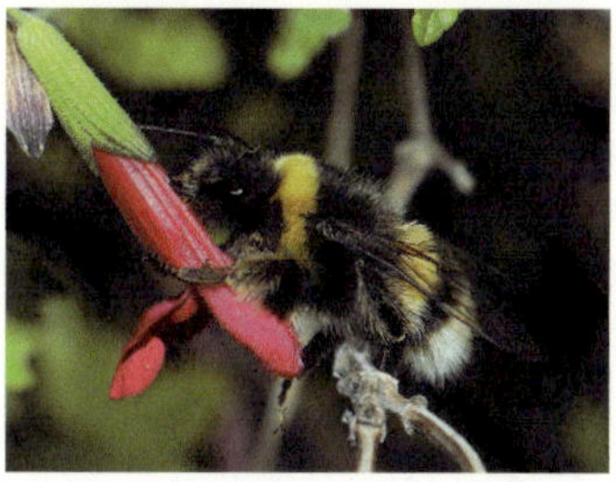

Figure 77.
Bumblebee Bombus terrestris.

reactions [43] and serum sickness necessitating balance between treatment benefit and the risk of adverse reactions [42]. Failure of snake antivenin may be due to the fact that different snake venoms contain varieties of potent hemotoxins, neurotoxins, and other toxins [44]. Therefore, the viper venom is more toxic than elapine venom due to the nature and molecular weight of toxins. Geographical variability, the species of snakes, body weight, and the route of administration of antivenin are very vital to successful treatment [45]. Toxins with molecular weight (<7KDa) diffuse quickly into the blood stream [25], which may not affect efficacy of snake antivenin IgY elevated by ion exchange chromatography [46].

But antivenin affects pharmacokinetic and pharmacodynamic properties of venom. Hence, the quality of preparation and optimization of the use of antivenin must be standardized [47]. The amount of antivenin is determined by clinical signs, size of snake, and the known efficacy of available antivenin [9]. The route of administration of antivenin is controversial, but intravenous route has been considered the most efficient [47]. Polyclonal antibodies are more effective against *Cerastes cerastes* snake venoms in laying hens than in mammals [48]. Chicken immunoglobulin (IgY) is more sensitive, easy to assay, does not activate human complement system and does not react with human anti venomous IgG antibodies or human Fc receptors [49]. The immunoglobulin IgY offers protection against embryo infections [50]. The effective IgY dose required to prevent mortality in rabbit was four times the dose of injected venom using Lowy's protein assay [51]. Milk whey lactoferrin increased antibody levels and immune-stimulatory effects against snake venom [52] whereas adjuvant sustains the release of antigen, interacts with immune cells [53], activates nonspecific mediators of the immune system and enhance macrophage phagocytic activity. IgG antibody neutralized activity against *T. albolabris* venom [54]. Thai neuro polyvalent antivenin is considered second-line treatment for *Hydrophis schistosus* and *Hydrophis curtus* [55]. Both IgG and $F(ab')_2$ antivenins activated human complement system with IgG having significantly higher anti-complementary activity than $F(ab')_2$ antivenin [56]. *Agkistrodon halys* antivenin is more efficacious than green pit viper antivenin [30]. Anti-Cc and Anti-Mm $F(ab')_2$ cross reacted extensively with *Bitis arietans* venom, perhaps due to the presence of venom antigens common to the both snakes [57]. Gamma irradiated *Naja haje* antivenin showed higher neutralizing capacity [58]. Equine antivenom neutralized coagulant and hemorrhagic activities against *Rhabdophis tigrinus* snake venom [59]. *Pseudo naja* antivenin could not neutralize afbrinogenemia with serious consequences [60]. Hence clotting factor replacement therapy using fresh frozen plasma is associated with afibrinogenemia [61]. Gold nano-particle-based lateral flow assay is used for detection of snake envenomation [62]. Therefore, pharmacokinetics may be useful in design and optimization of antivenins [63]. Purification and characterization of new bioactive compounds in snake venoms would be of help in diagnosis and treatment of snake envenomation [64]. Sea snakes such as

Hydrophis schistosus and *Hydrophis curtus* produce venoms that could be neutralized by their neuropolyvalent antivenom (NPAV) and cross neutralization should serve as basis for antivenom purification [55]. Non-irradiated and gamma-irradiated polyvalent antivenoms could neutralize *Naja haje* [65]. Lack of potent monovalent and polyvalent antivenins could be responsible for gross disparity in the management of snakebite. Treatment of snake envenomation was introduced by Albert Calmette of the Institute Pasteur Saigon in the 1890s. The antivenom is either whole IgG or pepsin refined F(ab) fragments of IgG derived from plasma of horse, donkey, mule, sheep immunized with venom of one or more species of snakes lyophilized venoms that have shelf-life of about 5 years and should be stored at $\leq 25^{0C}$, whereas liquid antivenom have shelf-life of 2–3 years and should be stored at 2–8°C and not frozen. Antivenoms against *Naja naja*, *Bungarus caeruleus*, *Daboia russelli* and *Echis carinatus* are produced in India [66]. About 8–10 vials of antivenom against Russell's viper that injects 63 mg of venom is required. Each vial neutralizes 6 mg of the snake venom. Children should receive the same dose as adults, but should be observed closely for antivenin post administration reaction. Normalization of blood pressure in 15–30 minutes, stopping of coagulopathy in 6-hour, reversal of neurotoxicity in 30 minutes and recovery within 24–48 hours are the characteristics of effective snake antivenom. If there is coagulopathy, administration of anti-snake venom can be repeated every 6 hours or after 1–2 hours of the initial dose. Worsening of cardiovascular signs requires repeating dose of snake antivenom every 1–2 hours [67]. About 70% of all snakebites are by non-venomous snakes and 50% of bites by venomous species are dry bites [68]. Serum produced from irradiated *Naja haje* is more potent in venom neutralization than the serum produced from native venom. The two sera inhibit cardiotoxic and hepatotoxic effects [58]. *Crescentia cujete* fruit has significant neutralizing capacity against Vipera russelli venom [69]. Snake envenomation detection immune assay (SEDIA) is a potential diagnostic test for snake envenomation [52]. Milk whey (lactoferrin) could be an adjuvant to snake antisera [52]. Pharmacokinetics of venom from *Hypnale hypnale* are not changed by intramuscular injection of the venom, although may reduce systemic bioavailability of the venom [63]. Structures, cytotoxicities, and affinities to phospholipids of cytotoxins from the venom of *Naja haje* differ [70]. *Acorus calamus* and *Withania somnifera* root extract have neutralizing potential against venom of *Echis carinatus* [71]. Isolated chicken immunoglobulin (IgY) could neutralize viper venom [51]. Low dose snake antivenom with supportive treatment is effective, less cost, and has low level of adverse reactions [72]. IgY antibody could neutralize venom of *Trimeresurus albolabris* [54] and *Cerestes cerestes* venoms [48]. Indian snake antivenoms (VINS and BHARAT) are effective against *D. russelli*, *E. carinatus*, *B. caeruleus* and *N. naja* with VINS being more superior to BHARAT [37]. Serum harvested from polyvalent venom from different species of snakes could neutralize snake venom such as *Rhabdophis tigrinus* [59]. Too small initial doses of snake antivenom could not neutralize venom of *Pseudo naja*; hence the patient remains afribrinogenemic for long period of time [60]. Neutralizing potential of snake antivenom (IgY) could be improved by ion exchange chromatography. Therefore, IgG antivenom has significant complementary antivenom activity than F(ab')2 antivenom [56].

4.3 Medicinal plants and phytochemicals against ophidism

Andrographis paniculata and *Aristolochia indica* could neutralize venom of *Daboia russelli* [41]. Higher dose of Haffkine polyvalent antivenom could neutralize venom of *Naja sumatrana* [40]. *Calotropis gigantea* could neutralize venom of *Vipera russelli* [73]. Brown snake, *Pseudo naja* causes venom induced consumption coagulopathy with over one-third of patients having serious hemorrhagic collapse and microangiopathy. The venom is neutralized by one vial of antivenom [42]. *Androctonus crassicauda* antivenom could neutralize *Mesobuthus* venom found in Aegean region of Turkey [74]. Lectins from *Abrus precatorius* may be tried against snake and scorpion venoms. Because native and denatured agglutinin from the plant has immunomodulatory potential [75]. Hence, clinical studies of the effectiveness and safety of antivenoms have to be intensified because most currently marketed antivenoms were registered without any formal clinical or preclinical safety and effectiveness testing [76]. Change in amino acid sequence of a venom component can lead to a change of new compounds. Alpha bungarotoxin is cholinergic. Therefore, venom proteomics and genomics could lead to discovery of new therapeutic agents including antivenoms [77]. Natural and synthetic inhibitors of snake venom metalloproteinases are phenols and rosmarinic acid which inhibits hemorrhage caused by venoms of *Trimeresurus flavoviridis*, *Crotalus atrox* and *Gloydius blomhoffii*, *Agkistrodon bilineatus*, *Deinagkistrodon acutus* and *Bitis arietans*. Apigenin also inhibits venom of *Echis carinatus* and gallic acid inhibits venom of *Daboia russelli*, isoquercitrin, myricetin-B-O-glucoside and gallocatechin from *Schizolobium parahyba* leaves neutralized venoms of Bothrops species including *B. jararacussu* and *B. alternatus* [78, 79]. Matrix metalloproteinase inhibitors such as that of zinc-binding group, marimastat, prinomastat and tanomastat inhibit venom of *Echis ocellatus*. They are hydroxamic acid derivatives. Matrix metalloproteinases are grouped as astacins, serralysins and reprolysins under metzincins [80, 81]. Zinc containing endopeptidases and calcium ions could be chelated by ethylenediamine-tetraacetic acid, o-phenanthroline [82, 83], N,N,N,′N′-Tetrakis (2-pyridylmethyl) ethane-1,2-diamine (TPEN), diethylene triamine pentaacetic acid (DTPA), tetraethylthiuram disulfide (TID) in hemorrhage and myotoxicity caused by venom of *E. carinatus* [84]. Bisphosphonate clodronate, tetracycline and doxycydine inhibit hemorrhagic, proteolytic, coagulant and defibrigenotic effect of venom from *B. asper* [85]. A clerodane diterpenoid from *Baccharis trimera* caused inhibition of *B. neuwiedi* and *B. jararacussu* venoms [86]. Triacontyl p-coumarate from *Bombacopsis glabra* inhibited venom of *Bothropoides pauloensis*, *B. leucurus*, *B. jararaca* and *B. pautoensis* [87]. Macrolobin A and B (triterpnoid saponins) from *Pentaclethra macroloba* inhibited venom of Bothrops [88]. Linearol and isolinearol (secodolastane diterpenes) from *Canistrocarpus cervicornis* inhibited venom of *B. jararaca* [89]. Lupeol and lupeol acetate (terpenes) inhibited *E. carinatus*-venom induced damage [90]. Quinolones including 2-hydroxymethyl-6-methoxy-1,4-dihydro-4-equinolinone inhibited venoms of *B. jararacussu*, *B. moojeni* and *B. alternatus* [78]. N-acetyl cysteine inhibited gelatinase, hyaluronidase, hemorrhagic and defribrinogenating activities of *Vipera russelli* and *E. carinatus* venoms [91]. A derivative of citalopram (DFD) neutralized venoms of *E. carinatus*, *E. ocellatus*, *E. carinatus sochureki*, *E. carinatus leakeyi* and *Crotalus atrox* [92]. However, *Allium cepa*, *Securidaca longipedunculata*, *Carica papaya*, *Harrisonia abyssinica* and *Nicotiana tobaccum* are frequently used in treatment of snakebite. Low dose of snake antivenom is highly cost-effective as compared to the high dose [92].

4.4 Signs of scorpionism

Scorpion species of medical importance are represented by the genera *Androctonus*, *Tityus*, *Mesobuthus*, *Hottentotta*, *Parabuthus*, *Centruroides* and *Leiurus*. *Leiurus abdullahbayrami* caused hyperexcitability, agitation, aggressiveness, squeaking, fighting, tachypnea, weakness, convulsions and death due to cardiac and respiratory failure [93]. Envenomation of *Leiurus quinquestriatus* showed degranulation of eosinophils, fever, edema of cerebrum and myocarditis in rabbit [94].

Tityus pachyurus polock envenomation was characterized by sialorrhea, respiratory distress, profuse sweating, ataxia, restlessness, somnolence and hypoglycemia [95]. The toxicity of venom is relative to the maturity and weight of the scorpion [96]. *Tityus stigmurus* caused, cardiogenic shock, pulmonary edema, severe neurological symptoms and death [9]. Spontaneous glycinergic and glutamatergic post synaptic currents, suggest that scorpion toxin act on inhibitory and excitatory presynaptic nerves. *A. australis* venom is more toxic followed by *T. pachyurus*, *A. crassicauda*, *L. quinquestriatus*, *M. eupeus*, *L. abdullahbayrami* and *H. sauleyi* [93]. *A. crassicauda* scorpion venom could induce activation of human monocytes leading to promotion of expression of IL-12 [97] with molecular peptides (Acra 1 and Acra 2) that are similar to known sodium-channel specific toxins of other scorpions [98]. *M. gibbosus* endemic to Mediterranean area causes scorpionism characterized by pain, pulsating and gloving sensations, cold, sweat, paleness, excitation, occasional spasm of the affected part, tortuousness of the vein, which lasted for more than 4 years. Periodical tingling, and occasional muscle twitches were observed during night. The treatment was symptomatic [99].

4.5 Treatment of scorpionism

Local anesthetic is effective, while opioids are ineffective and increase the risk of respiratory depression. Non-steroidal anti-inflammatory drugs may be disappointing. Bio 10 ml of 10% calcium gluconate administered over 5–10 minutes relieves muscle pain and cramps and the effects last 20–30 minutes, hence safe limit dose is required. SA IMR scorpion venom antiserum is equine anti-scorpion globulin supplement in 5 ml per ampoule and 5–10 ml is required for adults and children. Its plateau effect is achieved in 2–6 hours, hence respiratory support is of paramount importance during the period. If case-response to first dose is inadequate, another 5 ml could be administered. The victim should be kept under close observation for at least a period of 6–12 hours. Electrolytes, pH, acid-base balance arterial blood gases, and electrocardiography should be used for assessment of scorpionism to avoid fatality. The rule of thumb is that scorpions with thick tails and slender pincers (e.g. Buthidae) produce more venoms than those with slender tails and large pincers. Hence speed of scorpion and a wave of potential neurotoxic effects are very important. Bioclon and Butantan are very effective antivenins against scorpionism [95]. Treatment of scorpion envenomation requires specific antiserum. Antiserum against *Buthus quinquestriatus* from immunization of horses with crude venom as antigen has been proven to be effective [100], and high amount of antivenins is required to achieve satisfactory neutralization [101]. *A. crassicauda* antivenin could prevent, neutralize and cure *M. eupeus* scorpionism if applied at optimum time, dose, and route [102]. The LD_{50} of *A. crassicauda* venom (1.1 mg/kg) and 39.19 mg/kg [103] make it highly toxic. The long half-life of venom in the body might require antivenin that has long half-life [101].

In Saudi Arabia, scorpionism is treated using 5 ml of antivenom diluted in 5–20 ml of saline and the solution was administered intravenously. Adjunct chemotherapy could be instituted when required. However, a 12-year-old boy inadequately treated with antivenom died from pulmonary edema, hematemesis, severe neurotoxicity, and circulatory failure. All the patients treated in Saudi Arabia stayed in hospitals for 1–2 days. The incidence of antivenom reaction was 1.7–6.6%, low protein level of antivenom, and high quality of catecholamine could lead to antivenom failure [101].

Two purified toxic fractions of *Mesobuthus eupeus* toxin were quickly eliminated from tissue [104] signifying that *M. eupeus* toxicity may not last long in the body. Dissociation of the toxin-channel complex during depolarization is determined by the difference between electrical energies of the activated states of normal and toxin-modified channels [105]. The partially purified toxic fractions, when injected to rabbits, gave rise to more potent antivenoms against whole venoms as compared to presently commercially available antivenoms [106]. *A. crassicauda* has LD_{50} of venom (15.45 μg/kg) in mice, making it one of the highly toxic species of scorpions in the world [103]. *A. crassicauda* antivenom could neutralize *M. gibbosus* venom (20 LD_{50}) in Aegean region of Turkey [107]. Thus, highly potent antivenom could be produced from about 238 telsons in 51 days [74].

Comparing the calculated ratio of $\frac{292}{13.6}$ and $\frac{330}{13.6}$ which gives equivalent weight of 21.5 kg and 24.3 kg respectively shows that Butantan (292 μg/ml) and Bioclon (330 μg/ml) can be used effectively in the treatment of human weighing 21.5 and 24.3 kg body weight, respectively. Signifying that age plays role on the disposition of *Tityus* toxin, the toxic principle of Tityus species. Therefore, the difference in severity of symptoms observed in children and adults may be due to difference in pharmacokinetics of the toxin. *Mesobuthus eupeus* venom can be neutralized by nanovalent, polyvalent and anti-idiotype antivenom, respectively. They are non-toxicants and can be used as a vaccine in people at the risk of scorpion stings [108]. Scorpion anti-venoms are specific antigens, detoxified venoms or toxins, purified venom fractions, natural toxoids, recombinant toxins, synthetic peptides, monoclonal and recombinant antibodies [100]. Using peptides derived from the sequence of scorpion toxins, the penetration of antipeptide antibodies can neutralize the cognate venom [109]. Turkish antivenom against *A. crassicauda* is effective against other species of scorpions. Minimum lethal dose and minimum effective dose were used to evaluate the effect of Turkish antivenom on *M. gibbosus* envenomation [96] suggesting applicability of the new formula for calculation of effective dose for antivenoms. Scorpion sting results in adult morbidity and pediatric mortality [110]. The most lethal species are *T. serrulatus*, *T. bahiensis* in Brazil, *Centruroides suffusus*, *C. lionpidus*, *C. sculpturatus* in Mexico, *Leiurus quinquestriatus*, *A. crassicauda*, *A. australis*, *A. amoreuni*, *Buthus occitanus* in Middle East and North Africa, *Parabuthus grauntatus* and *P. transvaalicus* in South Africa, *Mesobuthus tamulus* and *Palamneus swammerdance* in India [111], respectively. One milliliter of *Androctonus crassicauda* antivenom could neutralize *Mesobuthus eupeus* venom. The antivenom is monovalent with immune activity and neutralizing capacity. The venom is produced by Refik Saydam Hygiene Centre in Turkey [103]. Also *A. crassicauda* antivenom could neutralize *Mesobuthus gibbosus* venom [96]. Stings from *Leiurus abdullahbayrami* causes hyperexcitability, agitation, aggressive behavior, squeaking, fighting, tachypnea, weakness, convulsions, and death due to cardiorespiratory failure. However, the venom has two kinds of protein with molecular masses of 4 and 6 kDa, respectively [93]. The condition was treated by dipping the affected hand in ice water, adrenaline (1:1000) was injected around the site of the sting and chlorpheniramine was injected intramuscularly into the upper arm. Snake antivenom made by J. Wyeth and Brother Ltd., Canada was administered intramuscularly [112] and produced desired therapeutic effect against scorpionism. Scorpion envenomation may be more dangerous in pregnant woman [113]. However, Meu TxKα3, a scorpion toxin-like peptide could undergo mutation at site 30 and help improve its K^+ channel-blocking and antibacterial function [114]. The designed bispecific NbF12–10 neutralized AahI and AahII toxins and could be used in the treatment of *Androctonus australis* envenomation. About 100-kDa horse antivenom serum could neutralize 7 kDa scorpion toxin and 15 kDa antivenom could neutralize AahI toxin. The NbAch1′ F_{12} fully neutralized 100 LD_{50} of AahI toxin [115]. Children with abnormal electrocardiography may require high dose of antivenom [116]. Aminotoxin could activate T lymphocytes and may be used as immunomodulators in infection and cancer [117] whereas Ca^{2+}-activated K^+ channel (ISK_2) is sensitive to apamin [118]. Nevertheless alpha-KTx peptides from the venom of *Centruroides elegans* block Kv1.3 of T lymphocytes [119] whereas Tst26 peptide from *T. stigmurus block* Kv1.2 and Kv1.3 channels [120] respectively. *T. serrulatus* could be detected using molecular mass of the venom [121]. *Androctonus mauretanicus mauretanicus* toxin could cross-react with the serum of *Androctonus australis* [122]. *Androctonus mauretanicus* and *Buthus occitanus* contain mycotoxins and post synaptic neurotoxins with the first being more toxic. But the polyclonal antivenom prevented lethality from *A. mauretanicus, B. occitanus* and *A. crassicauda* venoms [123]. Venom of *A. mauretanicus* is more toxic than that of *A. australis* hector that is more toxic than that of *B. occitanus*. Lethality of scorpion venom in mammals is dependent on age and species of the animals [124]. That is why the pharmacokinetics of a *Tityus* toxin from *T. serrulatus* scorpion venom is dependent on the age of affected individuals [125]. Death due to scorpionism is secondary to cardiorespiratory failure [126]. Hence quick detection and quantification of venom is necessary for rational therapy, which is highly beneficial to reduce management costs and patients risk [127]. Equine F(ab′)2, IgG recombinant toxin, synthetic apitoxin, mAb, Fab, ScFv, chFab and rFab are of great benefit in treatment of scorpion and spider envenomation [128]. Minimum effective dose of antivenom is administered precociously by intravenous route to achieve efficient immunotherapy [129].

A. australis has complex venom that contains cytotoxic principles with very fast resultant fatal effects [130]. The effective monoclonal antibodies (mAbs) specific for the α-neurotoxin 1 (Aah1) from *A. australis* hector venom has been reported [131]. *A. australis* has recombinant toxin II with immunological and biological properties [132]. In addition, *Androctonus australis* hector (Aah) envenomation is mediated by cytokines and complement system, which in turn activate leukocyte to damage tissue [133]. But kinins are involved in cardiovascular toxicity and lethality of *L. quinquestriatus* venom in rabbits. *Androctonus australis garzonii* venom (100 μg/kg) was neutralized by 4 mg/kg of antivenom injected intravenously [128]. Antivenoms against a number of scorpion venoms have been reported [127], suggesting that the potency of antivenom should be investigated in relation to the scorpion venom [93] and both LD_{50} and ED_{50} should be determined paradoxically and canonically [134].

Intravenous LD_{50} of *Vipera berus berus* (0.4 μg/kg) with signs including head-drop, floppy neck, flaccid paralysis of limb, respiratory paralysis and death [135] and that of *Laticauda colubrine*, 0.05–0.13 μg/g [136], Sri Lankan *B. caeruleus* 0.07 μg/g [137], and *Naja sputatrix* [138] disagree with the reported LD_{50} (0.5 ng) of *Androctonus australis* [93] signifying that the venom of *V. berus berus* is less potent than with that of *A. australis*. Similar signs were observed for *V. nikolskii* venom (1.0 μg/kg) but the signs caused by phospholipase A_2 were lost after the mice were injected strontium [139], which may become antivenom against *V. berus berus* and *A. australis* venoms in future. The newly developed dot-ELISA for detection of venoms of Indian venomous snakes, *Naja naja*, *Bungarus caeruleus*, *Daboia russelli* and *Echis carinatus* [140] with comparative proteomic enzymes [141] may be also used to detect scorpion venoms. High level of toxicity of *Montivipera raddei* and *Montivipera bubjardahica* venoms is responsible for, high activity against A549 human lung carcinoma [142] signifying that scorpion venom may have anticancer activity. Lethal doses of *L. quinquestriatus* were 0.5 mg/kg i.v. and 3 μg/kg i.m. [143]. The LD_{50} of *T. pachyurus* venom in monogastric animals show that mouse (4.8 μg/kg) is highly sensitive to *T. pachyurus* venom, Hamster (3.48 μg/kg), guinea pig (2.40 μg/kg), rat (2.32 μg/kg), rabbit (1.16 μg/kg), monkey (1.11 μg/kg), marmoset (2.40 μg/kg), squirrel monkey (2.08 μg/kg), ferret (1.99 μg/kg), cat (0.74 μg/kg), dog and baboon (0.70 μg/kg), child (0.56 μg/kg), micro pig (0.52 μg/kg), mini pig (0.40 μg/kg) and adult human (0.37 mg/kg) respectively [103] indicating that *Tityus pachyurus* toxin is more toxic to all the species of animals [139] as compared to American pit viper venom [144]. The toxicity may be due to the presence of *Tityus* toxins that are also present in *Tityus pachyurus*, *T. stigmurus*, *Tityus obscurus* and *Tityus serrulatus* venom. The toxic principle acts via Na^+, K^+, Ca^{2+} and Cl^- channels signifying excitatory effects on heart, CNS and muscular fibers [142]. Hence, mini pig could be the best model for determination of LD_{50} and ED_{50} for *T. pachyurus* venom and antivenom respectively for human application [103].

5. Conclusion

The toxicity of snake and scorpion venom is dependent on the quantity of the venom, whereas apitoxicosis in human is dependent on the number of stings and dose of venom produced per sting. Snake and scorpion venoms are the most dangerous. However, venoms of some snakes and scorpions are equipotent and require 2 or more vials of antivenoms. LD_{50} of honeybee venom in adult man is 2.5 mg/kg which can be neutralized by 7.5 mg/kg ($3LD_{50}$) of antivenin. LD_{50} of honeybee venom in child is 1.41 mg/kg and can be neutralized by 11.2 mg/kg ($7.9LD_{50}$) antivenin. The venom can kill in less than 4 hours. Hence, children are more sensitive to honeybee toxicity than the adults are, and so may require higher dose of antivenom. Spider and wasp envenomation are less severe and could be treated symptomatically. All the organ systems could be affected and complications could follow multiple attacks. Hence treatment is by administration of antivenins, anti-inflammatory, analgesic and respiratory support. Neurological and cardiorespiratory signs may be considered as indices of therapeutic success or failure. Prompt therapeutic intervention and hospitalization of 1 or more days could either delay or avert death. In the cases of severe anemia, blood transfusion and fluid therapy may be evident.

Author details

Saganuwan Alhaji Saganuwan
Department of Veterinary Pharmacology and Toxicology, College of Veterinary Medicine, Federal University of Agriculture, Makurdi, Benue State, Nigeria

*Address all correspondence to: pharm_saga2006@yahoo.com

References

[1] Bieber AL. Metal and non-protein constituent in snake venom. In: Lee T, editor. Snake Venoms: Hardwork of Experimental Pharmacology. Berlin: Springer Verlag; 1979. pp. 295-3006

[2] Gilliam LL, Brunker J. North American snake envenomation in the dog and cat. Veterinary Clinics: Small Animal Practice. 2011;**41**:1239-1259

[3] Borges A, Miranda RJ, Pasale JM. Scorpionism in central America, with special reference to the case of Panama. Journal of Venomous Animals and Toxins Including Tropical Diseases. 2012;**18**(2):130-143

[4] Muller GJ, Modler H, Wium CA, Veale DJH. Scorpion sting in Southern Africa: Diagnosis and management. Continuing Medical Education. 2012; **30**(10):1-8

[5] Dehesa-Davila M, Possani LD. Scorpionism and serotherapy in Mexico. Toxicon. 1994;**32**(9):1015-1018

[6] Costa CLSDO, Fe NF, Sampaio I, Tadei WP. A profile of scorpionism, including the species of scorpions involved in the state of Amazonas. Revista da Sociedade Brasileira de Medicina Tropical. 2016;**49**(3):376-379

[7] Pajovic B, Radosavljevic M, Radosavljevic I, Vukovic M, Boricic S. Biogeographic and clinical review of *Mesobuthus gibbosus* scorpionism in Montenegro: Clinical cases of six patients. Medical Data. 2015;**7**(4):315-318

[8] Deghani R, Rafinejad J, Fathi B, Shehi MP, Jazayeri M, Hashemi A. A retrospective study on scorpionism in Iran (2002-2011). Journal of Arthropod-Borne Diseases. 2017;**11**(2):194-203

[9] Chippaux JP, Goyfton M. Producers of antivenom sera. Toxin. 1983;**21**: 739-752

[10] Ulug M, Yaman Y, Yapia F, Can-Ulug N. Scorpion envenomation in children: an analysis of 99 cases. The Turkish Journal of Pediatrics. 2012;**54**: 119-127

[11] Seiter N, Koc H, Ulrich A, Yagmur EA. The case history of a toxic sting of a *Leiurus abdullahbayrami* scorpion in Turkey. Arachnology Letters. 2016;**51**:64-66

[12] Bharath RV, Kumar MR, Subrahmanyam BV, Rammohan P, Agrawal A. Scorpion envenomation in children and its management. Archives of Medicine and Health Sciences. 2014; **2**(2):131-135

[13] Ferreira SR Jr, Almeida RA, Barraviera SR, Barravie B. Historical perspective and human consequences of Africanized bee stings in the Americas. Journal of Toxicology and Environmental Health, Part B: Critical Reviews. 2012;**15**:97-108

[14] Diniz AZQ, Belmino JFB, Arujo KAMD, Viera AT, Elite RDS. Epidemiology of honeybee sting cases in the state of Ceara, Northeastern Brazil. Revista do Instituto de Medicina Tropical de Sao Paulo. 2016;**58**:40

[15] Linard ATS, Barros RM, Sousa JA, Elite RS. Epidemiology of bee stings in Campina Grade, Paraiba State, Northeastern Brazil. Journal of Venomous Animals and Toxins Including Tropical Diseases. 2014;**20**:13

[16] Betten DP, Richardson WH, Tong TC, Clark RF. Massive honeybee envenomation-induced rhabdomyolysis in an adolescent. Pediatrics. 2006; **117**(1):231-235

[17] da Silva GAR, Pires KL, Soares DCDS, Ferreira MR, Ferry FRDA. RRH: Envenoming syndrome due to 200 stings from

Africanized honeybees. Revista do Instituto de Medicina Tropical de São Paulo. 2013;**55**(1):61-64

[18] Schumacher MJ, Schmidt JO, Egen NB, Lowry JE. Quantity analysis and lethality of European and Africanized honeybee venom. The American Journal of Tropical Medicine and Hygiene. 1990;**43**(1):79-86

[19] Schumacher MJ, Schmidt JO, Egen NB, Dilon KA. Biochemical variability of venoms from individual European and Africanized honeybees (*Apis mellifera*). The Journal of Allergy and Clinical Immunology. 1992;**90**:59-65

[20] Almeida RAMDB, Olivo TET, Mendes RP, Barraviera SRCS, Souza LDR, Martins JG, et al. Africanized honey bee stings: How to treat them. Revista da Sociedade Brasileira de Medicina Tropical. 2011; **44**(6):755-761

[21] Kluz-Zawadzka J, Hartman-Ksycinska A, Lewandowska B. Emergent management of scorpion sting. Przeglad Epidemiologiczny. 2014; **68**:655-688

[22] Platnick AI. The World Spider Catalog Version 12.0. New York, USA: American Nugarm of Natural History; 2011. Available from: http://research.amnh.org/ig/spiders/catalog

[23] Isbister GK, Gray MR, Balit CR, Raven RJ, Stokes BJ, Porges K, et al. Funnel-web spider bite; a systematic review of recorded clinical cases. The Medical Journal of Australia. 2015;**182**: 407-411

[24] Gibb TJ, Bennett GW. Spiders. Extension Entomologists. 2017;**72**:1-2. Available from: www.extension.purdue.edu

[25] Okkache N, El Jaoudi R, Ghalim N, Chgoury F, Bouhaouala B, Mdaghri NE, et al. Evaluation of the lethal potency of scorpion and snake venoms and comparison between intraperitoneal and intravenous injection routes. Toxin (Basel). 2014;**6**(6):1873-1881

[26] Krifi MN, Marrakchi N, El Ayeb M, Dellagi K. Effect of some variables on the in vivo determination of scorpion and viper venom toxicities. Biologicals. 1998;**26**(4):277-288

[27] Krifi MN, El Ayeb M, Dellagi K. New procedures and parameters for better evaluation of *Androctonus australis* garzonii (Aag) and *Buthus occitanus* tunetanus (Bot) scorpion envenomation and specific scrotherapy treatment. Toxicon. 1996;**34**(2):252-266

[28] Wang JD, Tsan YT, Mao YC, Wag LM. Venomous snake bites and antivenom, treatment according to a protocol for pediatric patients in Taiwan. Journal of Venomous Animals and Toxins Including Tropical Diseases. 2009;**15**(4):667-679

[29] Chich-Fan C, Tzeng-Jih L, Wen-Chi H, Hua-Wei Y. Appropriate antivenom doses for six-types of envenomations caused by snakes in Taiwan. Journal of Venomous Animals and Toxins Including Tropical Diseases. 2009;**15**(3): 479-490

[30] Fung HT, Yung WH, Crow P, Lam KW, Tan KS, Gironi A, et al. Green viper antivenom from Thailand and *Agkistrodon halys* antivenin from chiria compared in treating *Cryptelytrops albolabris* envenomation of mice. Hong Kong Medical Journal. 2012;**18**:40-45

[31] Khaddach FZ, Benaji B, Djebari FL, Chgoury F, Boussada L, Wadi A, et al. Assessment of preclinical efficacy of antivenoms produced in rabbit by immunological methods and neutralization assays. Journal of Chemical and Pharmaceutical Research. 2014;**6**(12):446-455

[32] Vivas J, Ibarra C, Salazar AM, Neves-Ferreira AGC, Sanchez EE,

Perales J, et al. Purification and characterization of tener-plasoninin-1, a serine peptidase inhibitor with antiplasmin activity from the coral snake (*Micrurus tener* tener) venom. Comparative Biochemistry and Physiology Part C. 2016;**179**:107-115

[33] James TRJ, Danesh M, Vadivelan R, Shrestha A, Shanmugan V. In vivo and in vitro neutralizing potential of *Rauwolfia serpentina* plant extract against *Daboia russelli* venom. Biology. 2013;7(6):276-281. ID 58940648

[34] Silverstein D, Hopper K. Small Animal Critical Care Medicine. 2nd ed. Amsterdam: Elsevier Health Science; 2008. p. 1000

[35] Fry BG. Venomous Reptiles and Their Toxins: Evolution, Pathophysiology and Biochemistry. Oxford: Oxford University Press; 2015. p. 546

[36] Gleen JJ, Straight RC. Mojave rattlesnake (*Crotalus scutulatus* scutulatus) venom variation in toxicity with geographical origin. Toxicon. 1978; **18**:81-84

[37] Maduwager K, Siva A, Oleavy MA, Hodgson WC, Isbister GK. Efficacy of Indian polyvalent snake antivenoms against Sri Lankan snake venoms: Lethality studies or clinically focused in vitro studies. Scientific Reports. 2016; **6**:1-11

[38] Isbister GK, Brown SG, MacDonald E, White J, Alcurine BJ. Current use of Australian snake antivenoms and frequency of immediate-type hypersensitivity reactions and anaphylaxis. The Medical Journal of Australia. 2008;**188**:473-476

[39] Abubakar IS. Randomized controlled double-blind non-infirmity trial of two antivenins for saw-scaled or old carpet viper (*Eschris ocellatus*) envenoms in Nigeria. PLoS Neglected Tropical Diseases. 2010;**4**:e767

[40] Cham G, Lim F, Earnest A, Gopalakrishnakone P. Cross-reactivity against *Naja sumatrana* (black spitting cobra) envenoming from the Haffkine antivenom in a mouse model. ISRN Toxicology. 2013;**247645**:1-6

[41] Meenatchisundaram S, Parameswari G, Michael A. Studies on antivenom activity of *Andrographis paniculata* and *Aristolochia indica*. Indian Journal of Science and Technology. 2009;**2**(4):76-79

[42] Allen GE, Brown GA, Buckley NA. Clinical effects and antivenom dosing in brown snake (*Pseudonaja* spp.) envenoming Australian snakebite project (ASP-14). PLoS One. 2012;**7**(12):1

[43] Isbister GK. Antivenom efficacy or effectiveness. The Australian experience. Toxicology. 2010;**268**: 148-154

[44] Birell GW, Isbister GK, Masci PP, de Jersey J, Wallis TP. Molecular diversity in venom from the Australian brown snake, *Pseudonaja textilis*. Molecular & Cellular Proteomics. 2006; **5**:379-389

[45] Segura A, Herreva M, Vargars M. Intra specific variation and cross neutralization by antivenom. Toxicon. 2012;**59**:158-162

[46] Liu W, Wang WD, Wang W, Bai S, Dybowski C. Influence of structure on the spectroscopic properties of the polymorphs of piroxicam. The Journal of Physical Chemistry. 2010;**114**(49): 16641-16649

[47] Riviere G, Choumet V, Audebert F, Saboraud A, Debray M, Scherrmann JN, et al. Effect of antivenom on venom pharmacokinetics in experimentally envenomed rabbits towards an optimization of antivenom therapy. The Journal of Pharmacology and Experimental Therapeutics. 1997; **281**(1):1

[48] Moussa IN, Hassan AM, Alesisa AM, Al Arfaj AA, Salem BMM, Alrejai SA. Protective efficacy of immunoglobulins Y prepared against *Cerastes cerastes* snake venom in the kingdom of Saudi Arabia. Saudi Medical Journal. 2012;**33**(8):846-851

[49] De Almeda CN, da Silva CL, Couto HP, Escocard RC, da Rocha DG, Sentinelli I. Development of press to produce polyvalent IgG antibodies anti-African snake venom. Toxin. 2008;**52**: 293-301

[50] Larsson A, Sjoquist J. Chicken IgY utilizing evolutionary difference. Comparative Immunology, Microbiology & Infectious Diseases. 1990;**13**:199-201

[51] Krishnan LK, Saroja JB, Rajalingam M, John V, Valappil MP, Sreelathal V. Rabbit snake bite model to assess safety and efficacy of anti-viper chicken antibodies (IofG). American Journal of Clinical and Experimental Medicine. 2015;**3**(1):32-38

[52] Elaraby AK, El-Jakee J, Fahmy A, Kandid MM, Mahmood Z, Saida AA. Lactoferrin: a novel strategy for antivenom therapy. International Journal of Pharmaceutical Research and Allied Sciences. 2016;**5**(1):50-57

[53] Mahan T, Venom P, Rav DN. Novel adjuvants and delivery vehicles for vaccines development: a road ahead. The Indian Journal of Medical Research. 2013;**138**(5):779-795

[54] Duan HL, He Q-Y, Zhuu B, Wang WW, Li B, Zhang YZ, et al. Anti-*Trimeresurus albolabris* efficacy antibodies: Preparation, purification and neutralization efficacy. Journal of Venomous Animals and Toxins Including Tropical Diseases. 2016; **22**(23):1-6

[55] Tan C, Tan NH, Tan KY, Kong KO. Antivenom cross-neutralization of the venoms of *Hydrophis schistosus* and *Hydrophis curtis*, two common sea snakes in Malaysian waters. Toxin. 2015; **7**:572-581

[56] Pakmanee N, Noiphrom J, Kay A, Pormuttakun D, Sakolparp L, Hemmale W, et al. Comparative abilities of phospholipase A2, and coagulant activities induced by *Daboia siamensis* venom and their antiinflammatory activity. Science Asia. 2013;**39**:160-166

[57] Khaddah FZ, Benaiji B, Djebari FL, Chgoury F, Boussadda L, Wadi A, et al. Assessment of preclinical efficacy antivenoms produced in rabbit by immunological methods and neutralization assays. Journal of Chemical and Pharmaceutical Research. 2014;**6**(12):446-455

[58] Karam HM, Shaaban EA, Mohamed AF, Zaki HF, Kenawy SA. New approach for improving production of *Naja haje* snake antivenom. International Journal of Scientific and Research Publications (IJSRP). 2015;**5**(3):1-11

[59] Morokuma K, Kobori N, Fukuda T, Takashira M. Experimental manufacture of equine antivenom against yamakagashi (*Rhabdophis tigrinus*). Japanese Journal of Infectious Diseases. 2011;**64**(5):397-402

[60] Yeung JM, Little M, Murray LM, Jelinek GA, Daly FFS. Antivenom dosing in 35 patients with severe brown snake (*Pseudonaja*) envenoming in Western Australia over 10 years. The Medical Journal of Australia. 2004;**181**: 703-705

[61] Jelinek GA, Tweed C, Lynch D, Celenza T, Bush B, Michalopoulos N. Cross reactivity between venomous, mildly venomous, and non-venomous snake venoms with the Commonwealth Serum Laboratories Venom Detection Kit. Emergency Medicine Australasia. 2004;**16**(5–6):384-386

[62] Pawode BS, Sivi NC, Shaikh IK, Waghmare AB, Jalhar ND, Wagh VB, et al. Rapid and selective detection of experimental snake envenomation-use of gold nanoparticle based literal flow assay. Toxicon. 2016;**119**(1):299-306

[63] Tan CH, Sim SM, Gnanathasan CA, Fung SY, Tan NG. Pharmacokinetics of the Sri Lankan hump-nosed pit viper intramuscular injections of the venom into rabbits. Toxicon. 2014;**79**:37-44

[64] Fatima LD, Fatah C. Pathophysiological and pharmacological effects of snake venom components: molecular targets. Clinical Toxicology. 2014;**4**(2):1-9

[65] Shaban EA, Hafez MN. Ability of gamma-irradiated polyvalent antivenom to neutralize the toxicity of the Egyptian cobra (*Naja haje*) venom. Egyptian Journal of Hospital Medicine. 2003;**13**:135-152

[66] Chaudhary S, Singh S, Chaudhary N, Mahato SK. Snake-bite in Nepal. Journal of Universal College of Medical Sciences. 2014;**2**(3):45-53

[67] Ahmed SM, Ahmed M, Nadeem A, Mahajan J, Choudhary A, Pal J. Emergency treatment of a snake bite. Pearls from literature. Journal of Emergencies, Trauma, and Shock. 2008; **1**(2):97-105

[68] Theakston RD, Warrell DA, Griffiths E. Report of a WHO workshop on the standardization and control of antivenoms. Toxicon. 2003;**41**:541-547

[69] Shastry CS, Aswathanarayana BJ, Maulik MB. Antivenom activity of ethanolic extract of *Crescentia cujete* fruit. International Journal of Phytomedicine. 2012;**4**(1):108-114

[70] Suzuki-Matsubara M, Athanda SBP, Suzuki Y, Matsubara K, Moriyama A. Comparison of the primary structures, cytotoxicities, and affinities to phospholipids of five kinds of cytotoxins from the venom of Indian cobra. *Naja haje*. Comparative Biochemistry and Physiology Part C. 2016;**179**:158-164

[71] Meanatchisasudaram S, Parameswari G, Michael A. Studies on antivenom activity of *Andrographis paniculata* and *Aristolochia indica* plant extracts against *Daboia russelii* venom by in vivo and in vitro methods. Indian Journal of Science and Technology. 2009;**2**(4):76-79

[72] Hodek P, Trefil P, Simunek J, Hudecek J, Stiborova M. Optimized protocol of chicken antibody (IgY) purification providing electrophoretically homogenous preparations. International Journal of Electrochemical Science. 2013;**8**:113-124

[73] Chacko N, Ibrahim M, Shetty P, Shastry CS. Evaluation of antivenom activity of *Calotropis gigantea* plant extract against *Vipera russelli* snake venom. International Journal of Pharmaceutical Sciences and Research. 2017;**3**(7):2272-2279

[74] Ozkan O, Adiguzel S, Yakistiran S, Filazi A. Study of the relationship between *Androctonus crassicauda* (Oliver, 1807; Scorpiones, Buthidae), venom toxicity and telson size weight and storing condition. Journal of Venomous Animals and Toxins including Tropical Diseases. 2006;**12**(2):297-309

[75] Tripathi S, Maiti TK. Immunomodulatory role of nature and denatured agglutinin from *Abrus precatorius*. The International Journal of Biochemistry & Cell Biology. 2005;**37**: 451-462

[76] Williams DJ, Habib AG, Warrell DA. Clinical studies of the effectiveness and safety of antivenoms. Toxicon. 2018;**150**:1-10

[77] Utkin YN. Animal venom studies: Current benefits and future

development. World Journal of Biological Chemistry. 2015;**6**(2):28-33

[78] Preciado LM, Pereanez JA. Low molecular mass natural and synthetic inhibitors of snake venom metalloproteinases. Toxin Reviews. 2018;**37**(1):19-26

[79] do Vale FLH, Mendes MM, Fernandes RS, Costa TR, Hage-Melim LI, Sousa MA, et al. Protective effect of *Schizolobium parahyba* flavonoids against snake venoms and isolated toxins. Current Topics in Medicinal Chemistry. 2011;**11**: 2566-7577

[80] Rucavado A, Escaknte T, Gulierrez JM. Effect of the metalloproteinase inhibitors batimastat in the systemic toxicity induced by *Bothrops asper* snake venom: Understanding the role of metalloproteinases in envenomation. Toxicon. 2004;**43**:417-424

[81] Bode W, Gomis-Ruth FX, Stockler W. Astacins, serralysins, snake venom and matrix metalloproteinases exhibit identical zinc-binding environment (HEXXHXXGXXH) and met-turn, and topologies and should be grouped into a common family, the 'metzincin'. FEBS Letters. 1993;**331**(1–2):134-140

[82] Patino AC, Pereanez JA, Nunez V, Benjumea DM, Fernandez M, Rucavado A, et al. Isolation and biological characterization of Batx-1, a weak haemorrhagic and fibrinogenolytic PI metalloproteinase from Colombian *Bothrops atrox* venom. Toxicon. 2010;**56**: 936-943

[83] Mazzi MV, Marcussi S, Carlos GB, Stabeli RG, Frano JJ, Ticli FK, et al. A new haemorrhagic metalloprotease from *Bothrops jararacussu* snake venom: Isolation and biochemical characterization. Toxicon. 2004;**44**: 215-223

[84] Patra A, Kalita B, Chanda A, Mukherjee AK. Proteomics and antivenomics of *Echis carinatus* venom: Correlation with pharmacological properties and pathophysiology of envenomation. Scientific Reports. 2017; **7**:1-17

[85] Rucavado A, Henriquez M, Garcia J, Gutierrez JM. Assessment of metalloproteinase inhibitors clodronate and doxycycline in the neutralization of hemorrhage and coagulopathy induced by *Bothrops asper* snake venom. Toxicon. 2008;**52**:754-759

[86] Januario AH, Maraisa S, Santos SL, Mazzi MV. Neoderodane diterpenoid, a new metalloprotease snake venom inhibitor from *Bacharis trimera* (Asteraceae): Anti-proteolytic and anti-haemorrhagic properties. Chemico-Biological Interactions. 2005;**150**(3): 243-251

[87] Mendes MM, Vieira SAPB, Gomes MSR, Paula VF, Alcantara TM, Homsi-Brandeburgo MI, et al. Triacontyl p-coumarate: an inhibitor of snake venom metalloproteinases. Phytochemistry. 2013;**86**:72-82

[88] da Silva JO, Fernandes RS, Ticli FK, Oliveira CZ, Mazzi MV, Franco JJ, et al. Triterpenoid saponins, new metalloproteinase snake venom inhibitors isolated from *Pentaclethra macroloba*. Toxicon. 2007; **50**:283-291

[89] Domingos TFS, Vallim MA, Cavalcanti DN, Sanchez EF, Teixeira VL, Fuly AL, et al. Effect of diterpenes isolated of the marine alga *Canistrocarpus cervicornis* against some toxic effects of the venom of the *Bothrops jararaca* snake. Molecules. 2015;**20**:515-526

[90] Katkar GD, Sharma RD, Vishalakshi GJ, Naveenkumar SK, Madhur G, Thushara RM, et al. Lupeol derivative mitigates *Echis carinatus* venom induced tissue destruction by neutralizing venom toxins and

protecting collagen and angiogenic receptors on inflammatory cells. Biochimica et Biophysica Acta. 2015; **185**(12):2393-2409

[91] Sunitha K, Hemshekhar M, Santhosh MS, Kumar MS, Kemparaju K, Girish KS. Inhibition hemorrhagic activity of viper venoms by N-acetyl and thiol groups. Current Topics in Medicinal Chemistry. 2011;**11**(2): 2589-2600

[92] Ramaswamy M, Solaimuthu C, Duraikannu S. Medicinal plants for the treatment of snakebites among the rural populations of Indian subcontinent; an indication from the traditional use to pharmacological confirmation. Journal of Drug Delivery and Therapeutics. 2018;**8**(5):62-68

[93] Ozkan O, Yagmur EA, Ark M. A newly described scorpion species *Leiurus abdullahbayrami* (Scorpion: Buthidae), and the lethal potency and in vivo effects of its venom. Journal of Venomous Animals and Toxins Including Tropical Diseases. 2011;**17**(4): 414-421

[94] Afifi SH, Elkashef R, Seddek AS, Salem DA. Light and transmission election microscopical changes associated with *Leiurus quinquestriatus* venom in rabbits. Macedonian Veterinary Review. 2010;**39**(1):51-57

[95] Barona J, Otero R, Núñez V. Toxicological and immunological aspects of scorpion venom (*Tityus parachyurus*) neutralizing capacity of antivenom produced in Latin America. Bidondica. 2004;**24**(1):42-49

[96] Ozkan O, Adiguzel S, Kar S, Yakistiran S, Cesaretli KY, Karaer KZ. Determination of potency and paraspecific effects of *Androctonus crassicauda* (Oliver, 807) antivenom against *Mesobuthus gibbosus* (Brulle, 1832) venom (Scorpiones: Buthidae). Journal of Venomous Animals and Toxins Including Tropical Diseases. 2007;**13**(2):500-508

[97] Saadi S, Assarehzadegan MA, Pipelzadeh MH, Hadaddezfuli R. Induction of IL-12 from human monocytes after stimulation with *Androctonus crassicauda* scorpion venom. Toxicon. 2015;**106**:117-121

[98] Caliskan F, García BI, Coronas FI, Batista CV, Zamudio FZ, Possani LD. Characterization of venom components from the scorpion *Androctonus crassicauda* of Turkey. Toxicon. 2006;**48**(1):12-22

[99] Nazari M, Hassan R. Study on distribution of scorpions to provide prevention and interventions in combating scorpionism in Poldokhtar county, Lorestan Province, Iran. Journal of Clinical and Diagnostic Research. 2016;**10**(12):05-09

[100] Carno AO, Chatzaki M, Horta RCC, Mogalhaes BF, Oliveira-Mendes BBR, Chavez-Olortegui C, et al. Alternative methodologies of scorpion antivenomous production. Toxicon. 2015;**97**:64-74

[101] Ismail M, Abdelsalam MA, Ahaidisb MS. *Androctonus crassicauda* (Olivier), a dangerous and unduly neglected scorpion-1. Pharmacological and clinical studies. Toxicon. 1994; **32**(12):1599-1618

[102] Zayerzadeh E, Kooh MK, Mirakabadi AZ, Fardipoor A, Kassaian SE, Rabbani S, et al. Amelioration of cardio-respiratory perturbations following *Mesobuthus eupeus* envenomation in anaesthetized rabbits with commercial polyvalent $F(ab')_2$ antivenom. Toxicon. 2012;**59**(2):249-256

[103] Saganuwan SA. Determination of median effective dose fifty (ED_{50}) of scorpion antivenom against scorpion envenomation using a newly developed formula. Animal Models and Experimental Medicine. 2018;**1**:1-7

[104] Shirmardi SP, Shamsaei M, Gandomkar M, Sarie E, Ghannadi M, Zare A. Comparison of two purified toxic fractions from *Mesobuthus eupeus* scorpion. Journal of Venomous Animals and Toxins Including Tropical Diseases. 2010;**16**(4):639-646

[105] Mozhaeva GN, Naumov AP. Knietics of interaction of scorpion with sodium channels on the Ranvier node membrane. Neurophysiology. 1980; **12**(6):619-626

[106] Delari P, van Rietschoten J, Rochat H. Scorpion venoms and neurotoxins: An immunological study. Toxicon. 1981;**19**(3):393-407

[107] Ozkan O, Carhan A. The neutralization capacity of *Androctonus crassicauda* antivenom against *Mesobuthus eupeus* scorpion venom. Toxicon. 2008;**52**(2):375-379

[108] Khoobdel M, Zahraei-Salehi T, Nayeri-Fasaei B, Khosravi M, Omidian Z, Motedayen MH, et al. Purification of the immunogenic fractions and determination of toxicity in *Mesobuthus eupeus* (Scorpionida: Buthidae) venom. Journal of Arthropod-Borne Diseases. 2013;**7**(2):139-146

[109] Alvarenga LM, Dining CR, Grainer C, Chávez-Olórtegui C. Induction of neutralizing antibodies against *Tityus serrulatus* scorpion toxins by immunization with a mixture of defined synthetic epitopes. Toxicon. 2002;**40**(1):89-95

[110] Santo KS, Stephano MA, Marcelona JR, Ferreira VMR, Rocha T, Carricati C, et al. Production of the first effective hyperimmune equine serum antivenom against Africanized bees. PLoS One. 2013;**8**(11):e79971

[111] Salama MW, Sharshar KM. Surveillance study on scorpion species in Egypt and comparison of their crude venom protein files. Journal of Basic and Applied Zoology. 2013;**66**(2): 76-86

[112] Wyshynski PE, Little JA. Scorpionism: The first case reported in Canada. Canadian Medical Association Journal. 1962;**87**:974-975

[113] Kamalak Z, Kosus N. Scorpion sting during pregnancy: a case report accompanied by literature. Cumhuriyet Medical Journal. 2013;**35**:605-607

[114] Wang X, Gao B, Zhu S. A single-point mutation enhances dual functionality of scorpion toxin. Comparative Biochemistry and Physiology - Part C. 2016;**179**:72-78

[115] Hmila L, Saerens D, Abderrazek RB, Vincke C, Abidi N, Benlasfar Z, et al. A bispecific nanobody to provide full protection against lethal scorpion envenoming. FASEB Journal. 2010

[116] Abimannane A, Rameshkumar R, Satheesh P, Mahadevan S. Second dose of scorpion antivenom in children with Indian red scorpion (*Mesobuthus tamulus*) sting envenomation. Indian Pediatrics. 2018;**55**:315-318

[117] Casella-Martins A, Ayres LA, Burin SM, Morais FR, Pereira JC, Faccioli LH, et al. Immunomodulatory activity of *Tityus serrulatus* scorpion venom in human T lymphocytes. Journal of Venomous Animals and Toxins including Tropical Diseases. 2015;**21**:1-8

[118] Jager H, Grissmer S. Characterization of the outer pore region of the apamin-sensitive Ca^{2+}-activated K^+ channel rsk2. Toxicon. 2004;**43**(8):951-960

[119] Olamendi-Portugal T, Somodi S, Fernandez JA, Zamudio FZ, Bererril B, Varga Z, et al. Novel alpha-KTx peptides from the venom of the scorpion *Centruroides elegans* selectively blockade Kv1.3 over IKCa1 K^+ channels of T cells. Toxicon. 2005;**46**(4):418-429

[120] Papp F, Batista CV, Varga Z, Herceg M, Roman-Gonzalez SA, Gasper R, et al. Tst26, a novel peptide blocker of Kv1.2 and kv1.3 channels from the venom of *Tityus stigmurus*. Toxicon. 2009;**54**(4):379-389

[121] Pimento AM, Stocklin R, Favreau P, Bouqis PE, Martina Eauclaire MF. Moving pieces in a proteomic puzzle: mass finger printing of toxic fractions from the venom of *Tityus serrulatus* (Scorpiones, Buthidae). Rapid Communications in Mass Spectrometry. 2001;**15**(17):1562-1572

[122] Okkache N, Rosso JP, Alami M, Ghalim N, Saile R, Hasar M, et al. New analysis of the toxic compounds from the *Androctonus mauretanicus* mauretanicus scorpion venom. Toxicon. 2008;**51**(5):835-852

[123] Okkache N, Ahmad RMR, Othman I, Ghalim N, Chgoury F, Boussadda L, et al. Comparison of the neurotoxic and myotoxic effects of two Moroccan scorpion venoms and their neutralization by experimental polyclonal antivenom. Life Sciences. 2015;**124**:1-7

[124] Tiwari AK, Desphande SB. Toxicity of scorpion (*Buthus tamulus*) venom in mammals is influenced by the age and species. Toxicon. 1993;**31**(12):1619-1622

[125] Nunan EA, Arya V, Hocchaus G, Cardigo VN, Moraes-Santos T. Age effects on the pharmacokinetics of tityustoxin from *Tityus serrulatus* scorpion venom in rats. Brazilian Journal of Medical and Biological Research. 2004;**37**:385-390

[126] Das-Lopes C, Paiva AL, Querra-Duarte C, Molina F, Felicori L. Venomous arachnid diagnosis assays, lessons from past attempts. Toxin. 2013; **10**(365):1-26

[127] Laustsen AH, Solà M, Jappe EC, Oscoz S, Lauridsen LP, Engmark M. Biotechnological trends in spider and scorpion antivenom development. Toxins (Basel). 2016;**8**(8):1-33

[128] Krifi MN, Savin S, Debray M, Bon C, El Ayeb M, Choumet V. Pharmacokinetic studies of scorpion venom before and after antivenom immunotherapy. Toxicon. 2005;**45**(2): 187-198

[129] Nafie MS, Daim MMA, Ali IAI, Abdel-Rahman MA, Nabil ZI. Proteomic and biochemical characterization of the Egyptian scorpion "*Androctonus australis*" venom. In: Abstract of 6th International Conference on Natural Toxins; December 2014; Ismailia. 2014. pp. 1-2

[130] Clot-Faybesse O, Juin M, Rochat H, Devaux C. Monoclonal antibodies against the *Androctonus australis* hector scorpion neurotoxin 1: Characterization and use for venom neutralisation. FEBS Letters. 1999;**458**(3):313-318

[131] Bougis PE, Rochart H, Smith LA. Precursors of *Androctonus australis* scorpion neurotoxins. Structures of precursors, processing outcomes, and expression of a functional recombinant toxin II. The Journal of Biological Chemistry. 1989;**264**(32):19259-19265

[132] Adi-Bessalem S, Hammoudi-Triki D, Laraba-Djebari F. Pathophysiological effects of *Androctonus australis* hector scorpion venom: Tissue damages and inflammatory response. Experimental and Toxicologic Pathology. 2008;**60**(4–5):373-380

[133] Fatani AJ, Furman BL, Zeitlin IJ. The involvement of plasma kinins in the cardiovascular effects of *Leiurus quinquestriatus* scorpion venom in anaesthetized rabbits. Toxicon. 1998; **36**(3):523-536

[134] Saganuwan SA, Onyeyili PA. The paradox of human equivalent dose formula: A canonical case study of *Abrus*

precatorius aqueous leaf extract in monogastric animals. Macedonian Veterinary Review. 2016;**39**(1):23-32

[135] Malina T, Krecsák L, Westerström A, Szeman-Nagy G, Gyemant G, Hamvas MM, et al. Individual variability of venom from the European adder (*Vipera berus* berus) from one locality in Eastern Hungary. Toxicon. 2017;**135**:59-70

[136] Tan CH, Wong KY, Tan KY, Tan NH. Venom proteome of the yellow-lipped sea krait, *Laticauda colubrina* from Bali: insights into subvenomic diversity venom antigenicity and cross-neutralization by antivenom. Journal of Proteomics. 2017; **166**:48-58

[137] Amf O, Tan CH, Ariaranee GC, Quraishi N, Tan NH. Venomics of *Bungarus caeruleus* (Indian krait): comparable venom profiles, variable immune re-activities among specimens from Sri Lanka, India and Pakistan. Journal of Proteomics. 2017;**164**:1-18

[138] Tan NH, Wong KY, Tan CH. Venomics of *Naja sputatrix*, the Javan-spitting cobra: a short neurotoxin-driven venom needing improved antivenom neutralization. Journal of Proteomics. 2017;**157**:18-32

[139] Shaikh IK, Dixit PP, Pawade BS, Waykar IG. Development of dot-ELISA for the detection of venoms of major Indian venomous snakes. Toxicon. 2017; **139**:66-73

[140] Choudhury M, McCleary RJR, Kesherwani M, Kini RM, Velmurugan D. Comparison of proteomic profiles of two of the big four snakes of India, the Indian cobra (*Naja naja*) and the common krait (*Bungarus caeruleus*) and analyses of their toxins. Toxicon. 2017;**135**:33-42

[141] Nalbantsoy A, Hempel BF, Petras D, Heiss P, Gocmen B, Igci N, et al. Combined venom profiling and cytotoxicity screening of the Radde's mountain viper (*Montivipera raddei*) and Mount Bulgar viper (*Montivipera bulgardaghica*) with potent cytotoxicity against human A549 lung carcinoma cells. Toxicon. 2017;**135**:71-83

[142] Batista CV, Román-González SA, Salas-Castillo SP, Zamudio FZ, Gómez-Lagunas F, Possani LD. Proteomic analysis of the venom from the scorpion *Tityus stigmurus*: biochemical and physiological comparison with other *Tityus* species. Comparative Biochemistry and Physiology, Part C: Toxicology & Pharmacology. 2007;**146** (1–2):147-157

[143] Chippaux JP. Epidemiological investigation on envenomation: From theory to practice. Journal of Venomous Animals and Toxins Including Tropical Diseases. 2012;**18**(4):446-450

[144] Saganuwan SA. Calculation of effective dose fifty (ED_{50}) of antivenom for American pit viper envenomation. Comparative Clinical Pathology. 2018a; **27**:1321-1325

Chapter 6

Toxicosis of Snake, Scorpion, Honeybee, Spider, and Wasp Venoms: Part 2

Saganuwan Alhaji Saganuwan

Abstract

Toxicosis is a poisoning caused by venomous animals such as snake, scorpion, honeybee, spider and wasp. Their poisons contain amino acids, peptides, proteins, enzymes and metallic ions that are responsible for neurotoxicity, hemotoxicity and myotoxicity. Because of in vivo therapeutic challenges posed by toxicosis, there is need for ideal therapeutic agents against envenomation caused by venomous animals. Findings have shown that toxicosis could be treated symptomatically. Snake and scorpion antivenins could be used for treatment of poisoning caused by snake, scorpion, honeybee, spider and wasp. The amount of antivenin is dependent on the quantity of venom injected into the affected individuals. Moreso, sympotomatic treatments are also done according to the systems affected. Hospitalization is necessary for assessment of therapeutic success.

Keywords: toxicosis, snake, scorpion, toxin, antivenin, lethality, hemotoxicity, neurotoxicity, myotoxicity, hospitalization

1. Introduction

Venomous animals such as snake, scorpion, honeybee, spider and wasp constitute very significant health hazard in the world. The snake venom contains many toxic and non-toxic molecules [1]. Fourty-seven out of 50 US States have venomous snakes. Southwestern US are mostly affected. About 4700 venomous snakes bite human and 150,000 primarily dogs and cats are bitten by venomous snakes every year in the US, with human mortality of 0.06% and that of dog is 1–30% [2]. Scorpionism is caused by many poisonous scorpions including Tityus species endemic to Panama whereas latruroides are endemic to Guatemala, Belize, El Salvador, Nicaragua, and Costa Rica. They are wildly toxic via unchannel active toxins. In Panama the incidence was 52 cases per 100, 000 in 2007 and 28 deaths were recorded between 1998 and 2006 respectively. Tityus species present in the Atlantic coast of Costa Rica is responsible for fatalities in Panama. *Tityus pachyurus* [3] and *Parabutus granulatus* are of the most medical importance in the Western Cape of South Africa. *P. transvaalicus* venom is used for production of *P granulatus* venom [4]. About 200, 000 cases of scorpionism are reported in Mexico and cause 310 deaths every year and 20, 000 out of 38, 068 affected persons were successfully treated using equine antiserum (serotherapy) and no life was lost [5]. The first case of scorpionism was reported in Canada in a 36 year old man in 1962. The rate of scorpionism in Amazon region of Brazil is 8.14–273 cases per 100,000. Most species involved in envenomation belong to the genus of Tityus [6]. *M. gibbosus* is endemic to a small geographic area of Erbalj on terra rossa soil [7]. The incidence of scorpion sting in Iran was 61.2 per 100,000 populations [8], as against 1.2 million people with estimated 3250 death per year. The mean annual rate was 17.4 per woman population [9]. The highest rate of sting occurred in Iran among individuals of 25–34-year-old [8]. The global mortality rate was 10 per 1000 cases. Most of the stings were seen on lower limbs (58.6%) and upper limbs (34.3%) during the hot season [10]. The scorpion that had envenomated for the first time may have less toxic envenomation for the second time as reported in the case of sting from *Leiurus abdullahbayrami* [11]. In India envenomation was more common in males than in females [12].

Honeybee (*Apis mellifera*) constitutes a significant nuisance and of medical importance in Africa, Europe and other parts of the world. Other subspecies are *A. mellifera carnica*, *A. mellifera ligustica* and *A. mellifera scutellata* [13]. Honeybee stings reported in Ceare, Brazil showed 1307 cases affecting men between 20 and 29 years of age [14] translating to 19 cases per 100,000 in Campina Grade [15]. Bee envenomation is a problem in India, China, Latin America, Middle East, North and South Africa [16]. About 200 stings from *Apis mellifera* could cause envenoming syndrome in children and elderly [17] as multiple stings, not increased venom potency or delivery cause serious reactions [18]. Bee venoms differ in weight, concentrations of phospholipase and melittin [19]. Unfortunately, no specific anti-venom for bee envenomation, hence proper removal of stings, first aid treatment and chemotherapy should be considered as medical emergency [20]. Administration of hydrocortisone, calcium, analgesic, 0.9% sodium chloride and application of ice to the site of stung pregnant woman resulted in recovery from the pain and the fetus was stable and delivered 3 months after treatment without sequela [21]. There are 42,473 species of spiders grouped into 110 families (Platnick,) [22]. *Hadronyche formidabilis* and *H. cerberea* have very high envenoming rates [23]. Black widow spider (*Latrodectus mactans*), brown recluse spider (*Loxosceles reclusa*) are of most concern [24]. In view of the increased challenges and negligence of envenomotion caused by venomous snake, scorpion, spider, wasp and bee, there is need for thorough search for their therapeutic regimens with a view to having lasting solution against fatality.

2. Methodology

Literatures were searched on venomous snakes, scorpions, honeybees, spiders and wasps with an intent to identifying their toxicity potentials, epidemiology of their toxicosis, signs of toxicity, treatment and development of vaccines against their venoms. Sought also are information on medicinal plants, phytochemicals and other therapeutic agents, structures of some chemicals present in the venoms, their medical applications and medicinal uses. Mathematical formulas were also derived for calculation of body weight, body surface area, packed cell volume, hemoglobin, total blood volume, lost blood volume, median lethal dose (LD_{50}),median effective dose (ED_{50}), number of bee stings, total dose of bee venom and relationship between renotoxicity and haemotoxicity.

3. Results

Findings have shown that venoms from poisonous species of snakes, scorpions, honeybees, spiders and wasps are highly toxic and could cause various degrees of hemotoxicity, myotoxicity, and neurotoxicity including death (**Tables 1** and **2**).

Animal	Weight (kg)	Number of stings	Dose of stings (mg)	LD_{50} (mg/kg)	ED_{50} (mg/kg)	Lethal time (hr)
Child	10	94	28.2	1.41	11.2	2.10
Adult	60	1000	300	2.5	7.5	3.72

Table 1.
Calculated median lethal dose and effective dose fifty of honeybee venom and antivenom in human.

System	Age (yr)	Sting(s)	Sex	Signs	Treatment
Nervous	6,70 70	Each 1	Female Male	Axonal polyneuropathy, seizure brachial plexitis, Parkinsonism	Immunoglobulin I.V., anti-inflammatory, Oxygen
Muscular	34	3	Male	Rhadbomyolysis, muscle pain, allergy	Analgesic, anti-inflammatory
Circulatory	35–42	Many	Male	Myocardial infarction, ischemic attack, cardiac arrest, anaphylaxis, kounis syndrome	Angioplasty, steroids, antihistaminics
Renal	2	1	Male	Nephrotic syndrome, anasarca, acute renal failure	Corticosteriod
Ocular	21–50	1	Male Female	Cataract, glaucoma	Surgery, keratoplasty, antibiotics, corticosteroid
Miscellaneous	40	Multiple	Male	Intravascular coagulopathy, coma	Hydrocortisone, analgesic, pheniramine

Table 2.
Toxicity signs of honeybee sting in human.

4. Discussion

4.1 Treatment of scorpion envenomation requires body weight

Recently Abimannane *et al reported* that treatment of children showing autonomic symptoms from Indian red scorpion envenomation that could lead to myocardial infarction required second dose of 30 mg (3 ml) [25]. However, reference was not made to the weight of the children. Hence, the scorpion antiserum against Indian red scorpion (*Mesobuthus tamulus*) was reassessed using a child that weighed 20 kg body weight. Findings have shown that 12 mg (1.2 ml) should be given to the affected child (20 kg). Therefore, administration of the scorpion antivenin should be dose dependent to avoid death and hypersensitivity reaction that could be caused by *M. tamulus* venom and antivenin. The newly derived formula by Saganuwan is very relevant in the present context. Venom-antivenin neutralization factor of 1:2 to 1:25 could be tried. Fatal scorpionism is caused by members of Buthidae and Mesobuthus species is highly poisonous in human. The LD_{50} and ED_{50} of venom and antivenin of Mesobuthus species in mice are 0.18 mg/kg and 2.82 mg/kg respectively. High doses of venom and antivenin cause death and hypersensitivity reactions [26]. Therefore, there is need to reassess treatment of *Mesobuthus tamulus* envenomation in children. The formula developed by Saganuwan [26] was used to determine the LD50 and ED_1 of *Mesobuthus tamulus* venin and antivenin in a 20 kg weighed child.

$LD_{50} = ED_{50}^{1/3} X\ W_h x10^{-4.}$
LD_{50} = $ED_{50}{}^{1/3}$ X Wh x 10^{-4} (Wh = Weight of human).
LD_{50} = $30^{1/3}$ x 20,000x 10^{-4} (Ikg = 1000 g).
LD_{50} = $30^{1/3}$ x 20x 10^{4}x 10^{-4}.

$= 30^{1/3}$ x 2.
= 3.11 x 2 = 6.22 mg/20 kg.
30 mg → 50 children.
X → 1child

$$x = \frac{30x1}{50} = \frac{3}{5} = 0.6\, mg/kg$$

:. 20 x 0.6 = 12 mg should be given instead of 30 mg.

The calculated LD_{50} (6.22 mg) per 20 kg weighed child translating to 0.31 mg/kg shows that *M. tamulus* venom is very toxic. Moreso the calculated effective dose (0.6 mg/kg) of *M. tamulus* antivenin shows that neutralization dose of the antivenin should be twice the dose of venom. The obtained 12 mg (1.2 ml) of the scorpion antivenin disagrees with the report of Abimannane *et al* [25] indicating that the initial dose of the antivenin should be 30 mg (3 ml) followed by 60 mg (6 ml) of the second dose. The second dose should be 24 mg (2.4 ml). Amelioration of cardio-respiratory perturbations caused by *M. eupeus* envenomation in mice using polyvalent F $(ab^1)_2$ antivenin proves that neutralization factor is 1:2 to 1:25 in mice [26]. Cardio-respiratory activity modifying agents including prazosin could be administered [27]. *Buthus quinqestriatus* venom was neutralized by an effective serum obtained from horses immunized with crude venom [28, 29]. High amount of antivenin is required for satisfactory neutralization. *Mesobuthus gibbosus* venom could be neutralized by *Androctonus crassicauda* antivenin [30]. Scorpionism affects severely children of up to 24.3 kg body weight [31]. *Mesobuthus* venom could be neutralized by non-toxicant antivenins which could be used as vaccines against scorpion envenomation [32]. The efficacy of the treatment depends on species of scorpion, dose, potency and route of administration of antivenin [33].

4.2 The role of exponent and lethality time in determination of death caused by toxins in animal models of experiment

Drugs, chemicals, plant extracts and venoms from snake, scorpion and honeybee could cause death when introduced in large quantities and the toxicity signs affect all the organ systems and, in many occasions, culminating in death. The use of large number of animals for determination of median lethal dose (LD_{50}) has been discouraged worldwide. Therefore based on the principle of R3 (Reduction, Refinement and Replacement), the number of animals for LD_{50} determination has been reduced to 2–6 and yielded good results in monogastric animals. The traditional method that involves the use of 40 animals was applied in the production of vaccine made from silicate against *Crotalus atrox*, *Agkistrodon contortrix contortrix* and *Agkistrodon piscivorus leucostoma*. The LD_{50} software was generated on the NNTRC home page (ntrc.tamuk.edu/LD50calculator.xls) based on the Saganuwan's method [34] unfortunately it is not accessible. Hence I am appealing to NNTRC to make it available for scientific use. Newly devised LD_{50} formulas were used to determine LD_{50} and ED_{50} for snake, scorpion and honeybee venoms and antivenoms respectively using 6 mice each. The modified LD_{50} formulas used comprised effective dose fifty (ED_{50}) divided by the denominator (3) for snake and raised to exponent (0.33) for scorpion and honeybee showing that the relationship between snake venom and scorpion or honeybee venom is the difference between the denominator (3) and exponent (0.33). Hence snake venom is more toxic than the scorpion and honeybee venoms. The toxicity effect of scorpion is much higher than that of honeybee whose toxicity depends on the number of stings; hence death may be delayed giving rise to lethality time that has exponent (0.33). Median lethal time (LT_{50}) is LD_{50} over D^P whereas D (dose) and P (exponent) are integral parts of the formula [26, 34, 35].

4.3 Hematological and renal parameters of animals envenomated by snakes

Hemotoxic and renotoxic effects of ophidiotoxicity have made quick treatment of snake envenomation difficult [36]. However, Saganuwan and Onyeyili reported that total volume of animal blood was 8% of its weight [36]. Saganuwan also reported relationship between ED_{50}, LD_{50} and body weight as a function of effective snake antivenom therapy as proven by neutralization of American pit viper envenomation [35]. Relationship between age, body weight, serum creatinine, plasma creatinine, ED_{50}, LD_{50} and safety factor has been established [37]. Hence, the formulas have been integrated for calculation of hemotoxic and renotoxic parameters of snake envenomation.

4.4 Relationship between renotoxicity and hemotoxicity of toxins

The formula established for calculation of ED_{50} and LD_{50} with safety factor in animals is:

$$\mathrm{LD}_{50} = \frac{ED_{50}}{3} \; x \; W_a \; x \; 10^{-4} \tag{1}$$

$$0.08(W_a) = \mathrm{TBV} \tag{2}$$

$$\mathrm{W_a} = \frac{TBV}{0.08} \tag{3}$$

Substitute for W_a in equation (1)

$$\therefore \mathrm{LD}_{50} = \frac{ED_{50}}{3} \; x \; \frac{TBV}{0.08} \; x \; 10^{-4} \tag{4}$$

$$\text{But TBV} = \mathrm{PV} + \mathrm{EV} \tag{5}$$

Substitute for TBV in equation (4)

$$\therefore \mathrm{LD}_{50} = \frac{ED_{50}}{3} \; x \; \frac{PV + EV}{0.08} \; x \; 10^{-4} \tag{6}$$

$$\mathrm{LD}_{50} = \frac{ED_{50}}{3} \; x \; (PV + EV) \; x \; 8 \; x \; 10^{-2} \tag{7}$$

$$\text{But Hb} = 0.33\;(\mathrm{EV}) \tag{8}$$

$$\therefore \mathrm{EV} = \frac{Hb}{0.33} \tag{9}$$

Substitute for EV in equation (7)

$$\therefore \mathrm{LD}_{50} = \frac{ED_{50}}{3} \; x \left(PV + \frac{Hb}{0.33}\right) x \; 8 \; x \; 10^{-2} \tag{10}$$

$$\text{However, CrCl} = \frac{K \; x \; (140 - age) x \; W_a}{D \; x \; Scr \; x \; 72} \tag{11}$$

$$\mathrm{W_a} = \frac{CrCl \; x \; D \; x \; Scr \; x \; 72}{K \; x \; (140 - age)} \tag{12}$$

Substitute for W_a in equation (1)

$$\therefore \mathrm{LD}_{50} = \frac{ED_{50}}{3} \; x \; \frac{CrCl \; x \; D \; x \; Scr \; x \; 72}{K \; x \; (140 - age)} \; x \; 10^{-4} \tag{13}$$

Equate equation (3) and (12)

$$\frac{TBV}{0.08} = \frac{CrCl\ x\ D\ x\ Scr\ x\ 72}{K\ x\ (140 - age)} \tag{14}$$

$$\text{TBV}(\text{K x }(140\text{–age}) = 0.08(CrCl\ x\ D\ x\ Scr\ x\ 72) \tag{15}$$

$$\text{TBV} = \frac{0.08(CrCl\ x\ D\ x\ Scr\ x\ 72)}{K\ x\ (140 - age)} \tag{16}$$

$$\text{But D} = \frac{Pcr}{Scr}\ x\ 144 \tag{17}$$

Substitute for D in equation (14)

$$\text{TBV} = \frac{0.08\left(CrCl\ x\ \left(\frac{Pcr}{Scr}\ x\ 144\right)\ x\ Scr\ x\ 72\right)}{K\ x\ (140 - age)} \tag{18}$$

Equate equation (10) with equation (13)

$$\text{LD}_{50} = \frac{ED_{50}}{3}\ \text{x}\ \left(PV + \frac{Hb}{0.33}\right)\ x\ 8\ x\ 10^{-2} = \frac{ED_{50}}{3}\ x\ \frac{CrCl\ x\ D\ x\ Scr\ x\ 72}{K\ x\ (140 - age)}\ x\ 10^{-4} \tag{19}$$

$$\left(PV + \frac{Hb}{0.33}\right)\ x\ 8\ x\ 10^{-2} = \frac{CrCl\ x\ D\ x\ Scr\ x\ 72}{K\ x\ (140 - age)}\ x\ 10^{-4} \tag{20}$$

$$\left(PV + \frac{Hb}{0.33}\right) = \frac{CrCl\ x\ D\ x\ Scr\ x\ 72}{K\ x\ (140 - age)}\ x\ 12.5 \tag{21}$$

$$\text{PV} = \left(\frac{CrCl\ x\ D\ x\ Scr\ x\ 72}{K\ x\ (140 - age)}\right)\ x\ 12.5 - \left(\frac{Hb}{0.33}\right) \tag{22}$$

$$\left(\frac{Hb}{0.33}\right) = PV - \left(\frac{CrCl\ x\ D\ x\ Scr\ x\ 72}{K\ x\ (140 - age)}\right)\ x\ 12.5 \tag{23}$$

$$\text{Hb} = PV - \left(\frac{CrCl\ x\ D\ x\ Scr\ x\ 72}{K\ x\ (140 - age)}\right)\ x\ 12.5\ x\ \frac{1}{0.33} \tag{24}$$

$$\text{Amount of Required Donor Blood} = \text{Required Recipient Wt(kg)} \times 80\text{ml/kg} \times \frac{Desired\ PCV - Recipient\ PCV}{Donor\ PCV} \tag{25}$$

TBV = Total blood volume; PV = Plasma volume; EV = Erythrocyte volume; Hb = Hemoglobin; CrCl = Creatinine clearance; D = Depuration; K = Constant (male = 1.0, female = 0.85); Scr = Serum creatinine; Pcr = Plasma creatinine; PCV = Packed cell volume.

4.5 Apitoxicosis

Honeybee is a social insect that feeds on nectar of plant and serves as source of beneficial and harmful effects (**Table 2**) which include Parkinsonism, allergy, brachial plexitis, intravascular coagulopathy, rhabdomyolysis, acute renal failure, nephrotic syndrome, anaphylaxis, fatality, acute ischemic stroke, corneal decomposition, cataract, glaucoma, seizure, ischemic attack, heart attack and acute axonal polyneuropathy [38–50]. *Apis mellifera* constitutes a significant problem of medical importance. Other important medical subspecies are *A. mellifera carnica, A. mellifera ligustica and A. mellifera scutellata* [13]. In India, honeybee sting affects human beings of all ages. But cases of honeybee stings affect human between 20 and 29 years of age in Brazil [14]. However, bee envenomation is a problem in India, China, Latin America, Middle East, North and South Africa [51] and should be listed by WHO as neglected tropical disease. The venom contains alkaloids, terpenes, histamine, formic acid [52], apamin and melittin that meditate their actions via ion channels and intracellular calcium of heart cells [53] causing myocardial infarction and cardiac arrest. The venom also contains heptanone, a local anesthetic [54], which causes nausea, vomiting, diarrhea, headache, vertigo, CNS depression, incoordination, cardiorespiratory failure and hypotension [55–58]. However, *A. mellifera* venom also contains phospholipase A_2, hyaluronidase, adrenaline and serotonin, therefore causing allergic reaction, edema, skin inflammation, headache, weakness and dizziness [59] which is treated using serum [60]. But apamine, secapine, pamine, minimine, adolapine, procamine A&B, protease inhibitor, tertiapine, cardiopep, phosphatase, α-glucosidase, phospholipase B, dopamine, noradrenaline, aminobutyric acid, α-amino acids, and complex esthers produced by honeybees are used in treating a myriad of diseases [61]. Postmortem findings caused by honeybee envenomation are edema of brain, larynx, trachea as well as congestion of all other internal organs. The cause of death may be due to anaphylactic reaction [62]. The honeybee envenomation could also lead to focal neurological deficit 5 hrs post multiple stings causing acute ischemic stroke [63] and acute renal failure [64]. Immunotherapy when instituted on time is quite helpful. It involves secretion of cytokines and stimulation of T cells which indicate immune response. There is a switch from the abnormal Th_2 cytokine response to a Th_1 response by down regulation of Th_2 response or immune deviation in favor of Th_1 response, thereby producing interleukins 3–5 leading to IgE synthesis activating eosinophils and mast cells. The overall effects are venom neutralization or immunization [39].

4.6 Calculation of lethal dose of honeybee antivenom

Development of a new formula for calculation of LD_{50} of honeybee venom and antivenom is as follow:

i. If one (1) sting produced one (1) dose of venom,

ii. 1000 stings would produce 1000 x dose per sting

Therefore; NS = No of stings.

DS = Dose per sting

iii. Total Dose (TD) = NS x DS = Toxic dose

If the toxic dose (TD) can kill one hundred mice, how much can kill 50 mice?

Hence TD $\longrightarrow$ 100 mice.

$LD_{50} \longrightarrow$ 50 mice

iv. $TD = \frac{LD_{50}\ x\ 100}{50}$

$TD = 2LD_{50} = 2MLD$.

TD = Dose that kills all the mice and may not be specific because of the factors (age, sex, potency of toxin etc.) that determine toxicity level of a toxin.

v. Also TD = NS x DS = 2 x MLD

vi. Therefore, MLD = $\frac{NS \ x \ DS}{2} = LD_{50}$

Bee venom may be as poisonous as scorpion venom. Therefore, the LD_{50} formula for scorpion envenomation is applied.

vii. LD_{50} = $ED_{50}^{1/3} \ x \ Wa \ x \ 10^{-4}$ (formula for calculation of scorpion venom) [56].

Equate vi and vii.

$LD_{50} = \frac{NS \ x \ DS}{2} = \frac{ED_{50}^{1/3} x \ Wa \ x \ 10^{-4}}{1.}$

$2(ED_{50}{}^{1/3} \text{ x Wa x } 10^{-4}) = \text{NS x DS}$

viii. $NS = \frac{2\left(ED_{50}^{1/3} \ x \ Wa \ x \ 10^{-4}\right)}{DS}$

ix. $DS = \frac{2\left(ED_{50}^{1/3} \ x \ Wa \ x \ 10^{-4}\right)}{NS}$

x. Lethal time 50 (LT_{50}) = $\frac{LD_{50}}{D^{p}}$ whereas D = dose of toxin; p = power law exponent ($^{1}/_{3}$).

xi. Potency of antivenom (PA) = Total venom used – $1EC_{50}/EC_{50}$

$1EC_{50}$ = One effective concentration fifty; EC_{50} = Effective concentration fifty.

xii. Honeybee can only sting once and dies because its sting and the venom apparatus are avulsed from its abdomen, unlike bumble bee that can sting several times as its sting is not barbed.

4.7 Application of the formula

Q1.An adult man who weighed 60 kg received 1000 stings from honey bees at the rate of 0.3 mg per sting.

i. Calculate LD_{50} and ED_{50} of the honeybees venom and the likely antivenom that should have been used prior to the man's death.

Q2. A child weighed 10 kg and received 94 stings, but eventually died before antivenom therapy.

i. Calculate the dose of venom received by the child on the condition of 0.3 mg per sting

ii. Calculate LD_{50} and ED_{50} of the venom and antivenom, respectively.

Solution 1;

Total dose (TD) of venom = Number of stings x Dose per sting

TD = 1000 x 0.3 mg = 300 mg

TD = $2LD_{50}$

$LD_{50} = \frac{TD}{2} = \frac{300}{2} = 150mg/60kg$

But if 150 mg $\longrightarrow$ 60 kg

Xmg $\longrightarrow$ 1 kg

$X = \frac{150 \ x \ 1}{60} = 2.5mg/kg = LD_{50}$

But $LD_{50} = ED_{50}^{1/3} \times Wa \times 10^{-4}$

$$2.5 = ED_{50}^{1/3} \times 60 \times 10^{-4}$$

$$ED_{50}^{1/3} = \frac{2.5}{60 \times 10^{-4}} = \frac{2.5 \times 10^{4}}{60}$$

$$= \frac{2.5 \times 10^{3}}{6} = \frac{2500}{6} = 416.66$$

$$ED_{50} = \sqrt[3]{416.66} = 7.5 mg/kg$$

$$ED_{50} = 7.5 \text{ mg/kg}$$

Solution 2:

$$TD = NS \times DS$$

$$TD = 94 \times 0.3 = 28.2 \text{ mg}$$

$$TD = 2LD_{50}$$

$$28.2 = 2LD_{50}$$

$$LD_{50} = \frac{28.2}{2} = \frac{14.1mg}{10kg}$$

$$LD_{50} = 1.41 \text{ mg/kg}$$

But $LD_{50} = ED_{50}^{1/3} \times Wa \times 10^{-4}$

$$1.41 = ED_{50}^{1/3} \times 10 \times 10^{-4}$$

$$ED_{50}^{1/3} = \frac{1.41}{10 \times 10^{-4}} = \frac{1.41}{10^{-3}} = \frac{1.41 \times 10^{3}}{1}$$

$$ED_{50}^{1/3} = 1410$$

$$ED_{50} = \sqrt[3]{1410} = 11.2mg/kg$$

Calculation of lethal time

Adult

$$\text{Lethal time } (LT_{50}) = \frac{LD_{50}}{D^{P}}$$

$$= \frac{2.5}{0.3^{1/3}} = 3.72 \text{ hr.}$$

Child

$$\text{Lethal time } (LT_{50}) = \frac{LD_{50}}{D^{P}}$$

$$= \frac{1.41}{0.3^{1/3}} = 2.10 \text{ hr.}$$

The weight of child and adult human, the number of honeybee stings, total dose of venom from stings, LD_{50}, LT_{50} and ED_{50} of honeybee venom and antivenom are presented in **Table 1**.

4.8 Toxic principles of honeybees

Honeybee venom contains phosphohpase A_2, melittins and antigen is found in swasp venom. The two venoms contain hyaluronidase making patients allergic to wasp venom and rarely allergic to bee venom [39]. However, 2 heptanone secreted from mandibular glands of honeybee could serve as pheromone and local anesthetic [54]. Some toxins such as saxitoxin, piratoxin-1, batrachotoxin and grayanotoxin, are specific fast sodium (Na^{+}) channel blockers. Whereas charybdotoxin, apamin, dendrotoxin and gaboon viper venom are specific for different types of potassium (K^{+}) channels. Some toxins activate L-type calcium (Ca^{2+}) and Na^{+} channels in heart muscle, w-conotoxin blocks the L-type and N-type Ca^{2+} channels in neurons and maitotoxin activates voltage-independent Ca^{2+} channel in heart cells [53].

4.9 Signs of apitoxicosis

Signs of honeybee envenomation include intense local pain, erythema, 1 cm diameter of edema, local and generalized allergic reactions [39], pruritus, urticaria, facial or generalized angioedema, sense of impending doom, dyspnea due to laryngeal edema, or asthma, hypotension, light-headedness, giddiness, fainting, abdominal pain, incontinence, chest pain, visual disturbance and loss of consciousness which may happen within 10 minutes of sting [39]. Honeybee venom is highly vasoactive, inflammatory and thrombogenic. Multiple stings could cause multiple organ dysfunctions called Kounis syndrome. The treatment is by steroid, antihistaminic and angioplasty to left anterior descending artery [49]. Occasional death is due to anaphylactoid shock [62]. Generally, the venom of wringed hymenoptera include acetylcholine, dopamine, histamine, norepinephrine, serotonin, polypeptides (protein toxins) such as apamin and melittin. Death could be due to dysfunction of immune system in which venom allergen reacts with cell bound immunoglobulin E [65].

The circulatory, dermal, respiratory and gastrointestinal systems react to sting after one or more sensitizing stings (Type 1 hypersensitivity reaction), 58% die in 6 hours [65]. Autopsy revealed that 75% of dead patients showed obstruction of airway. LD_{50} of the venom is caused by 19 stings which should be removed. Bee venom being relatively acidic should be neutralized by base. Cold pack should be applied locally to reduce pain [62]. Bee sting could cause immediate or delayed hypersensitivity reaction, leading to motor-predominant axonal polyneuropathy associated with acute inflammatory demyelination. Intravenous immunoglobulin was effective [66]. Bee sting causes increased creatinine, interstial eosinophilia, nephritis, acute tubular necrosis, anuria, decreased creatinine kinase, altered sensorium, leukocytosis and doll's eye [43]. The reported median lethal dose (LD_{50}) of bee venom is 2.8 mg/kg [61] making it extremely toxic [67]. Bee and wasp could cause acute ischemic neurological deficits 5 hours after multiple stings. Stings of 100–200 bees could be responsible for stroke [63]. Vomition, diarrhea, dyspnea, myocardial infarction, and cerebral infarction are rare [68]. Seizure, hemiparesis, aphasia, apraxia, ataxia, dysphagia and coma are also associated with wasp and bee stings [69]. Cerebral ischemia could be secondary to biogenous amine, adrenaline, platelete aggregation, thromboxane and leucotrienes [70, 71], which may lead to disseminated intravascular coagulation and death caused by 25–30 stings [41]. Parkinsonism, an extrapyramidal abnormality could be caused by an immune-mediated delayed hypersensitivity which responds to aggressive treatment using immunosuppressants [38]. Brachial plexitis, rhabdomyolysis with generalized body and muscle pain, acute renal insufficiency and liver dysfunction characterized by alkaline enuresis are signs of apitoxicosis [42]. Nephrotic syndrome secondary to hypersensitive reaction which disappeared after corticosteroid treatment (prednisolone 2 mg/kg) that reappeared after one year, hypoproteinemia, proteinuria [44], acute renal failure and cardiac arrest were also observed [45].

4.10 Diagnosis of apitoxicosis

Diagnosis is by detection of venom-specific 1gE antibodies, CAP-RAST and radio adsorbent test [39]. Intravenous administration of 125 mg of *Vipera aspis* venom was redistributed in 7 hours and neutralized by antibody 15 min after antivenom injection. Lower doses of antivenom failed to yield complete neutralization. $F(ab')_2$ and Fab could be used as antidotes [72]. Multiple organ failure and acute renal failure could be caused by wasp sting, acute tubular necrosis secondary to hemolysis; rhabdomyolysis and thrombotic microangiopathy have also been reported [46]. With supportive care, victims should survive hundreds of wasps or approximately 1000 honeybee stings [73]. Early renal biopsy is vital for patients who do not respond to supportive measures. Hence timely dialysis and steroid may improve survivability [74]. Atropine sulphate, dexamethasone, neuroxine-B, multivitamin and electrolyte therapy led to recovery of passive respiration [75]. Similar treatment may be effective in human. $F(ab)_2$- based antivenom raised in horse may lead to production of specific high 1gC titer, counter hemolysis, myotoxicity and cytotoxicity [76]. Polyclonal antibodies against *Apis indica* reversed a lot of toxic effects in experimental mice [77], hence may be tried in human. Acute renal failure without hemolysis could be treated successfully using low dose of dopamine, fluid therapy and hemodialyis [64]. Apitoxin 1 (77.8%) and apitoxin 2 (51.9%) with LD_{50} (71.5 μg/ml) and LD_{50} (191.6 μg/ml) respectively are affected by moisture and protein content [78]. Lethal dose of snake venom could be neutralized by antidote equal to one-third of lethal dose with reference to body weight of the affected animal and safety of 10^{-4} [35]. Treatment of scorpion envenomation requires antivenom that is 66.6% of median lethal dose of scorpion venom [26]. In both cases treatments shall continue until the patients recover from the toxicity. Since kidney is affected, creatinine clearance, volume of urine, creatinine, plasma creatinine, serum creatinine and urine volume should be determined to assess the extent of renal damage, using the formulas reported by Saganuwan et al. [37]. Level of hemolysis should be assessed and quantity of hematonics and plasma expanders should be calculated. *Abrus pracatorius* could be used as hematonic [36]. Since the toxins cause neurological signs, their atomic weight may be less than 600 daltons. Hence the transport of the toxin to the brain may be by protonation or deprotonation or damage to meninges [79].

4.11 Treatment of apitoxicosis

Pheniramine maleate (1 mg/kg) and methyl prednisolone (1 mg/kg) in 100 cc physiologic serum should be administered parenterally. A loading dose of phenytoin administered against convulsion, supply of oxygen, adrenaline (0.5 mg i.m.) repeated at 10–15 min intervals, diphenhydramine, prednisolone and aminophylline for bronchospasm are highly beneficial [80]. Treatment is by administration of antihistamine for several days, steroids, chlorpheniramine, hydrocortisone, adrenaline, and inhaled B_2 agonist [81]. Bee sting could cause polyneuritis, Parkinsonism, encephalitis, acute disseminated encephalomyelitis, Guillam-Barre Syndrome, Glasgow Coma Score (GCS) of 11, myocardial infarction, pulmonanary edema, hemorrhage, hemolytic anemia, renal diseases and tonic–clonic seizure [48]. Climatic seasonal and feeding factors could qualitatively or quantitatively affect the potency of melittin and phosphohpase A2 of *Apis mellifera* [60]. The similarity in the calculated LD_{50} (2.5 mg/kg) of honeybee venom in the present study as compared to the reported value (2.8 mg/kg) in human [82] shows that honeybee venom is very toxic. The fact that 7.5 mg/kg ($3LD_{50}$) of the honeybee antivenom could neutralize 2.5 mg/kg of the venom agrees with the report indicating that antivenom of 3 folds venom LD_{50} could neutralize honey bee venom. Our findings are corroborated by the report that the dose of apilic antivenom is determined by number of stings. The higher the number of stings, the higher the dose of apilic antivenom is used [83]. The F $(ab)_2$ – based antivenom contain 1gG that prevented hemolysis, cytotoxicity and myotoxicity [84]. However, polyclonal antibody against honeybee envenomation could neutralize 40% of LD_{50} venom [76]. Venom produced by bees (apitoxin) is of two types; type I has LD_{50} of 71.5 microgram/ml and type II has LD_{50} of 191.6 microgram/mL, respectively [77] and 0.5 mg of *A. mellifera* venom can severely damage kidney of rabbit, signifying that mechanisms of lethality in animals may involve kidney failure. Change in living conditions of honeybee can lead to change in composition of their toxins [78]. The calculated LD_{50} (1.41 mg/kg) for child that weighed 10 kg in the present study agrees with the report that children, elderly and underweight people can be affected and a multiple stings of more than 500 can yield large quantity of the venom [85] which can produce more severe reactions in allergic patients [19]. Relatively higher ED_{50} (11.2 mg/kg) for the honeybee antivenom shows that the children are severely affected and as such require relatively large volume of the antivenom for neutralization of the venom. In the present study about 7.9 LD_{50} of antivenom is required in children of 10 kg. The calculated LT_{50} of 2.10 and 3.72 hr for child and adult human respectively, agree with the report indicating that honeybee venom from over 50 stings can kill within short period of time [86]. The fact that 200 stings could cause envenoming syndrome in adult with type 2 diabetes and prostate cancer [87] and non-diseased human [83] shows the newly derived formula may be used for determination of effective dose of honeybee antivenin for all the population segments. The calculated LD_{50} (2.5 mg/kg) for honeybee venom is comparable to that of scorpion (*Mesobuthus eupeus*) venom (0.18–4.5 mg/kg). This indicates that, there is relationship between the two venoms. Majority of deaths is caused by airway obstruction and anaphylactic shock [62] and 58% of the affected humans can die in less than 1 hr and over 75% can die in less than 6 hr [65]. However, stings of 600–1500 can be survived depending on therapeutic intervention [88]. Therefore, the preliminary efficacy and safety of Africanized honeybee antivenin predicts its clinical validity [83]. Dentar bee stung patient may require keratoplasty and removal of cataract and glaucoma which may require antibiotic /steroid. Moxifloxacin (0.5%) or tobramycin (0.3%) with dexamethasone (0.1%) 6 times daily for up to 4–6 weeks are highly beneficial. Oral prednisolone (40–50 mg) may be used in place of dexamethasome [89].

4.12 Medical uses of honey

The use of raw honey, royal jelly, pollen, propolis, bee venom and wax for treatment of various medical conditions is known as apitherapy. Conditions usually treated are arthritis, multiple sclerosis, and skin diseases among others. Melittin (40–50%) is the major component of honey used as antiviral, antimicrobial, and anti-inflammatory as apamin (2–3%) increases production of cortisol in adrenal gland, adolapine (0.5–1%) is anti-inflammatory and analgesic, acting via cyclooxygenase. Nevertheless histamine (0.5–2%) cause pain and swelling, dopamine (0.2–1%), serotonin (0.5–1%) and norepinephrine (0.1–0.5%) are all neurotransmitters for mood balance. Hyaluronidase (1–2%), and phosphohpase A2 (10–12%) are enzymes for activation of immune cells, production of immunoglobulin E (1 g E) and degranulation of mast cells. The sting and bite cause fluid exudation and protease inhibitor (0.1–0.8%) act as anti-inflammatory and antihemorrhagic [89].

4.13 Spider envenomation

Eggs of black widow spider (Latrodectus), family (Theridiidae) are toxic to mammals. Species of spiders belonging to Agelenidae, Tetragnathidae, Pimoidae and Linyphiidae are also toxic [90]. Brazilian spider (*Sicarius ornatus*, Araneae, Scicariidae) venom contains active sphingomyelinase D that causes hemolysis and keratinocyte death similar to the South American loxosceles species [91]. Methyl ketones (2 –tridecanone, 2-undecanone) from tomato (*Lycopersicon hirsutum f. glabratum* are lethal to insects [92]. Black widow spiderling extract caused apoptosis and death of HeLa cell lines [93]. Spider venoms contain toxic proteins and peptides in varying compositions. Sphingomyelinase causes varying degree of dermonecrosis from American *Sicarius loxosceles* and African Sicarius [94]. However, scorpion, spider and wasp could be controlled using pesticide [95]. Spiders such as Callobius (Amaurobiidae), Antrodiaetus (Antrodiaetidae), yellow sac spider (*Cheiracanthium mildei*), erb-weaver of the genus Araneus and hobo spider bites, result in pain, redness of stung sites and muscle twitching which disappear in 12 hr [96]. Pesticides confidor and Buctril-M are used against agrobiont spiders, *Lycosa terrestris* Butt and *Oxyopes javanus* [97]. New Zealand spiders, *Latrodectus katipo* and *L. atritus* are being threatened [98]. Latrotoxin though unique to black widow spider can be transferred to other spiders and bacteria via symbiosis. Latrodectin venom genes originate from ecdysozoan ion transport peptide (ITP) and crustacean hyperglycemic hormone (CHH) neuropeptide super family. The lower presence of latrotoxins in house spiders relative to black widow spiders, in the absence of a vertebrate alpha-latrotoxin in the house spider genome account for high potency of black widow venom [99]. Latrodectism caused by *Latrodectus spp* is manifested by local, regional or generalized pain, associated with non-specific symptoms and autonomic effects. Loxoscelism caused by *Loxosceles spp* has continuous manifestation characterized by pain and erythema that can develop into a necrotic ulcer. Systemic loxoscelism is characterized by intravascular hemolysis and renal failure. *Atran spp*, *Hadronyche spp* and *Phoneutria spp* from Brazil are also harmful. Antivenoms have been less successful in the treatment of their toxicoses [100].

4.14 Treatment of spider envenomation

Extracts of *Capsicum chinense*, *C. frutescence*, *C. baccatum*, *C. annuum* and *C. pubescens* could be used to repel spiders. *Solanum habrochaites* has methyl ketones (2-undecanone; 2-dodecanone; 2-tridecanone; 2-pentadecanone) with high acaricidal potential and may be used in control of harmful spiders. *Cheiracanthium punctorium* caused mild necrosis and dermonecrosis (necrotic arachnidism) [73]. Venoms of *Tityus serrulatus* (scorpion) and *Loxosceles gaucho* (spider) including *Apis mellifera* are highly toxic [101]. Atracotoxins targeting calcium channels blockers should be considered as conventional pesticides [102]. Sulfur induces release of cortisol from adrenal glands that protects the body from infection. Bee venoms could cause heart failure and suffocation [82]. Imidaclopid (insecticide) causes delayed and time-cumulative toxicity to bees, ants and termites [84].

5. Conclusion

The toxicity of snake and scorpion venom is dependent on the quantity of the venom, whereas apitoxicosis in human is dependent on the number of stings and dose of venom produced per sting. Snake and scorpion venoms are the most dangerous. However, venoms of some snakes and scorpions are equipotent and require 2 or more vials of antivenoms. LD_{50} of honeybee venom in adult man is 2.5 mg/kg which can be neutralized by 7.5 mg/kg ($3LD_{50}$) of antivenin. LD_{50} of honeybee venom for child is 1.41 mg/kg and can be neutralized by 11.2 mg/kg ($7.9LD_{50}$) antivenin. The venom can kill in less than 4 hr. Hence, children are more sensitive to honeybee toxicity than the adults are, and so may require higher dose of antivenom. Spider and wasp envenomation are less severe and could be treated symptomatically. All the organ systems could be affected and complications could follow multiple attacks. Hence treatment is by administration of antivenins, antiiflammatory, analgesic and respiratory support. Neurological and cardiorespiratory signs may be considered as indices of therapeutic success or failure. Prompt therapeutic intervention and hospitalization of 1 or more days could either delay or avert death.In the cases of severe anemia, blood transfusion and fluid therapy may be evident.

Author details

Saganuwan Alhaji Saganuwan
Department of Veterinary Pharmacology and Toxicology, College of Veterinary Medicine, Federal University of Agriculture P.M.B. 2373, Makurdi, Benue State, Nigeria

*Address all correspondence to: pharm_saga2006@yahoo.com

References

[1] Bieber AL. Metal and non-protein constituent in snake venom. In: Lee T (ed) Snake Venoms: Hardwork of Experimental Pharmacology, Springer Verlag, Berlin. 1979: 295–3006

[2] Gilliam LL, Brunker J. North American snake envenomation in the dog and cat. Vet Clin Small Anim. 2011; 41: 1239–1259

[3] Borges A, Miranda RJ, Pasale JM. Scorpionism in central America, with special reference to the case of Panama. J Venom Anim Toxins incl Trop Dis. 2012; 18(2): 130–143

[4] Muller GJ, Modler H, Wium CA, Veale DJH. Scorpion sting in Southern Africa: diagnosis and management. Contin Med Educ. 2012; 30(10): 1–8

[5] Dehesa-Davila M, Possani LD. Scorpionism and serotherapy in Mexico. Toxicon. 1994; 32(9): 1015–1018

[6] Costa CLSDO, Fe NF, Sampaio I, Tadei WP. A profile of scorpionism, including the species of scorpions involved in the state of Amazonas, Brazil. Rev Soc Bras Med Trop. 2016; 49 (3): 376–379

[7] Pajovic B, Radosavljevic M, Ivava RI, Vukovic , Boricic S. Biogeographic and clinical review of Mesobuthus gibbosus scorpionism in Montenegro: clinical cases of six patients. MD. 2015; 7(4): 315–318

[8] Deghani R, Rafinejad J, Fathi B, Shehi MP, Jazayeri , Hashemi A. A retrospective study on scorpionism in Iran (2002–2011). J Arthropod-Borne Dis. 2017; 11(2): 194–203

[9] Chippaux JP Goyfton M. Producers of antivenom sera. Toxin. 1983; 21: 739–752

[10] Ulug M, Yaman Y, Yapia F, Can-Ulug N. Scorpion envenomation in children: an analysis of 99 cases. York J Phediatr. 2012; 54: 119–127

[11] Seiter N, Koc H, Ulrich A, Yagmur EA. The case history of a toxic sting of a Leiurus abdullahbayrami scorpion in Turkey. Arachnol Lett. 2016; 51: 64–66

[12] Bharath RV, Kumar MR, Subrahmanyam BV, Rammohan P, Agrawal A. scorpion envenomation in children and its management. Arch Med Health Science. 2014; 2(2): 131–135

[13] Ferreira SR. Jr, Almeida RA, Barraviera SR, Barravie B. Historical perspective and human consequences of Africanized bee stings in the Amerias. Toxicol Environ Health B Crit Rev. 2012; 15: 97–108

[14] Diniz AZQ, Belmino JFB,Arujo KAMD, Viera AT, Elite RDS. Epidemiology of honeybee sting cases in the state of Ceara, Northeastern Brazil. Rev Inst Med Trop Sao Paulo. 2016; 58: 40

[15] Linard ATS, Barros RM, Sousa JA, Elite RS. Epidemiology of bee stings in Campina Grade, Paraiba State, Northeastern Brazil. J Venom Anim Toxin Inclu Trop Dis. 2014; 20: 13

[16] Betten DP, Richardson WH, Tong TC, Clark RF. Massive honeybee envenomation-induced rhabdomyolysis in an adolescent. Paediatrics. 200; 117 (1): 231–235

[17] da Silva GAR, Pires KL, Soares DCDS, Ferreira MR, Ferry FRDA. RRH: envenoming syndrome due to 200 stings from Africanized honeybees. Rev Insitut Med Trop Sao Paulo. 2013; 55(1): 61–64

[18] Schumacher MJ, Schmidt JO, Egen NB, Lowry JE. Quantity analysis and lethality of European and Africanized honeybee venom. Am J Trop Med Hyg. 1990; 43(1): 79–86

[19] Schumacher MJ, Schmidt JO, Egen NB, Dilon KA. Biochemical variability of venoms from individual European and Africanized honeybees (*Apis mellifera*). J Allergy Clin Immunol. 1992; 90: 59–65

[20] Almeida RAMDB, Olivo TET, Mendes RP, Barraviera SRCS, Souza LDR, Martins JG, Hashimoto M, Fabris VE, Junior RSF, Barraviera B. Africanized honey bee stings: how to treat them. Rev Soc Bras Med Trop. 2011; 44 (6): 755–761

[21] Kluz-Zawadzka J, Hartman-Ksycinska A, Lewandowska B. Emergent management of scorpion sting. Pergl Epidemiol. 201; 68: 655–688

[22] Platnick AI. The World Spider catalog version 12.0. American Nugarm of Natural History. Available: http://research.amnh.org/ig/spiders/catalog

[23] Isbister GK, Gray MR, Balit CR, Raven RJ, Stokes BJ, Porges K, Tankel AS, Turner E, White J, Fisher MM. Fuunel-web spider bite: a systematic review of recorded clinical cases. Med J Aust. 2015; 182: 407–411

[24] Gibb TJ, Bennett GW. Spiders. Entension Entomol. www.extension.purdue.edu. 2017; 72: 1- 3

[25] Abimannane A, Rameshkumar R, Satheesh P, Mahadevan S. Second dose of Scorpion antivenom in children with Indian red scorpion (Mesobuthus tamulus) sting envenomation. Indian Pediatric. 2018; 55: 315–318

[26] Saganuwam SA. Determination of median effective dose (ED_{50}) of scorpion antivenom against scorpion envenomation using a newly developed formula. Animal Model Exp Med. 2018; 1: 228–284

[27] Pandi K. Krishnamurthy S, Srinvasaraghavan R. Mahaderan S. Efficacy of scorpion antivenom plus prazosin versus prazosin alone for Mesobuthus tamulus scorpion sting-envenomation in children: a randomized controlled trial. Arch Dis Child. 2014; 99: 575–580

[28] Carno AO, Chatzak N. Horta CC, Magalhaes BF, Olivera-Mendes BBR, Chavez-Olortegui C, Kalapothakis E. Alternative methodologies of scorpion antivenomous production. Toxicon. 2015; 97: 64–74

[29] Ozkan, O. Carhan A. The neutralization capacity of Androctonus crassicauda antivenom against *Mesobuthus eupeus* scorpion vernom. Toxicon. 2008; 52(2): 375–379

[30] Ozkan O, Adiguzel S, Yakistiran S, Filazi A. Study of the relationship between Androctonus crassicauda (Oliver, 1807; Scorpiones, Burhidae), venom toxicity and telson size weight and storing condition. Venom Anim Toxin Incl Trop Dis. 2006; 12(2): 297–309

[31] Vazirianzadeh B, Farhadpour F, Hosseinzadeh M, Zarean M, Morawej SA. An epidemiological and clinical study on scorpionism in hospitalized children in Khuzeska, Iran J Arthropod-Borne Dis. 2012; 6(1): 62–69

[32] Khoobdel M, Zahraei –Salehi T, Nayeri-Fasaei B, Khosravi M, Omidian Z, Motedayen MH, Akbari A. Purification of the immunogenic fractions and determination of toxicity in Mesobuthus eupeus (Scorpionida: Buthidae) venom. J Anthropod Borne Dis. 2013; 7(2):139–146

[33] Hmila I, Saerens D, Abderrazak RB, Vicke C, Abidi N, Benlasfar Z, Govaect J, El Ayeb M, Boy haouala-Zahar B, Muyldermans S. A bio specific nanbody to provide full protection against lethal scorpion envenoming. FASEB Journal. 2010; 24(9): 3479 -3489

[34] Saganuwan SA. A modified arithmetical method of Reed and Muench for determination of a

relatively ideal median lethal dose (LD_{50}). Afr J Pharm Pharmacol. 2011; 5 (12): 1543–1546

[35] Saganuwan SA. Calculation of effective dose fifty (ED_{50}) of antivenom for American pit viper envenomation Comp Clin Pathol. 2018; 27: 1321–1325

[36] Saganuwam SA. Hematonic and plasma expander effects of aqueous leaf extract of Abreus Precatorius in *Mus musculus*. Comp Clin Pathol. 2012; 21: 1249–1255

[37] Saganuwam SA. The use of body surface area for determination of age, body weight, urine creatinine, plasma creatinine, serum creatinine, urine volume, and creatinine clearance: the reliable canomical method of assessing renotoxicity in animals. Comp Clin Pathol. 2018; 27: 1531–1536

[38] Leopold NA, Bara- Jimenez W, Hallett M. Parkinsonism after a wasp string. Movement Disorder. 2001; 14(1): 122–127

[39] Ewan PW. Venom allergy. BMJ. 1998; 316: 1365–1368

[40] Jithendranath P, Byju N, Saifudkeen K, Jose J. Brachial plexitis following bee sting. Ann Indian Acad Neurol. 2012; 15 (3): 234

[41] Dharma RV, Bodepudi SK, Krishna M. Disseminated intravascular coagulation after multiple honeybee sting. Natl Med J India. 2014; 23(3): 141–143

[42] Akdur O,Lan S, Atacan G. Rhabdomyolysis secondary to bee sting. Case Rep Emerg Med. 2013: ID258451

[43] Desphande PR, Ahsan FKK, Bairy M, Prabhu RA. Acute renal failure and/ or rhabdomyolysis due to multiple bee sting: a retrospective study. North Am J Med Sci. 2013; 5(3): 235–239

[44] Kaarthigeyan K, Sivanandam S, Jothilakshmi K, Mathal J. Nephrotic syndrome following a single bee sting in a child. Indian J Nephrol. 2018; 22(1): 57–58

[45] Valisethy R, Venkatarathbamma PN, Rrasad BNR, Gupta U. A rare case of massive envenomation of honeybees with anaphylaxis. J Evol Med Dent Sci. 2014; 3(54): 12512–12516

[46] George P, Pawar B, Calton N, Mathew P. Wasp sting: An unsual fatal outcome. Saud J Kidney Dis Transplant. 2008; 19(6): 969–972

[47] Qudiseva H, Uddaraju N, Pradhan S, Das N, Mascatenhas J, Srinisan M, Prajna NV. Ocular manifestations of isolated corneal bee sting injury, management strategies, and clinical outcomes. Indian J Ophthamol. 2018; 66: 262–268

[48] Turtseven A, Guvenc T. Seizure and ischaemic attack following bee sting. Turk J Neurol. 2015; 21: 138–140

[49] Shetty K, Shetty R, Chandra GSN, Pai U, Kiran A, Mohan NK. Bee alert I. Multiple honeybee stings lead to heart attack: a case report. IJPSRR. 2016; 41 (18): 83–85

[50] Saini A, Sankhyan N, Suthar R, Singhi P. Acute axonal polyneuropathy following honeybee sting: a case report. J Child Neurol. 2014; 29(5): 674-676

[51] Betten DP, Richardson WH, Tong TC, Clark RF. Massive honeybee envenomation-induced rhabdomyolysis in an adolescent. Pediatrics. 2000; 117 (1): 231–235

[52] Schmidt JD. Chemistry, pharmacological and chemical ecology of venoms In: Piek T (ed.) Venoms of the Hymenoptera, Academic Press, Londoners. 2006: 425–508

[53] Bkaily G, Sperelakis N, Renaud JF, Payer MD. Apamin, a high specific Ca2+

blocking agent in heart muscle. Am J Physiol. 1985; 248: 961–965

[54] Papachristoforous A, Kagiava A, Papaefthimiou C, Termentzi A, Fokialakis N, Skaltsounis AL, Watkins M, Arnold G, Theophilidis G. The bite of the honeybee: 2-heptanone secreted from honeybee mandibles during a bite acts as a local anesthetic in insects and animals. Plos One. 2012; 7(10): e47432

[55] Schumacher M, Egen N. Significance of Africanized bees for public health: a review. Arch Intern Med. 1995; 155: 2038–2044

[56] Winston ML. The Africanized killer bee: biology and public health. Q J Med. 1994; 87: 263–267

[57] Tunget CL, Clark RF. Invasion of the killer bees: separating facts from fiction. Postgrad Med. 1993; 94: 92–102

[58] Greenberg MI, Hendrickson RG, Silverberg M. Greenberg's Text Atlas of Emergency Medicine, Lippincott, Philadelphia, USA

[59] Hider RC. Honey bee venom: a rich source of pharmacologically active peptides. Endeavour. 1988; 12: 60–65

[60] Junior RSF, Sciani JM, Marques-Porto R, Junior AL, Orsi RDO. Barraviera B, Pimenta DC. Africanized honeybee (*Apis mellifera*) venom profiling: seasonal variation of melittin and phospholipase A2 levels. Toxicon. 2010; 56(3): 355–362

[61] Eze OBL, Nwodo OFC, Ogugua VN. Therapeutic effect of honeybee venom. J Pharmaceut Chem Biol. 2016; 4(1): 48–53

[62] Sethi SS, Jena MK. Bee sting envenomation: rare fatality. J Indian Acad Forensic Med. 2015; 37(2): 202–203

[63] Rachaiah NM, Kalegowda RH, Krishnaswamy RB. An acute ischaemic stroke after multiple bee stings in an elderly patient. Asian J Med Sci. 2013; 4 (2): 55–58

[64] Lin HC, Chen HH, The JC. Acute renal failure complicated by multiple bee stings: a case report and literature review. Acute Nephrol. 2000; 15: 20–22

[65] Karalliedde L. Animal toxins. Br J Anaesthes. 1995; 74: 319–327

[66] Saini AG, Sankhyan N, Suther R, Songhi P. Acute axonal polyneuropathy following honeybee sting: a case report. J Child Neurol. 2014; 29(5): DOI.101177/0883073813517262

[67] Saganuwan SA. Principles of Pharmacological Calculation, 1st ed., Ahmadu Bello University Press. 2012;529

[68] Rajendiran C, Puvanalingam A, Thangam I, Ragunanthanan S, Ramesh D, Venkatesan S, Sundar C. Stroke after multiple bee sting. J Assoc Physicians India. 2012; 60: 44–45

[69] Schiffman JS, Tang RA, Ulysses E, Dorotheo N, Singh SS, Bahrani HM. Bilateral ischaemic optic neuropathy and stroke. Br. J Ophthamol. 2004; 88: 1596–1598

[70] de Toledo LFM, Moore DCBC, Caixeta DMDL, Salu MDS, Farias CVB, de Azevedo ZMA. Multiple bee stings, multiple organs involved: a case report. Rev Soc Bras Med Trop. 2018; 51(4): 560–562

[71] Riggs JE, Ketonen LM, Wymer JP, Barbano RL, Valanne LK, Bodensteiner JB. Acute and delayed cerebral infarction after wasp sting anaphylaxis. Clin Neuropharmacol. 1994; 17(4): 384–388

[72] Riviere G, Choumet V, Audebert F, Saboraud A, Debray M, Scherrmann JN, Bon C. Effect of antivenom on venompharmakinetics in experimentally envenomed rabbits

towards an optimization of antivenom therapy. J Pharmacol Exp Ther. 1997; 281(1): 1

[73] Vetter RS, Isbister GK, Bash SP, Boutin LJ. Verified bites by yellow Sac spiders (genus cheiracanthium) in the United States and Australia: where is the necrosis? Am J Trop Med Hyg. 2006; 74 (6): 1043–1048

[74] Dhanapriya J, Dineshkumar T, Sakthirajan R, Shamkar P, Gopalakrishan N, Balasubramaniyan T. Wasp sting-induced acute kidney injury. Clin Kidney J. 2016; 9(2): 201–204

[75] Savaliya KB, Parikh SS. A unique case of honeybee sting in Gir cow and its therapeutic management. Sch J Agric Vet Sci. 2015; 2(4A): 285–286

[76] Santo KS, Stephano MA, Marcelona JR, Ferreira VMR, Rocha T, Carricati C, Higashi HG, Moro AM, Kalil JE, Malaspino O, Castro FMM, Palma MS. Production of the first effective hyperimmune equine serum antivenom against Africanized bees. Plos One. 2013; 8(11): e79971

[77] Ahmad S, Upadhyay RK. Production of polyclonal antibodies against Indian honey bee (*Apis mellifera*) venom toxins and its efficacy in reversal of toxic effects. Afr J Biotechnol. 10 (53): 10991–11003

[78] Abrantes AF, Rocha TCD, Lima ABSD, Cavalcanti MI. Honey bee venom: influence of collection on quantity and cytotoxicity. Cinencia Rural Santa Maria. 2017; 47(10): e20160486

[79] Saganuwan SA. Physicochemical and structure-activity properties of piroxicam- amini review. Comp Clin Pathol. 2016; 25: 941–945

[80] Hatano S. Experience from a multicentre stroke register. A preliminary report. Bull World Health Organ. 1980; 58: 113–130

[81] Pakmanee N, Noiphrom J, Kay A, Pormuttakun D, Sakolparp L, Hemmale W, Akesowan S, Khomvilar S, Sitparija V. Comparative abilities of phospholipase A2, and coagulant activities induced by Daboia sianensis venom and their antiinflammatory activity. Sci Asia. 2013; 39: 160–166

[82] Ali MAM. Studies on bee venom and its medical uses.Int J Adv Res Technol. 2013; 1(2): 1–15

[83] Barbosa AN, Boyer L, Chippaux J-L, Medolago NB, Caramon CA, Paixao AG, Poli JPV, Mendes MB, dos Santos LD, Ferreira RS, Barraviera B. A clinical trial protocol to treat massive africanized honeybee (*Apis mellifera*) attack with a new apilic antivenom. J Venom Anim Toxin Inclu Trop Dis. 2017; 23(14): 1–10

[84] Rondeau G, Sanchez-Bayo F, Tennekes HA, Decourtye A, Ramirez-Romero R, Desneux N. Delayed and time-cumulative toxicity of imidacloprid in bees, ants and termites. Sci Report. 2014; 4: 1–8

[85] Utkin YN. Animal venom studies: current benefits and future development. World J Biol Chem. 2015; 6(2): 28–33

[86] Anolry N, Arslan MN, Kumral B, Buyuk Y. Death caused by honeybee stings: case report. Med Sci. 2014; 3(2): 1305–1314

[87] Silva GARD, Pires KL, Soares DCDS, Ferreira MR, Ferry FRDA, Motta RN, Azevedo MCVMD. RRH: envenoming syndrome due 200 stings from Africanized honeybees. Rev Inst Med Trop Sau Paulo. 2013; 55(1): 61–64

[88] Daher EDF, da Silva Junior GB, Benzerra GP, Pontes LB, Martins AMC, Guimares JA. Acute renal failure after massive honeybee stings. Rev Inst Med Trop S Paulo. 2003; 45(1): 45–50

[89] Gudiseva , Uddaraju M, Pradhan S, Das M, Mascarenhas J, Srinivasan, Prajna NV. Ocular manifestations of isolated corneal bee sting injury, management strategies and clinical outcomes. Indian J Ophthamol. 2018; 66 (2): 262–268

[90] Schmidt JO, Vetter RS, Howe AK. Egg toxicity in diverse spider taxa. J Arachnol. 2017; 45(2): 209–212

[91] Lopes PH, Bertani R, Goncalves-de-Andrade, RM, Nagahama RH, Ven den Berg CW, Tamburgi DV. Venom of the Brazilian spider Sicarius ornatus (Araneae, Sicarridae) contains acive sphingomyelinase D: potential for toxicity after envenomation. Plos Negl Trop Dis. 2013; 7(8): 12394

[92] Chatzivasileiadis EA, Sabelis MW. Toxicity of methyl ketones from tomato trichomes to Tetranychus urticae Koch. Exp Appl Acarol. 1997; 21: 473–488

[93] Peng X, Dai Z, Lei Q, Liang L, Tan S, Wang X. Cytotoxic and apoptotic activities of black widow spiderling extract against Hela cells. Exp Therapeutic Med. 2017; 13: 3267–3274

[94] Zobel-Thropp P, Bodner MR, Binford GJ. Comparative analyses of venoms from American and African Sicarius spiders that differ in sphingomyelinase D activity. Toxicon. 2010; 55(7): 1274–1282

[95] Stoytcheva M. Pesticides in the Modern World-Pests Control and Pesticides Exposure and Toxicity Assessment. IntechOpen. 2011: 614

[96] Mckeown N, Vetter RS, Hendrickson RG. Verified spider bites in Oregon (USA) with the intent to assess hobo spider venom toxicity. Toxicon. 2014; 84: 51–55

[97] Sherawat SM, Butt A, Tahir HM. Effects of pesticides on agrobiom spiders in laboratory and field. Pakistan J. 2001 2015; 47(4): 1089–1095

[98] Vink CJ, Sirvid P, Malumbres-Olarte J, Griffiths JW, Paguin P, Paterson AM. Species status and conservation issues of New Zealandis endemic latrodectus spider species (Araneae; Theridiidae). Invert Syst. 2008; 22(6): 589–604

[99] Gendreau KL, Haney RA, Schwager EE, Wierschin T, Stanke M, Richards S, Oarb JE. House spider genome uncovers evolutionary shifts in the diversity and expression of black widow venom proteins associated with extreme toxicity. BMC Genomics. 2017; 18(178): 1–14

[100] Isbister GK, Fan HW. Spider bite. Lancet. 2011; 378(9808): 2039–2047

[101] Manzoli-Palma MF, Gobbi N, Palma S. Insects as biological models to assay spider and scorpion venom toxicity. J Venom Anim Toxin incl Trop Dis. 2013; 19(2): 1–6

[102] Wang X, Smith R, Fletcher JI, Wilson H, Wood CJ, Howden ME, King GF. Structure-function studies of omega-atracotoxin, a potent antagonist of insect voltage-gated calcium channels. Eur J Biochem. 1999; 264(2): 488–494

Section 3

Toxins

Chapter 7

Scorpion Toxins from *Buthus martensii* Karsch (BmK) as Potential Therapeutic Agents for Neurological Disorders: State of the Art and Beyond

Xiaoli Wang, Shuzhang Zhang, Yudan Zhu, Zhiping Zhang, Mengyao Sun, Jiwei Cheng, Qian Xiao, Guoyi Li and Jie Tao

Abstract

Scorpions are fascinating creatures which became residents of the planet well before human beings dwelled on Earth. Scorpions are always considered as a figure of fear, causing notable pain or mortality throughout the world. Their venoms are cocktails of bioactive molecules, called toxins, which are responsible for their toxicity. Fortunately, medical researchers have turned the life-threatening toxins into life-saving therapeutics. From Song Dynasty in ancient China, scorpions and their venoms have been applied in traditional medicine for treating neurological disorders, such as pain, stroke, and epilepsy. Neurotoxins purified from Chinese scorpion *Buthus Martensii* Karsch (BmK) are considered as the main active ingredients, which act on membrane ion channels. Long-chain toxins of BmK, composed of 58–76 amino acids, could specifically recognize voltage-gated sodium channels (VGSCs). Short-chain BmK toxins, containing 28–40 amino acids, are found to modulate the potassium or chloride channels. These components draw attention as useful scaffolds for drug-design in order to tackle the emerging global medical threats. In this chapter, we aim to summarize the most promising candidates that have been isolated from BmK venoms for drug development.

Keywords: scorpion toxins, BmK, neurological disorders, VGSCs, potassium channels, chloride channels

1. Introduction

Recent advances underlying medical studies have illuminated that several neurological disorders such as epilepsy, chronic pain, multiple sclerosis, stroke, brain tumor etc. are induced by dysfunction of membrane ion channels [1–3]. Up to now, multiple drugs specifically targeting ion channels have been designed to treat the diseases [4]. Some clinical studies and trials have also been initiated to discriminate therapeutic potentials of natural toxins and their derivatives such as scorpion toxins, spider toxins, snake toxins, sea anemone toxins, and toad venom, which could recognize relevant ion channels [5].

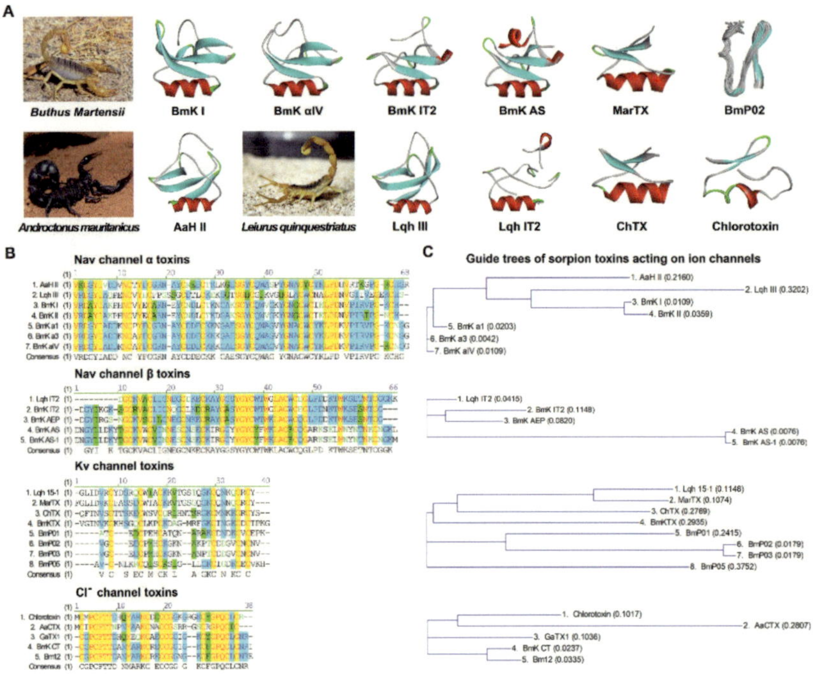

Figure 1.
Structures of scorpion toxin peptides. (A) The α/α-like scorpion toxins BmK I (PDB: 1SN1) [6] and BmK αIV [7–9] (using LQQ III, PBD: 1LQQ; BmK I, chimera Lqh αIT/AaH II, PBD: 1SEG; BmK $\alpha 2$, PDB: 2KBJ as templates) isolated and purified from Buthus martensii *Karsch, AaH II [10] (PDB: 1PTX) isolated and purified from* Androctonus mauritanicus, *Lqh III [11] (PDB: 1BMR) isolated and purified from* Leiurus quinquestriatus. *The β/β-like scorpion toxins BmK IT2 [7, 12–14] (using Lqh IT2, PBD: 2I61; LQQ III, PBD: 1LQQ; Lqh αIT A39L, PDB: 2YEO; Kurtoxin, PDB: 1T1T as templates), BmK AEP (using the same templates as BmK IT2), and BmK AS/AS-1 [9, 12, 14–16] (using Kurtoxin, PDB: 1T1T; Lqh IT2, PBD: 2I61; CsE-V, PBD: 1NRB; Ts3, PBD: 5CYo; BmK $\alpha 2$, PDB: 2KBJ as templates) isolated and purified from* Buthus martensii *Karsch. Lqh IT2 [12] (β-sheet not shown) isolated and purified from* Leiurus quinquestriatus. *The short-chain scorpion toxins acting on K^+ channels. The toxins MarTX [17] (PDB: 1M2S) and BmP02 [18] (PDB: 1DU9) isolated and purified from* Buthus martensii *Karsch. ChTX [9] (PDB: 2CRD) isolated and purified from* Leiurus quinquestriatus. *The short-chain scorpion toxins acting on Cl^- channels. The toxin chlorotoxin [19] (PDB: 2CRD) isolated and purified from* Leiurus quinquestriatus. *Sequence homology comparison is obtained by using PSI-Blast, and homology modeling of scorpion toxins is acquired by using Discovery Studio 2017 R2. (B) Top, multiple sequence alignment of α/α-like scorpion toxins. Middle, the second one in figure B, multiple sequence alignment of β/β-like scorpion toxins. Below, the third one in figure B, multiple sequence alignment of toxins acting on K^+ channels. Bottom, multiple sequence alignment of toxins acting on Cl^- channels. Conserved residues and cysteines formatting intrachain disulfide bonds are in red and shadowed in yellow; residues conserved in most of the peptides are shadowed in blue; residues with same charge in most of the peptides are shadowed in green. The species of toxins are mentioned above, except for Lqh 15–1 [20] and GaTX1 [21] isolated and purified from* Leiurus quinquestriatus *hebraeus; BmK II, BmK a1, BmK a3, BmKTX, BmP01, BmP03, BmK CT, and Bm12 isolated and purified from* Buthus martensii *Karsch [22]; AaCTX [23] isolated and purified from* Androctonus australis. *(C) The guide tree is constructed by ALIGNX, a component of the VECTOR NTI 11.0 software suite. Scores in the brackets are based on the identity of the amino acids' chemical properties. Top, the guide tree of α/α-like scorpion toxins. Middle, the guide tree of β/β-like scorpion toxins. Below, the guide tree of short-chain K^+ channel toxins. Bottom, the guide tree of short-chain Cl^- channel toxins.*

BmK scorpion, used as a drug which is also known as "Quan Xie" (whole scorpion body), can be traced to almost 2000 years ago since the Song Dynasty (A.D. 960–1279) of China. Based on the traditional Chinese medicine theories of "Xi Feng Zhi Jing, Gong Du San Jie, Tong Luo Zhi Tong" (suppressing the epileptic seizure, inhibiting growth and metastasis of tumor, dredging blood vessels and analgesia), BmK scorpion has been widely used to treat epilepsy, apoplexy, spasm, migraine, tetanus etc. [24]. The venom of BmK scorpion, considered as the main effective component, is a rich source of bioactive toxin polypeptides that regulate the activity of ion channels [25, 26] (**Figure 1**). According to the length of these peptides, scorpion toxins are classified into long-chain toxins and short-chain toxins. The long-chain scorpion toxins composed of 58–76 amino acid residues mainly act on voltage-gated sodium channels (VGSCs), while the short-chain scorpion toxins containing 28–40 amino acid residues generally target K^+ or Cl^- channels [27] (**Figure 1B**). Based on their physiological effects on VGSC gating and binding properties, the long-chain toxins can be further classified into two categories: α-toxins, such as BmK I, a 64-residue α-like toxin isolated from BmK [2], and BmK αIV, a novel cloned 68-residue polypeptide, binding to neurotoxin receptor site 3 of the VGSC, with inhibitory effects on the fast inactivation of VGSCs (**Figure 2**). β-toxins, which bind to receptor site 4 such as BmK IT2 as well as BmK AEP, two 64-residue inhibitory β-toxins [28], and BmK AS, a 66-residue β-like toxin, could shift the threshold of VGSCs activation to more negative membrane potentials [29–32] (**Figure 2**). By sequence alignment and phylogenetic trees, it could be found that the primary structure of BmK I is similar to that of the classical α-like toxin Lqh III, while the structural properties of BmK αIV are more similar to that of the classical α-toxin AaH II (**Figure 1C**). In addition, the structure of BmK IT2 and BmK AEP are similar to that of the classical β-toxin Lqh IT2, but it is quite different from the structure of BmK AS which is also separated from BmK (**Figure 1C**). Among short-chain toxins, martentoxin and BmP02 are considered as the specific blockers of BK channel (α + β4) and Kv1.3, respectively [33–35]. From sequence alignment and phylogenetic trees, martentoxin have low homology with the classical BK channel blocker charybdotoxin (ChTX), isolated and purified from

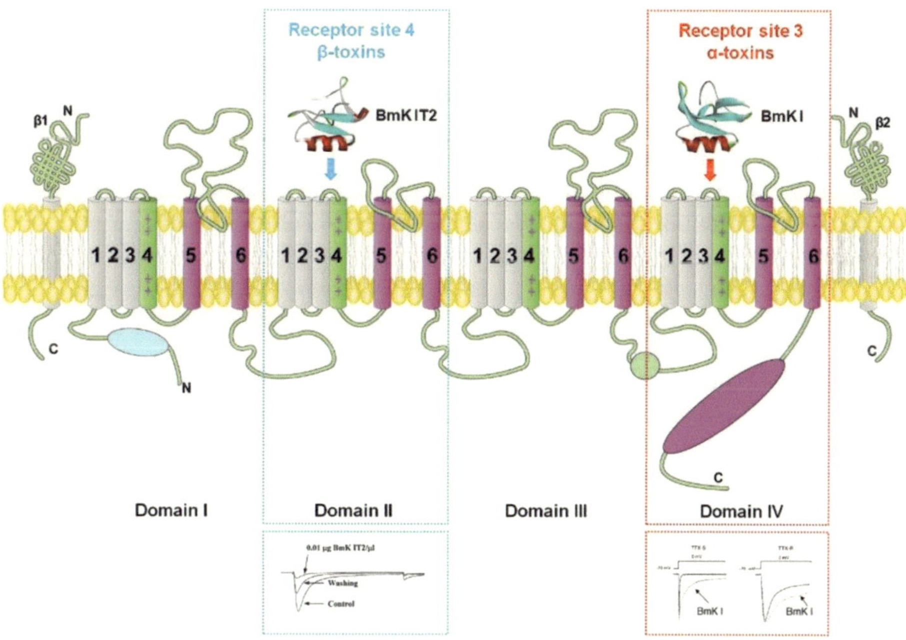

Figure 2.
Structure of VGSC and its pharmacological characterization modulated by α/α-like or β/β-like scorpion toxins. Schematic representation of Nav channels' α and β subunits. The α subunit of Nav channels is illustrated along with not only β1 but also β2 subunits; the β subunits' extracellular domains are exhibited to be an immunoglobulin-like fold that interacts with the loops in α subunits. The domains of the α subunit are represented by Roman numerals; segments 5 and 6 (exhibited in violet) are pore-lining segments, and S4 helices (green) constitute the voltage sensors. The green circle in the domains III and IV intracellular loop represents the inactivation-gating IFM motif. The α/α-like toxin BmK I delaying the inactivation of VGSCs by targeting the receptor site 3. The β toxin BmK IT2 suppressing transient currents of VGSCs by targeting the receptor site 4.

Leiurus quinquestriatus, but have high homology with Lqh 15–1 (ChTX2), another BK channel blocker from *Leiurus quinquestriatus* (**Figure 1B** and **C**). BmK CT could recognize the glioma-specific chloride channels. In this chapter, we aim to describe the most promising candidates for drug development that have been isolated from BmK venoms, with categorization according to their biological activity.

2. Analgesic effects of BmK toxins against VGSCs

Pain seriously damages human health and quality of life, so it is of importance to find effective analgesic targets and drugs. Nav channels (VGSCs) are transmembrane proteins responsible for generation and conduction of APs (action potentials) in excitable cells [1–3]. Of the nine functional α subunits (Nav1.1–1.9), Nav1.1, Nav1.3, Nav1.6, Nav1.7, Nav1.8, and Nav1.9 are distributed in primary sensory neurons, playing a crucial role in nociception and chronic pain [4]. In detail, mechanical pain is mainly caused by Nav1.6 [5]. Functional acquired mutations in Nav1.7 cause severe thermal hyperalgesia [24], while Nav1.7 with loss-of-function mutations leads to pain insensitivity [25]. Nav1.8 contributes to the APs generation in peripheral system and Nav1.9 plays a role in persistent Na+ currents in small-diameter dorsal root ganglia (DRG) neurons [26]. Because of the critical roles of VGSC subtypes in pain signal conduction [36, 37], natural products, specifically inhibiting VGSCs, might reveal the potential for treating chronic pain symptoms [38]. The neurotoxins of scorpion BmK are an excellent source of sodium channel modulators [22]. Among them, β/β-like scorpion toxins, binding to VGSC receptor site 4 such as BmK IT2 and BmK AS, show anti-nociceptive effects in *in vivo* experiments [39, 40].

BmK AS, polypeptide composed of 66 amino acid residues purified from BmK venom, was a unique β-like scorpion toxin with many distinct functions [41]. In the peripheral nervous system (PNS), BmK AS-induced antinociceptive effect on inflammation-induced thermal as well as spontaneous pain and mechanical hyperalgesia [30, 42]. Peripheral or spinal delivery of BmK AS significantly suppressed formalin-induced nociceptive behaviors and c-Fos expression in spinal cord [30, 43]. In order to clarify the mechanisms underlying antinociceptive effects of receptor site 4 toxins on VGSCs, the primary sensory neurons (dorsal root ganglion, DRG) isolated from the L4-L6 of adult rats are usually chosen for investigation. Patch clamp recording showed that BmK AS could significantly decrease excitability of small DRG neurons, by depressing the peak tetrodotoxin-resistant (TTX-R) and tetrodotoxin-sensitive (TTX-S) Na^+ currents of DRG neurons, and causing a negative shift of voltage-dependent activation [30]. Furthermore, BmK AS reduces the peak currents, facilitates steady-state activation, and inhibits slow inactivation of the Nav1.3 channels [44]. Through testing the VGSCs endogenously expressed in the DRG neuroblastoma ND7–23 cells as well as heterologously expressed Nav1.2 in *Xenopus* oocytes, it exhibited a U-shaped modulation of gating kinetics by BmK AS over a wide range of concentrations. BmK AS could suppress the peak currents, facilitate steady-state activation of VGSCs endogenously expressed in ND7–23 cells, while it did not affect the voltage-dependent activation and persistent currents of Nav1.2 [45]. These results provide a better understanding of the peripheral anti-injury sensation of BmK, which selectively inhibited the activity of Nav1.3 and DRG subtypes of VGSCs.

BmK IT2, consisting of 61 amino acid residues, contains 4 disulfide bonds, and could induce strong insect toxicity [28]. Like other depressant toxins, such as LqhIT2 [46, 47], BmK IT2 possesses two non-interacting binding sites (the high/low-affinity binding sites) on insect nerve membranes [48, 49]. But a previous study also found that formalin-induced spontaneous pain behavior and spinal c-Fos expression could be effectively suppressed by either pre- or post-treatment with intrathecal BmK IT2 [50], which strongly implied that BmK IT2 could not only bind to insect VGSCs, but also recognize mammal VGSC subtypes. In fact, the inhibition of BmK IT2 on total Na^+ currents was observed in small DRG neurons [31]. By testing VGSC subtypes in *Xenopus* oocytes expression system, Nav1.2, Nav1.3, and Nav1.6 display insensitive property to BmK IT2, suggesting that other isoforms, especially Nav1.7–1.9, might be involved in the suppressive activity of BmK IT2 in rat pathological models [51]. The results illuminated that BmK IT2 can be developed as a novel analgesic peptide with therapeutic potential.

3. Antiepileptic activity of BmK toxins

3.1 Antiepileptic activity of BmK Na^+ channel toxins

VGSCs play a critical role in the generation and propagation of neuroexcitibilty. Genetic alterations in VGSC genes are considered to be associated with epileptogenesis. The SCN1A (Nav1.1 gene) is the most relevant VGSC gene for epilepsy in clinical tests. More than 1200 Nav1.1 mutants have been characterized to be associated with epilepsy, most of variants mutations lead to febrile seizures [52]. Nav1.2 subunits are mainly distributed in the Ranvier node and axon-initiating segment (AIS). The mutation of Nav1.2 (SCN2A) is relevant to various epilepsies, such as Dravet's syndrome (DS), benign familial neonatal seizures (BFNIS), hereditary epilepsy with febrile seizures plus (GEFS+), and other stubborn childhood epileptic encephalopathies [53]. Another VGSC subtype widely distributed in CNS is Nav1.6, which is mainly distributed to the soma and synaptic origins. Mutations of Nav1.6 could induce severe epileptic encephalopathy exhibiting autistic features, early onset seizures, intellectual disability, ataxia, or sudden unexpected death in epilepsy (SUDEP) [54]. Therefore, this evidence strongly implies that natural products inhibiting VGSCs could also have the potential for suppressing the epileptic seizure.

BmK AEP, composed of 61 residues with 4 disulfide bonds, is the first anti-epilepsy peptide purified from scorpion venom. BmK AEP was less toxic to mice and insects, while it had forceful anticonvulsant effects on epileptic rats, and is thus named as BmK anti-epilepsy peptide (BmK AEP) [55]. BmK AEP has been reported to display anti-epileptic activity in a coriaria lactone-induced epileptic model in the rat with comparable efficacy to diazepam [56]. Recent studies demonstrated that BmK AEP concentration-dependently suppresses the Na^+ currents of Nav1.3 and Nav1.6, heterologously expressed in HEK293 cells, and shifts the voltage-dependent activation to the hyperpolarized direction, with minimal effects on steady-state inactivation [32].

Through intrahippocampal injection, β scorpion toxin BmK AS produced obviously anticonvulsant activity on the pentylenetetrazol (PTZ)-induced epileptic rodents. It could not only suppress the duration and number of high-amplitude, high-frequency discharges (HAFDs) in electroencephalography (EEG), but also obviously reduce the peak Na^+ currents of hippocampal pyramidal cells [57, 58]. By contrast, BmK AS did not regulate the epileptiform EEG of pilocarpine model over the same dose range [57]. Intrahippocampal injection of BmK AS obviously reduced the increase of c-Fos expression evoked by pilocarpine, implying that neuronal hyperactivity is decreased during the epileptic state [43].

Injection of BmK IT2 at hippocampal CA1 region could dose-dependently inhibit PTZ-induced epilepsy-like behavior as well as reduce the number and duration of HAFD on PTZ-induced epileptic EEG components. Similarly, BmK IT2 significantly prolonged the incubation period of status epilepticus (SE) onset, reduced the severity of SE, and inhibited the expression of c-fos in the hippocampus during SE of pilocarpine-induced epileptic rodents [59]. BmK IT2, which relieves epileptic symptoms, is thought to inhibit the activity of VGSC subtypes. Binding experiments showed that BmK IT2 could recognize neuronal synaptosome membranes. The patch-clamp experiment also proved that BmK IT2 can inhibit the persistent sodium current of hippocampal pyramidal neurons [59]. However, previous studies have found that BmK IT2 had no significant inhibitory effect on the peak Na^+ currents of Nav1.2, 1.3, and 1.6 heterologous-expressed in oocytes [51]. It is suggested that BmK IT2 might act on Nav1.1 or Nav1.7 in the central nervous system (CNS).

3.2 Antiepileptic activity of BmK K^+ channel toxins

BK channels, widely expressed in CNS, are voltage- and Ca^{2+}-activated K^+ channels with large conductance [60–62] (**Figure 3**). They have been shown to modulate fast afterhyperpolarization (fAHPs) and rapid spike repolarization in a number of types of neurons [63–65]. Under pathological state, it interacted the inactivation of Nav channels, with inducing neuronal spike shortening and increasing in firing rate as well as excitatory transmitter release, which could exacerbate seizure bursts [66–68].

Pentylenetetrazol (PTZ)-induced generalized tonic-clonic seizures give rise to a BK channel gain-of-function, characterized by increased BK currents as well as neuronal firing in the somatosensory cortex [69]. Interestingly, the BK channel blocker, paxilline, suppressed generalized tonic-clonic seizures in picrotoxin or

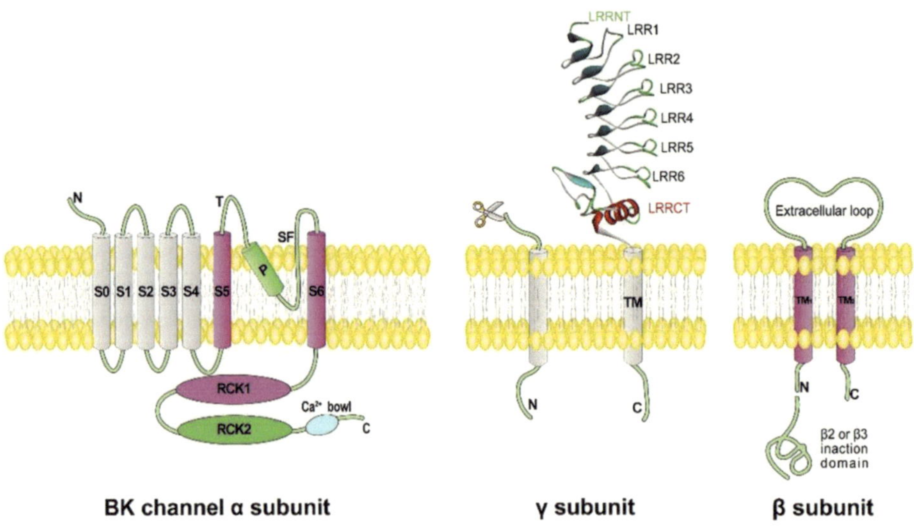

Figure 3.
Structure of BK channel and its auxiliary subunits. BK channel topology predicted by the hydrophilicity profiles (left). The α helices are represented by a cylindrical shape and S0 to S4 segments (gray column) make up the voltage sensor domain. The turret (T) is the loop joining S5 with the pore helix (P) (green column). The selective filter (SF) and S6 form the pore internal entryway. N terminal is located at the extracellular, and C terminal is located at cytosolic. Intracellular domain forms a pair of RCK domains including a Ca^{2+} bowl (light blue ellipse), one of the intracellular calcium-binding regions. Topology of auxiliary β subunits (right). NH_2 and COOH terminus facing intracellular side, two transmembrane domains linked by an extensive extracellular loop. At the NH_2 terminus, β2 and β3 subunits contain additional amino acids that constitute the particle of inactivation. The topological structure shared by all subtypes of γ subunits: after selective cleavage, the γ subunits only have one transmembrane segment, with LRRC domains and the NH2 terminus facing the extracellular side. The homology model of LRRC domain was established by using the crystal structure underlying the LRR domain from lymphocyte receptor B59 of hagfish variable (PDB ID: 2O6S) [70]. The homology modeling of LRRC domain is acquired by using Discovery Studio 2017 R2.

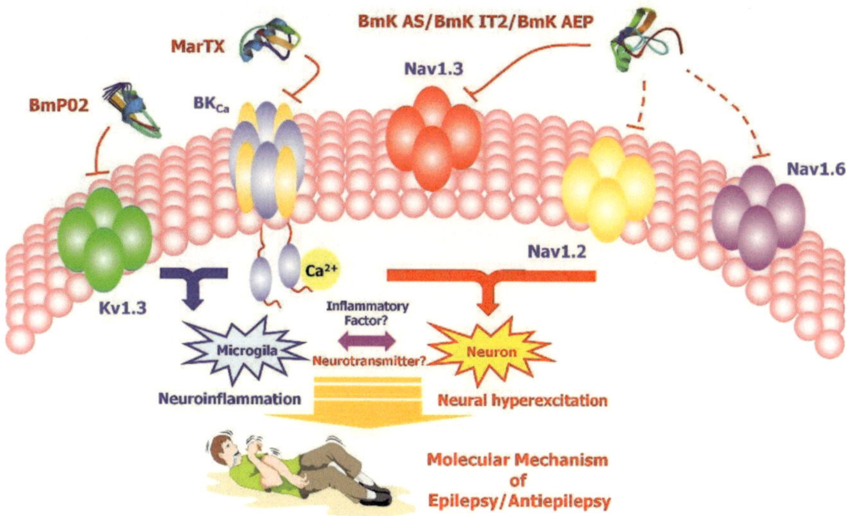

Figure 4.
Antiepilepsy effects of BmK venom toxins by targeting Na^+/K^+ channels. Long-chain β toxins BmK IT2/BmK AS/BmK AEP could reduce the epileptic seizure by inhibiting the activities of VGSCs. The specific BK channel blocker MarTX, a short-chain BmK toxin, suppressed the epilepsy by acting on the fAHPs and rapid spike repolarization of neurons, which might affect the activation of microglia through BK channels. BmP02, a Kv1.3 inhibitor, has potential antiepileptic effects also by regulating the activation of microglia.

PTZ-induced epileptic animal models, and reversed the elevated neuronal firing which follows tonic-clonic seizures [69, 71].

Martentoxin, a polypeptide consisting of 37 residues isolated from the venom of BmK, could selectively block iberiotoxin-insensitive BK channel subtye (α + β4) [33, 72], with no obvious effects on BK channels with α subunit alone. In animal model experiments, martentoxin could prolong the latency and decrease the duration, as well as seizure numbers, especially the high stage seizure, of seizures induced by PTZ. The attitude and the duration of epileptic discharge are both decreased by intra-hippocampal injection with martentoxin [73] (**Figure 4**).

4. Anti-multiple sclerosis and stroke via Kv1.3

4.1 Anti-multiple sclerosis effects of BmK Kv1.3 blockers

Multiple sclerosis (MS), a neuroinflammatory demyelinating disease, is the second most common neurological disease. The occurrence of multiple sclerosis is often accompanied by the destruction of the blood-brain barrier (BBB) and the infiltration of the central nervous system by reactive T cell [74]. These cells rapidly produce large amounts of pro-inflammatory cytokines, such as IFN-γ and IL-4, inducing sebaceous lesions or damage by targeting myelin basic proteins, thereby promoting shedding.

The potassium channel Kv1.3 was first discovered in human T-cells in 1984 [75]. Accumulated data display Kv1.3 in myelin-reactive T cells from the peripheral blood (PB) underlying MS patients is more highly expressed compared with healthy people [76]. In animal model of experimental autoimmune encephalitis (EAE), it has also been confirmed that the expression of Kv1.3 is significantly elevated [77]. Kv1.3 blocks membrane depolarization and maintains the driving force for Ca^{2+} entry by effluxing K^+, which in turn participates in T cell activation, Ca^{2+} activation signaling cascade, leading to T cell proliferation and cytokine production [78, 79]. These findings make Kv1.3 a valuable potential therapeutic target for immunosuppression in MS and EAE [80]. The therapeutic efficacy of Kv1.3 channel blockers has been evidenced by not only in *in vitro* assays on suppressing cytokine secretion and the proliferation of T cells, but also by *in vivo* experiments on diverse animal models of autoimmune diseases [81–85].

A variety of animal toxin peptides have been found to have the same channel target. The venoms of different species such as scorpions, anemones, snakes, and cone snails constitute a peptide damper for Kv1.3 [86–88]. Studies have shown that different toxin peptides have different affinities for the Kv1.3 channel and can inhibit Kv1.3 in the picomolar to nanomolar range [89].

BmKTX is an α-KTx toxin purified from the venom of BmK with 37 amino acids, which has an amidated C-terminal, and blocks Kv1.3 current with nanomolar concentration [90, 91]. However, in addition to being selective for Kv1.3, BmKTX also has affinity for other K+ channels, which promotes the design as well as appearance of highly selective BmKTX structural analogs [92]. The BmKTX D33H variant was produced by replacing the Asp33 residue with His in BmKTX. The selectivity of this novel BmKTX analog is 10,000-fold higher than wild-type BmKTX for targeting Kv1.3 [92, 93]. ADWX-1, a novel peptide based on the scorpion toxin BmKTX, replaces three residues of BmKTX (Gly 11, Ile 28, and Asp 33) with Arg 11, Thr 28, and His 33. The ADWX-1 peptide not only has a picomolar affinity (IC 50, 1.89 pm) for blocking Kv1.3, but its activity is increased 100-fold compared to the native BmKTX toxin [94]. More importantly, ADWX-1 also showed good selectivity on Kv1.3 compared to the related Kv1.1 and Kv1.2 channels. The data show that both BmKTX-D33H and ADWX-1 can effectively inhibit the activation and subsequent proliferation of human and rat CD4 + CCR7-TEM cells and the secretion of cytokines [93, 94]. It is similar to the pharmacological properties of ShK-186, an anemone toxin analog that has been used in clinical research as a novel drug for the treatment of autoimmune diseases [95]. In addition, ADWX-1 can selectively inhibit the activation of effector memory T cells by inhibiting Kv1.3, thereby significantly improving the symptoms of experimental autoimmune encephalomyelitis (EAE) in a rat model [84, 93]. The results above illuminated that BmKTX-D33H as well as ADWX-1 have the potential for clinical treatments of Kv1.3-related channel diseases.

BmP02, also referred to α-KTx9.1, is a short peptide toxin from the BmK scorpion. It is comprised of 28 amino acids, whose tertiary structure is stabilized by 3 disulfide bonds [21, 96]. It was found that it has nanomolar affinity for Kv1.3 [35, 97]. Functional characterization of BmP02 as a highly selective and potent Kv1.3-targeted peptide will help develop novel therapeutic agents for human autoimmune diseases.

4.2 Anti-stroke potential of BmK Kv1.3 blockers

Stroke is an acute cerebrovascular disorder that causes brain tissue damage, which is the second leading disease causing sudden death after ischemic heart disease and accounts for 9% of deaths worldwide [83]. Ischemic stroke is the most common type of stroke, usually occurring when the blood vessels in the neck or brain are blocked [98]. In the early stages of stroke, activated macrophages or microglial cells (M1 type) release a variety of inflammatory factors (TNF-α, IL-1-β, IL-23), trigger neuronal damage, and induce TEM cell-mediated further inflammatory responses [99]. A few days later, macrophages could change to M2-like functions, begin to clear various inflammatory factors, cell debris, and secrete anti-inflammatory as well as neurotrophic factors (IL-10, TGF-β, IGF-1) to promote injury recovery [99].

Kv1.3 plays important roles in microglia as well as macrophage activation by modulating Ca^{2+} signaling, oxidative burst, cytokine production, and neuronal killing [100–102], which is required for microglia or macrophage M1-like pro-inflammatory activation *in vivo* [103]. Activated microglia in the pathology of ischemic stroke significantly contributes to secondary expansion of the infarct, and Kv1.3 blockers are thought to be useful in ameliorating this condition [104, 105]. Studies have shown that while Kv1.3 inhibitors preferentially inhibit "M1-like" inflammatory microglia/macrophage functions they can preserve beneficial "M2-like" functions [106, 107].

BmP02 and BmKTX act as BmK K^+ channel toxins that can effectively inhibit Kv1.3. We speculate that they and their derivatives may also reduce pro-inflammatory factors and improve brain damage by inhibiting the M1-like function of microglia or macrophages.

5. Anti-glioma activity

Glioma shows the general characteristics of tumor cells, with the difference being that the specific chloride channel current (CCC) is a unique electrophysiological feature of glioma cells. The current intensity always increases with the increase of malignant degree of glioma [108]. The specific type of chloride channel on glioma cells can regulate the morphology and volume of cells, which are involved in the process of tumor cell proliferation and metastasis. Abnormal expression of chloride channel currents in glioma could be regarded as a kind of chloride channel disease, especially in glioma with high malignancy [109]. Therefore, it may provide a novel idea for the diagnosis and treatment of glioma by blocking its specific chloride channel current, from the perspective of ion channel disease.

BmK chloride channel toxins, BmK CT, are short-chain neurotoxin proteins composed of 36 amino acids and contain 4 pairs of disulfide bonds, which have 68% homology with chlorotoxin (CTX), a chloride channel toxin isolated from scorpion *Leiurus quinquestriatus*. BmK CT could not only specifically block the glioma chloride channels, but also recognize the matrix metalloproteinases-2 (MMP-2) for inhibiting glioma migration [110, 111]. The recombinant protein GST-BmK CT significantly suppresses on tumor growth in nude mice, with an inhibition rate of 86% *in vivo*. The tumor metastasis in the lung lesion area was only 38% in the BmK CT-treated group compared to 75% in the control group [112]. In addition, BmK CT could promote the sensitivity of chemotherapeutic drug temozolomide-induced cell apoptosis of glioma U251 cells *in vitro*, which is through inhibiting the AKT signaling pathway [113]. On the one hand, the specific inhibition of the proliferation and metastasis of glioma cells suggests BmK CT as an ideal candidate to treat glioma. On the other hand, due to the abundant expression of chloride channels in glioma cells, BmK CT is also used for imaging and treating glioma by conjugating it with Cy5.5, FND, or 131I/125I [114].

6. Proposal

Up to now, there are 15 venom-derived drugs used to treat a variety of diseases, including hypertension, pain, and diabetes, in clinic. As a result, many lives have been saved. In addition, 13 animal-derived toxins are considered to be drug candidates, and have entered clinical trials [115]. Among them, scorpion toxin chlorotoxin, isolated from *Leiurus* quinquestriatus, is under phase II clinical trial. It was reported that Iodine-131-chlorotoxin (TM-601) is a targeted drug candidate for the treatment of gliomas because it could cross the blood-brain as well as some tissue barriers and specifically bind to malignant brain tumor cells without influencing the function of normal cells [116]. ShK derivatives, ShK-186 and ShK-192, are mainly used to treat autoimmune diseases, including neuroinflammatory multiple sclerosis by targeting Kv1.3 channels. In this review, we discuss the possibility of BmK scorpion toxins for clinical treatment on ion channel-relevant neurological disorders. It is shown that long-chain scorpion toxins, such as BmK IT2 and BmK AS, could effectively suppress neuroexcitability in nociception and epileptic seizure via VGSCs. *In vivo* study demonstrated that inhibition of Kv1.3 is favorable for the reversion of neuroinflammatory diseases by BmKTX and BmP02. It is also found that BmK CT could specifically suppress proliferation as well as metastasis of glioma cells. This brings the dawn to the effective control of neurological diseases suspected of overcoming, such as chronic pain, MS, intractable epilepsy, and giloma.

However, it is still a challenge for BmK toxins used to the treatment of neurology disorders. The first problem underlying the application of these peptides is that they could not be taken orally, mainly because they are difficult to penetrate the intestinal mucosa. Due to their molecular size, polarity, hydrophilicity, and chargeability, the cell membrane penetration of BmK toxins is hampered. The second obstacle is that BmK toxins cannot cross the blood-brain barrier. Different from multiple sclerosis, the myelin and blood-brain barrier are not destroyed in other neurological diseases [117]. Clinical application of BmK toxins for treating these diseases will encounter difficulties. Fortunately, the situation is not unsolvable, we still have a glimmer of light. A few years ago, scientists at the Sunnybrook Health Science Center in Canada used focused ultrasound technology to successfully pass chemotherapy drugs across the blood-brain barrier in a non-invasive manner [118] and reach the location of the tumor, which is of great significance in the field of neuropharmacology. In addition, the cell penetrating peptide (CPP) [119] with a strong cell membrane penetration, could be used as a drug carrier to assist the passage of polypeptide drugs across the cell membrane [117]. The fusion protein consists of CPP and BmK toxin might be developed as an oral drug for treating neurological disorders. In short, finding suitable, safe, and efficient ways to promote the clinical use of BmK toxins are most valuable points to be solved.

Acknowledgements

This work was supported by National Science Foundation of China (Nos. 81603410 and 31771191); Youth Talent Promotion Project of China Association of Chinese Medicine; Shanghai Municipal Commission of Health and Family Planning Fund (Nos. 20184Y0086, 2016JP007 and 2018JQ003); Project for Capacity Promotion of Putuo District Clinical Special Disease; Project within budget of Shanghai University of Traditional Chinese Medicine (Nos. 18TS086 and 18-DX-06); the Key Speciality Program (No. 2016102A); and Research Project (Nos. 2016208A, 2018314 and 2018313) of Putuo Hospital, Shanghai University of Traditional Chinese Medicine.

Conflict of interest

The authors confirm that they have no conflict of interest with regard to this chapter's content.

Author details

Xiaoli Wang[1,2], Shuzhang Zhang[2], Yudan Zhu[1], Zhiping Zhang[2], Mengyao Sun[1], Jiwei Cheng[1], Qian Xiao[1], Guoyi Li[1] and Jie Tao[1*]

1 Department of Neurology and Central Laboratory, Putuo Hospital, Shanghai University of Traditional Chinese Medicine, Shanghai, China

2 Institute of Biomembrane and Biopharmaceutics, Shanghai University, Shanghai, China

*Address all correspondence to: jietao_putuo@foxmail.com

References

[1] Zhang S, Zhang Z, Shen Y, et al. SCN9A epileptic encephalopathy mutations display a gain-of-function phenotype and distinct sensitivity to oxcarbazepine. Neuroscience Bulletin. 2020;**36**(1):11-24. DOI: 10.1007/s12264-019-00413-5

[2] Zhou G, Jiao Y, Zhou Y, et al. Up-regulation of Akt and Nav1.8 in BmK I-induced pain. Neuroscience Bulletin. 2018;**34**(3):539-542. DOI: 10.1007/s12264-018-0222-x

[3] Hatta S, Sakamoto J, Horio Y. Ion channels and diseases. Medical Electron Microscopy. 2002;**35**(3):117-126. DOI: 10.1007/s007950200015

[4] Wulff H, Christophersen P. Recent developments in ion channel pharmacology. Channels (Austin, Tex.). 2015;**9**(6):335. DOI: 10.1080/19336950.2015.1077650

[5] Lewis RJ, Garcia ML. Therapeutic potential of venom peptides. Nature Reviews. Drug Discovery. 2003;**2**(10): 790-802. DOI: 10.1038/nrd1197

[6] He XL, Li HM, Zeng ZH, et al. Crystal structures of two alpha-like scorpion toxins: Non-proline cis peptide bonds and implications for new binding site selectivity on the sodium channel. Journal of Molecular Biology. 1999;**292**(1):125-135. DOI: 10.1006/jmbi.1999.3036

[7] Landon C, Cornet B, Bonmatin JM, et al. 1H-NMR-derived secondary structure and the overall fold of the potent anti-mammal and anti-insect toxin III from the scorpion *Leiurus quinquestriatus* quinquestriatus. European Journal of Biochemistry. 1996;**236**(2):395-404

[8] Karbat I, Frolow F, Froy O, et al. Molecular basis of the high insecticidal potency of scorpion alpha-toxins. The Journal of Biological Chemistry. 2004;**279**(30):31679-31686. DOI: 10.1074/jbc.M402048200

[9] Zhu J, Tong X, Cao C, et al. Solution structure of BmKalphaTx11, a toxin from the venom of the Chinese scorpion *Buthus martensii* Karsch. Biochemical and Biophysical Research Communications. 2010;**391**(1):627-633. DOI: 10.1016/j.bbrc.2009.11.110

[10] Housset D, Habersetzer-Rochat C, Astier JP, et al. Crystal structure of toxin II from the scorpion *Androctonus australis* Hector refined at 1.3 Å resolution. Journal of Molecular Biology. 1994;**238**(1):88-103. DOI: 10.1006/jmbi.1994.1270

[11] Krimm I, Gilles N, Sautiere P, et al. NMR structures and activity of a novel alpha-like toxin from the scorpion *Leiurus quinquestriatus* hebraeus. Journal of Molecular Biology. 1999;**285**(4):1749-1763. DOI: 10.1006/jmbi.1998.2418

[12] Karbat I, Turkov M, Cohen L, et al. X-ray structure and mutagenesis of the scorpion depressant toxin LqhIT2 reveals key determinants crucial for activity and anti-insect selectivity. Journal of Molecular Biology. 2007;**366**(2):586-601. DOI: 10.1016/j.jmb.2006.10.085

[13] Ye P, Hua L, Jiao Y, et al. Functional up-regulation of Nav1.8 sodium channel on dorsal root ganglia neurons contributes to the induction of scorpion sting pain. Acta Biochimica et Biophysica Sinica. 2016;**48**(2):132-144. DOI: 10.1093/abbs/gmv123

[14] Ye P, Jiao Y, Li Z, et al. Scorpion toxin BmK I directly activates Nav1.8 in primary sensory neurons to induce neuronal hyperexcitability in rats. Protein and Cell. 2015;**6**(6):443-452. DOI: 10.1007/s13238-015-0154-4

[15] Jablonsky MJ, Watt DD, Krishna NR. Solution structure of an old world-like neurotoxin from the venom of the new world scorpion *Centruroides sculpturatus* Ewing. Journal of Molecular Biology. 1995;**248**(2):449-458

[16] Dang B, Kubota T, Mandal K, et al. Elucidation of the covalent and tertiary structures of biologically active Ts3 toxin. Angewandte Chemie (International Ed. in English). 2016;**55**(30):8639-8642. DOI: 10.1002/anie.201603420

[17] Wang Y, Chen X, Zhang N, et al. The solution structure of BmTx3B, a member of the scorpion toxin subfamily alpha-KTx 16. Proteins. 2005;**58**(2):489-497. DOI: 10.1002/prot.20322

[18] Xu Y, Wu J, Pei J, et al. Solution structure of BmP02, a new potassium channel blocker from the venom of the Chinese scorpion *Buthus martensi* Karsch. Biochemistry. 2000;**39**(45):13669-13675. DOI: 10.1021/bi000860s

[19] Lippens G, Najib J, Wodak SJ, et al. NMR sequential assignments and solution structure of chlorotoxin, a small scorpion toxin that blocks chloride channels. Biochemistry. 1995;**34**(1):13-21. DOI: 10.1021/bi00001a003

[20] Norton RS, Chandy KG. Venom-derived peptide inhibitors of voltage-gated potassium channels. Neuropharmacology. 2017;**127**:124-138. DOI: 10.1016/j.neuropharm.2017.07.002

[21] Fuller MD, Thompson CH, Zhang ZR, et al. State-dependent inhibition of cystic fibrosis transmembrane conductance regulator chloride channels by a novel peptide toxin. The Journal of Biological Chemistry. 2007;**282**(52):37545-37555. DOI: 10.1074/jbc.M708079200

[22] Goudet C, Chi CW, Tytgat J. An overview of toxins and genes from the venom of the Asian scorpion *Buthus martensi* Karsch. Toxicon. 2002;**40**(9):1239-1258

[23] Rjeibi I, Mabrouk K, Mosrati H, et al. Purification, synthesis and characterization of AaCtx, the first chlorotoxin-like peptide from *Androctonus australis* scorpion venom. Peptides. 2011;**32**(4):656-663. DOI: 10.1016/j.peptides.2011.01.015

[24] Zhijian C, Feng L, Yingliang W, et al. Genetic mechanisms of scorpion venom peptide diversification. Toxicon. 2006;**47**(3):348-355. DOI: 10.1016/j.toxicon.2005.11.013

[25] Deuis JR, Mueller A, Israel MR, et al. The pharmacology of voltage-gated sodium channel activators. Neuropharmacology. 2017;**127**:87-108. DOI: 10.1016/j.neuropharm.2017.04.014

[26] Housley DM, Housley GD, Liddell MJ, et al. Scorpion toxin peptide action at the ion channel subunit level. Neuropharmacology. 2017;**127**:46-78. DOI: 10.1016/j.neuropharm.2016.10.004

[27] He Y, Zou X, Li X, et al. Activation of sodium channels by alpha-scorpion toxin, BmK NT1, produced neurotoxicity in cerebellar granule cells: An association with intracellular Ca^{2+} overloading. Archives of Toxicology. 2017;**91**(2):935-948. DOI: 10.1007/s00204-016-1755-2

[28] Ji YH, Hattori H, Xu K, et al. Molecular characteristics of four new depressant insect neurotoxins purified from venom of *Buthus martensi* Karsch by HPLC. Science in China Series B, Chemistry, Life Sciences and Earth Sciences. 1994;**37**(8):955-963

[29] Cestele S, Catterall WA. Molecular mechanisms of neurotoxin action on voltage-gated sodium channels. Biochimie. 2000;**82**(9-10):883-892

[30] Chen J, Feng XH, Shi J, et al. The anti-nociceptive effect of BmK AS, a

scorpion active polypeptide, and the possible mechanism on specifically modulating voltage-gated Na^+ currents in primary afferent neurons. Peptides. 2006;**27**(9):2182-2192. DOI: 10.1016/j.peptides.2006.03.026

[31] Tan ZY, Xiao H, Mao X, et al. The inhibitory effects of BmK IT2, a scorpion neurotoxin on rat nociceptive flexion reflex and a possible mechanism for modulating voltage-gated Na^+ channels. Neuropharmacology. 2001;**40**(3):352-357. DOI: 10.1016/s0028-3908(00)00168-4

[32] Zhang F, Wu Y, Zou X, et al. BmK AEP, an anti-epileptic peptide distinctly affects the gating of brain subtypes of voltage-gated sodium channels. International Journal of Molecular Sciences. 2019;**20**(3). DOI: 10.3390/ijms20030729

[33] Tao J, Zhou ZL, Wu B, et al. Recombinant expression and functional characterization of martentoxin: A selective inhibitor for BK channel (alpha + beta4). Toxins (Basel). 2014;**6**(4):1419-1433. DOI: 10.3390/toxins6041419

[34] Wu B, Zhu Y, Shi J, et al. BmP02 atypically delays Kv4.2 inactivation: Implication for a unique interaction between scorpion toxin and potassium channel. Toxins (Basel). 2016;**8**(10). DOI: 10.3390/toxins8100280

[35] Wu B, Wu BF, Feng YJ, et al. Mapping the interaction anatomy of BmP02 on Kv1.3 channel. Scientific Reports. 2016;**6**:29431. DOI: 10.1038/srep29431

[36] Cummins TR, Sheets PL, Waxman SG. The roles of sodium channels in nociception: Implications for mechanisms of pain. Pain. 2007;**131**(3):243-257. DOI: 10.1016/j.pain.2007.07.026

[37] Ji YH, Liu T. The study of sodium channels involved in pain responses using specific modulators. Sheng Li Xue Bao. 2008;**60**(5):628-634

[38] Krafte DS, Bannon AW. Sodium channels and nociception: Recent concepts and therapeutic opportunities. Current Opinion in Pharmacology. 2008;**8**(1):50-56. DOI: 10.1016/j.coph.2007.09.007

[39] Bai ZT, Zhang XY, Ji YH. Fos expression in rat spinal cord induced by peripheral injection of BmK I, an alpha-like scorpion neurotoxin. Toxicology and Applied Pharmacology. 2003;**192**(1):78-85

[40] Zhang XY, Zhang JW, Chen B, et al. Dynamic determination and possible mechanism of amino acid transmitter release from rat spinal dorsal horn induced by the venom and a neurotoxin (BmK I) of scorpion *Buthus martensi* Karsch. Brain Research Bulletin. 2002;**58**(1):27-31. DOI: 10.1016/s0361-9230(02)00752-9

[41] Ji YH, Li YJ, Zhang JW, et al. Covalent structures of BmK AS and BmK AS-1, two novel bioactive polypeptides purified from Chinese scorpion *Buthus martensi* Karsch. Toxicon: Official Journal of the International Society on Toxinology. 1999;**37**(3):519-536

[42] Chen B, Ji Y. Antihyperalgesia effect of BmK AS, a scorpion toxin, in rat by intraplantar injection. Brain Research. 2002;**952**(2):322-326

[43] Liu T, Pang XY, Jiang F, Bai ZT, Ji YH, et al. Anti-nociceptive effects induced by intrathecal injection of BmK AS, a polypeptide from the venom of Chinese-scorpion *Buthus martensi* Karsch, in rat formalin test. Journal of Ethnopharmacology. 2008;**117**(2):332-338

[44] Liu ZR, Tao J, Dong BQ, Ding G, Cheng ZJ, He HQ, et al. Pharmacological kinetics of BmK

AS, a sodium channel site 4-specific modulator on Nav1.3. Neuroscience Bulletin. 2012;**28**(3):209-221

[45] Zhu MM, Tao J, Tan M, Yang HT, Ji YH, et al. U-shaped dose-dependent effects of BmK AS, a unique scorpion polypeptide toxin, on voltage-gated sodium channels. British Journal of Pharmacology. 2009;**158**(8):1895-1903

[46] Cohen L, Gilles N, Karbat I, Ilan N, Gordon D, Gurevitz M, et al. Direct evidence that receptor site-4 of sodium channel gating modifiers is not dipped in the phospholipid bilayer of neuronal membranes. The Journal of Biological Chemistry. 2006;**281**(30):20673-20679

[47] Gordon D, Moskowitz H, Eitan M, Warner C, Catterall WA, Zlotkin E. Localization of receptor sites for insect-selective toxins on sodium channels by site-directed antibodies. Biochemistry. 1992;**31**(33):7622-7628

[48] Li YJ, Tan ZY, Ji YH. The binding of BmK IT2, a depressant insect-selective scorpion toxin on mammal and insect sodium channels. Neuroscience Research. 2000;**38**(3):257-264

[49] Chai ZF, Bai ZT, Liu T, Pang XY, Ji YH, et al. The binding of BmK IT2 on mammal and insect sodium channels by surface plasmon resonance assay. Pharmacological Research. 2006;**54**(2):85-90

[50] Bai ZT, Liu T, Pang XY, Chai ZF, Ji YH. Suppression by intrathecal BmK IT2 on rat spontaneous pain behaviors and spinal c-Fos expression induced by formalin. Brain Research Bulletin. 2007;**73**(null):248-253

[51] He H, Liu Z, Dong B, Zhang J, Shu X, Zhou J, et al. Localization of receptor site on insect sodium channel for depressant β-toxin BmK IT2. PLoS One. 2011;**6**(1):e14510

[52] Meng H, Xu HQ, Yu L, et al. The SCN1A mutation database: Updating information and analysis of the relationships among genotype, functional alteration, and phenotype. Human Mutation. 2015;**36**(6):573-580. DOI: 10.1002/humu.22782

[53] Liao Y, Deprez L, Maljevic S, et al. Molecular correlates of age-dependent seizures in an inherited neonatal-infantile epilepsy. Brain. 2010;**133**(Pt 5):1403-1414. DOI: 10.1093/brain/awq057

[54] Veeramah KR, O'Brien JE, Meisler MH, et al. De novo pathogenic SCN8A mutation identified by whole-genome sequencing of a family quartet affected by infantile epileptic encephalopathy and SUDEP. American Journal of Human Genetics. 2012;**90**(3):502-510. DOI: 10.1016/j.ajhg.2012.01.006

[55] Zhou XH, Yang D, Zhang JH, et al. Purification and N-terminal partial sequence of anti-epilepsy peptide from venom of the scorpion *Buthus martensii* Karsch. The Biochemical Journal. 1989;**257**(2):509-517. DOI: 10.1042/bj2570509

[56] Wang CG, He XL, Shao F, et al. Molecular characterization of an anti-epilepsy peptide from the scorpion *Buthus martensi* Karsch. European Journal of Biochemistry. 2001;**268**(8):2480-2485. DOI: 10.1046/j.1432-1327.2001.02132.x

[57] Zhao R, Weng CC, Feng Q, et al. Anticonvulsant activity of BmK AS, a sodium channel site 4-specific modulator. Epilepsy and Behavior. 2011;**20**(2):267-276. DOI: 10.1016/j.yebeh.2010.12.006

[58] Liu ZR, Zhang H, Wu JQ, et al. PKA phosphorylation reshapes the pharmacological kinetics of BmK AS, a unique site-4 sodium channel-specific modulator. Scientific Reports. 2014;**4**:3721. DOI: 10.1038/srep03721

[59] Zhao R, Zhang XY, Yang J, et al. Anticonvulsant effect of BmK IT2, a sodium channel-specific neurotoxin, in rat models of epilepsy. British Journal of Pharmacology. 2008;**154**(5):1116-1124. DOI: 10.1038/bjp.2008.156

[60] Blatz AL, Magleby KL. Ion conductance and selectivity of single calcium-activated potassium channels in cultured rat muscle. The Journal of General Physiology. 1984;**84**(1):1-23. DOI: 10.1085/jgp.84.1.1

[61] Marty A. The physiological role of calcium-dependent channels. Trends in Neurosciences. 1989;**12**(11):420-424

[62] Sah P, McLachlan EM. Potassium currents contributing to action potential repolarization and the afterhyperpolarization in rat vagal motoneurons. Journal of Neurophysiology. 1992;**68**(5):1834-1841. DOI: 10.1152/jn.1992.68.5.1834

[63] Adams PR, Constanti A, Brown DA, et al. Intracellular Ca^{2+} activates a fast voltage-sensitive K^+ current in vertebrate sympathetic neurones. Nature. 1982;**296**(5859):746-749. DOI: 10.1038/296746a0

[64] Storm JF. Action potential repolarization and a fast after-hyperpolarization in rat hippocampal pyramidal cells. The Journal of Physiology. 1987;**385**:733-759. DOI: 10.1113/jphysiol.1987.sp016517

[65] Lancaster B, Nicoll RA. Properties of two calcium-activated hyperpolarizations in rat hippocampal neurones. The Journal of Physiology. 1987;**389**:187-203. DOI: 10.1113/jphysiol.1987.sp016653

[66] Quirk JC, Reinhart PH. Identification of a novel tetramerization domain in large conductance K(ca) channels. Neuron. 2001;**32**(1):13-23

[67] Tseng-Crank J, Foster CD, Krause JD, et al. Cloning, expression, and distribution of functionally distinct Ca^{2+}-activated K^+ channel isoforms from human brain. Neuron. 1994;**13**(6):1315-1330

[68] Tian L, Duncan RR, Hammond MS, et al. Alternative splicing switches potassium channel sensitivity to protein phosphorylation. The Journal of Biological Chemistry. 2001;**276**(11):7717-7720. DOI: 10.1074/jbc.C000741200

[69] Amberg GC, Santana LF. Downregulation of the BK channel beta1 subunit in genetic hypertension. Circulation Research. 2003;**93**(10):965-971. DOI: 10.1161/01.res.0000100068.43006.36

[70] Kim HM, Oh SC, Lim KJ, et al. Structural diversity of the hagfish variable lymphocyte receptors. The Journal of Biological Chemistry. 2007;**282**(9):6726-6732. DOI: 10.1074/jbc.M608471200

[71] Watanabe I, Zhu J, Sutachan JJ, et al. The glycosylation state of Kv1.2 potassium channels affects trafficking, gating, and simulated action potentials. Brain Research. 2007;**1144**:1-18. DOI: 10.1016/j.brainres.2007.01.092

[72] Shi J, He HQ, Zhao R, et al. Inhibition of martentoxin on neuronal BK channel subtype (alpha+beta4): Implications for a novel interaction model. Biophysical Journal. 2008;**94**(9):3706-3713. DOI: 10.1529/biophysj.107.122150

[73] Zhu Y, Zhang S, Feng Y, et al. The Yin and Yang of BK channels in epilepsy. CNS and Neurological Disorders Drug Targets. 2018;**17**(4):272-279. DOI: 10.2174/1871527317666180213142403

[74] Huang J, Han S, Sun Q, et al. Kv1.3 channel blocker (ImKTx88) maintains blood-brain barrier in experimental autoimmune encephalomyelitis. Cell and Bioscience. 2017;7:31. DOI: 10.1186/s13578-017-0158-2

[75] DeCoursey TE, Chandy KG, Gupta S, et al. Voltage-gated K+ channels in human T lymphocytes: A role in mitogenesis? Nature. 1984;**307**(5950):465-468. DOI: 10.1038/307465a0

[76] Wulff H, Calabresi PA, Allie R, et al. The voltage-gated Kv1.3 K+ channel in effector memory T cells as new target for MS. The Journal of Clinical Investigation. 2003;**111**(11):1703-1713. DOI: 10.1172/jci16921

[77] Rus H, Pardo CA, Hu L, et al. The voltage-gated potassium channel Kv1.3 is highly expressed on inflammatory infiltrates in multiple sclerosis brain. Proceedings of the National Academy of Sciences of the United States of America. 2005;**102**(31):11094-11099. DOI: 10.1073/pnas.0501770102

[78] Bozic I, Tesovic K, Laketa D, et al. Voltage gated potassium channel Kv1.3 is upregulated on activated astrocytes in experimental autoimmune encephalomyelitis. Neurochemical Research. 2018;**43**(5):1020-1034. DOI: 10.1007/s11064-018-2509-8

[79] Wulff H, Castle NA, Pardo LA. Voltage-gated potassium channels as therapeutic targets. Nature Reviews. Drug Discovery. 2009;**8**(12):982-1001. DOI: 10.1038/nrd2983

[80] Beeton C, Wulff H, Standifer NE, et al. Kv1.3 channels are a therapeutic target for T cell-mediated autoimmune diseases. Proceedings of the National Academy of Sciences of the United States of America. 2006;**103**(46):17414-17419. DOI: 10.1073/pnas.0605136103

[81] Tudor JE, Pallaghy PK, Pennington MW, et al. Solution structure of ShK toxin, a novel potassium channel inhibitor from a sea anemone. Nature Structural Biology. 1996;**3**(4):317-320

[82] Kalman K, Pennington MW, Lanigan MD, et al. ShK-Dap22, a potent Kv1.3-specific immunosuppressive polypeptide. The Journal of Biological Chemistry. 1998;**273**(49):32697-32707. DOI: 10.1074/jbc.273.49.32697

[83] Schmitz A, Sankaranarayanan A, Azam P, et al. Design of PAP-1, a selective small molecule Kv1.3 blocker, for the suppression of effector memory T cells in autoimmune diseases. Molecular Pharmacology. 2005;**68**(5):1254-1270. DOI: 10.1124/mol.105.015669

[84] Li Z, Liu WH, Han S, et al. Selective inhibition of CCR7− effector memory T cell activation by a novel peptide targeting Kv1.3 channel in a rat experimental autoimmune encephalomyelitis model. The Journal of Biological Chemistry. 2012;**287**(35):29479-29494. DOI: 10.1074/jbc.M112.379594

[85] Pennington MW, Chang SC, Chauhan S, et al. Development of highly selective Kv1.3-blocking peptides based on the sea anemone peptide ShK. Marine Drugs. 2015;**13**(1):529-542. DOI: 10.3390/md13010529

[86] Cao Z, Yu Y, Wu Y, et al. The genome of *Mesobuthus martensii* reveals a unique adaptation model of arthropods. Nature Communications. 2013;**4**:2602. DOI: 10.1038/ncomms3602

[87] Varga Z, Gurrola-Briones G, Papp F, et al. Vm24, a natural immunosuppressive peptide, potently and selectively blocks Kv1.3 potassium channels of human T cells. Molecular Pharmacology. 2012;**82**(3):372-382. DOI: 10.1124/mol.112.078006

[88] Rodriguez de la Vega RC, Schwartz EF, Possani LD. Mining on scorpion venom biodiversity. Toxicon: Official Journal of the International Society on Toxinology. 2010;**56**(7):1155-1161. DOI: 10.1016/j.toxicon.2009.11.010

[89] Mouhat S, Andreotti N, Jouirou B, et al. Animal toxins acting

on voltage-gated potassium channels. Current Pharmaceutical Design. 2008;**14**(24):2503-2518

[90] Romi-Lebrun R, Lebrun B, Martin-Eauclaire MF, et al. Purification, characterization, and synthesis of three novel toxins from the Chinese scorpion *Buthus martensi*, which act on K^+ channels. Biochemistry. 1997;**36**(44):13473-13482. DOI: 10.1021/bi971044w

[91] Gao B, Peigneur S, Tytgat J, et al. A potent potassium channel blocker from *Mesobuthus eupeus* scorpion venom. Biochimie. 2010;**92**(12):1847-1853. DOI: 10.1016/j.biochi.2010.08.003

[92] Chen Z, Hu Y, Hu J, et al. Unusual binding mode of scorpion toxin BmKTX onto potassium channels relies on its distribution of acidic residues. Biochemical and Biophysical Research Communications. 2014;**447**(1):70-76. DOI: 10.1016/j.bbrc.2014.03.101

[93] Ye F, Hu Y, Yu W, et al. The scorpion toxin analogue BmKTX-D33H as a potential Kv1.3 channel-selective immunomodulator for autoimmune diseases. Toxins. 2016;**8**(4):115. DOI: 10.3390/toxins8040115

[94] Han S, Yi H, Yin SJ, et al. Structural basis of a potent peptide inhibitor designed for Kv1.3 channel, a therapeutic target of autoimmune disease. The Journal of Biological Chemistry. 2008;**283**(27):19058-19065. DOI: 10.1074/jbc.M802054200

[95] Shen B, Cao Z, Li W, et al. Treating autoimmune disorders with venom-derived peptides. Expert Opinion on Biological Therapy. 2017;**17**(9):1065-1075. DOI: 10.1080/14712598.2017.1346606

[96] Romi-Lebrun R, Martin-Eauclaire MF, Escoubas P, et al. Characterization of four toxins from *Buthus martensi* scorpion venom, which act on apamin-sensitive Ca^{2+}–activated K^+ channels. European Journal of Biochemistry. 1997;**245**(2):457-464. DOI: 10.1111/j.1432-1033.1997.00457.x

[97] Zhu L, Gao B, Luo L, et al. Two dyad-free shaker-type K^+ channel blockers from scorpion venom. Toxicon. 2012;**59**(3):402-407. DOI: 10.1016/j.toxicon.2011.11.016

[98] Wallace AN, Kansagra AP, McEachern J, et al. Evolution of endovascular stroke therapies and devices. Expert Review of Medical Devices. 2016;**13**(3):263-270. DOI: 10.1586/17434440.2016.1143772

[99] Man SM, Karki R, Kanneganti TD. Molecular mechanisms and functions of pyroptosis, inflammatory caspases and inflammasomes in infectious diseases. Immunological Reviews. 2017;**277**(1):61-75. DOI: 10.1111/imr.12534

[100] Kirk J, Plumb J, Mirakhur M, et al. Tight junctional abnormality in multiple sclerosis white matter affects all calibres of vessel and is associated with blood-brain barrier leakage and active demyelination. The Journal of Pathology. 2003;**201**(2):319-327. DOI: 10.1002/path.1434

[101] Ortiz GG, Pacheco-Moises FP, Macias-Islas MA, et al. Role of the blood-brain barrier in multiple sclerosis. Archives of Medical Research. 2014;**45**(8):687-697. DOI: 10.1016/j.arcmed.2014.11.013

[102] Peelen E, Damoiseaux J, Smolders J, et al. Th17 expansion in MS patients is counterbalanced by an expanded $CD39^+$ regulatory T cell population during remission but not during relapse. Journal of Neuroimmunology. 2011;**240-241**:97-103. DOI: 10.1016/j.jneuroim.2011.09.013

[103] Di Lucente J, Nguyen HM, Wulff H, et al. The voltage-gated potassium channel Kv1.3 is required for microglial pro-inflammatory activation in vivo. Glia. 2018;**66**(9):1881-1895. DOI: 10.1002/glia.23457

[104] Macrez R, Ali C, Toutirais O, et al. Stroke and the immune system: From pathophysiology to new therapeutic strategies. The Lancet Neurology. 2011;**10**(5):471-480. DOI: 10.1016/s1474-4422(11)70066-7

[105] Iadecola C, Anrather J. The immunology of stroke: From mechanisms to translation. Nature Medicine. 2011;**17**(7):796-808. DOI: 10.1038/nm.2399

[106] Chen YJ, Nguyen HM, Maezawa I, et al. Inhibition of the potassium channel Kv1.3 reduces infarction and inflammation in ischemic stroke. Annals of Clinical Translational Neurology. 2018;**5**(2):147-161. DOI: 10.1002/acn3.513

[107] Murray PJ, Allen JE, Biswas SK, et al. Macrophage activation and polarization: Nomenclature and experimental guidelines. Immunity. 2014;**41**(1):14-20. DOI: 10.1016/j.immuni.2014.06.008

[108] Saberbaghi T, Wong R, Rutka JT, et al. Role of Cl^- channels in primary brain tumour. Cell Calcium. 2019;**81**:1-11. DOI: 10.1016/j.ceca.2019.05.004

[109] Ullrich N, Sontheimer H. Biophysical and pharmacological characterization of chloride currents in human astrocytoma cells. The American Journal of Physiology. 1996;**270**(5 Pt 1):C1511-C1521. DOI: 10.1152/ajpcell.1996.270.5.C1511

[110] Olsen ML, Schade S, Lyons SA, et al. Expression of voltage-gated chloride channels in human glioma cells. The Journal of Neuroscience. 2003;**23**(13):5572-5582

[111] Mamelak AN, Jacoby DB. Targeted delivery of antitumoral therapy to glioma and other malignancies with synthetic chlorotoxin (TM-601). Expert Opinion on Drug Delivery. 2007;**4**(2):175-186. DOI: 10.1517/17425247.4.2.175

[112] Fan S, Sun Z, Jiang D, et al. BmKCT toxin inhibits glioma proliferation and tumor metastasis. Cancer Letters. 2010;**291**(2):158-166. DOI: 10.1016/j.canlet.2009.10.011

[113] Du J, Wang R, Yin L, et al. BmK CT enhances the sensitivity of temozolomide-induced apoptosis of malignant glioma U251 cells in vitro through blocking the AKT signaling pathway. Oncology Letters. 2018;**15**(2):1537-1544. DOI: 10.3892/ol.2017.7483

[114] Cheng Y, Zhao J, Qiao W, et al. Recent advances in diagnosis and treatment of gliomas using chlorotoxin-based bioconjugates. American Journal of Nuclear Medicine and Molecular Imaging. 2014;**4**(5):385-405

[115] King GF. Venoms as a platform for human drugs: Translating toxins into therapeutics. Expert Opinion on Biological Therapy. 2011;**11**(11):1469-1484. DOI: 10.1517/14712598.2011.621940

[116] Mamelak AN, Rosenfeld S, Bucholz R, et al. Phase I single-dose study of intracavitary-administered iodine-131-TM-601 in adults with recurrent high-grade glioma. Journal of Clinical Oncology. 2006;**24**(22):3644-3650. DOI: 10.1200/JCO.2005.05.4569

[117] Li S, Hou H, Mori T, et al. Swedish mutant APP-based BACE1 binding site peptide reduces APP beta-cleavage and cerebral Abeta levels in Alzheimer's mice. Scientific Reports. 2015;**5**:11322. DOI: 10.1038/srep11322

[118] Burgess A, Shah K, Hough O, et al. Focused ultrasound-mediated drug delivery through the blood-brain barrier. Expert Review of Neurotherapeutics. 2015;**15**(5):477-491. DOI: 10.1586/14737175.2015.1028369

[119] Kristensen M, Birch D, Morck Nielsen H. Applications and challenges for use of cell-penetrating peptides as delivery vectors for peptide and protein cargos. International Journal of Molecular Sciences. 2016;**17**(2). DOI: 10.3390/ijms17020185

Chapter 8

Mechanisms of Cyanotoxin Toxicity—Carcinogenicity, Anticancer Potential, and Clinical Toxicology

Deyana Georgieva Vankova, Milena Gincheva Pasheva, Yoana Dimitrova Kiselova-Kaneva, Dobri Lazarov Ivanov and Diana Georgieva Ivanova

Abstract

Cyanoprokaryotes are distributed worldwide and they produce various bioactive compounds, including cyanotoxins. The major route of human exposure to cyanotoxins is the oral intake by using contaminated drinking water, by incidental intake of contaminated water during recreational and professional activities, and by consuming contaminated food or dietary supplements prepared from cyanobacteria. The prolonged chronic exposure to low concentrations of cyanotoxins provokes cell damage and may increase the risk for cancer development. Due to the variety of cyanotoxin chemical structures, different mechanisms of their toxic effects are known. At the same time, some of the natural compounds produced by cyanoprokaryotes have anticancer potential and are promising sources for the development of novel drugs. This chapter is dedicated to the target mechanisms behind the effects of the widely distributed cyanotoxins with an impact on human health, microcystins, nodularins, and cylindrospermopsin.

Keywords: cyanotoxins, microcystins, nodularins, cylindrospermopsin, toxicity mechanisms

1. Introduction

Cyanoprokaryotes are Gram-negative photosynthetic algae considered to have arisen approximately 3.5 billion years ago [1]. In nature, they are found as single cell species or as colonies rapidly growing in fresh water, all types of aquatic ecosystems, and terrestrial habitats. Cyanobacteria are photosynthetic organisms, and as such, they are considered primary first-level consumers in the food chains in water ecosystems. Blue-green algae play an important role in carbon and nitrogen balance in the biosphere [2]. They produce a high number of bioactive molecules, and certain species produce cyanotoxins that contribute as defense mechanisms against different ambient stress factors [3]. The growth of cyanobacteria at high blooming densities increases in expansion and frequency following anthropogenic activities and climatic change, globalization, and increasing commodity exchanges [4]. This, in turn, raises morbidity and death rates of wild and domestic animals [5, 6] and brings some risk to human health.

More than 90 microcystin isoforms, that are cyclic peptide cyanotoxins, have been described. The microcystin-leucine arginine (MC-LR) is known as the most toxic and the most abundant variant of microcystins [7]. Several authors have reported that MC-LR has been considered as the most widely spread microcystin in Portuguese waters [8]. However, Rodrigues et al. report similar results for microcystin MC-RR (a MC variant with the amino acid arginine in positions 2 and 4) [9]. MC-RR is the major toxin variant found in the rivers, lakes, and reservoirs in China [10] reaching concentrations of up to 93.5% in the cells of cyanoprokaryotes [11], thus associated with the contamination produced by intensive use of water sources and fast economic development [12]. In Bulgaria, a country rich in water reservoirs and natural water bodies, many cases of cyanoprokaryote blooms have been reported. Surveys conducted for a period of 15 years (2000–2015) in 120 Bulgarian water basins have recorded cyanobacteria blooms in 14 water bodies and have identified 16 cyanotoxins (microcystins LR, LA, RR, YR, nodularins, and saxitoxins) [13].

Cyanotoxins have various chemical structures; thus, their toxic effects are due to different mechanisms. Cyanotoxins are classified into three major groups according to their chemical structure: alkaloids (cylindrospermopsin, saxitoxin, lyngbyatoxin-a, and aplysiatoxin,), cyclic peptides (microcystins, MCs, and nodularins—NODs), and lipopolysaccharides [14]. Poisoning of humans with cyanotoxins is possible through various pathways, mainly by the consumption of contaminated food (vegetables, fish, seafood, and livestock), as well by bathing and recreational activities with contaminated water [15]. Different studies have reported high accumulation of cylindrospermopsin (CYN) in fish (up to 2.7 ng/g) [16], in mussels (up to 2.52 mg/g) [17], and in lettuce (up to 8.029 μg/kg) [18].

Along with the reports about the toxicity of cyanobacteria metabolites, there are studies describing their anticancer properties, hence, viewing them from a new perspective as novel potential sources for anticancer drug development [19]. However, to identify possible drug targets, the science about the mechanisms of the toxicity needs to be extracted out of the numerous scientific reports and review studies on cyanobacteria blooms, case studies and investigations on the effects of cyanotoxins described by different authors.

This review addresses the target mechanisms behind the effects of widely distributed groups of cyanotoxins with an impact on human health, the cyclic peptides microcystins and nodularins, and the alkaloid cylindrospermopsin.

Data collection was performed through keyword research, namely cyanotoxins, microcystins, nodularins, cylindrospermopsin, cyanotoxins/microcystins/nodularins/cylindrospermopsin molecular mechanisms/carcinogenicity/anticancer potential/clinical toxicology/poisoning incidence/clinical toxicology. ScienceDirect and PubMed databases were screened for the above-mentioned key words. More than 100 papers were examined and bibliography includes references dating back to 1878.

2. Water blooms, human and animal health

A great number of studies about cyanotoxins discuss their toxicity from different points of view. Clinical intoxication cases and epidemiological studies on reported cases of exposure to cyanobacteria and their toxins are described [20]. There are reports on acute poisonings of animals and humans due to exposure to cyanotoxins [21, 22]. Chronic intake of contaminated water; aerosolization, including respirable bioaerosols; consumption of contaminated seaborne food [23]; or even intake of dietary supplements containing blue-green algae are investigated and reported [24].

Observational studies on the correlation between clinical symptoms and contact with blooming water have been recorded throughout the centuries. The earliest report on such poisoning dates back 1000 years ago in China when green-colored river water consumption caused mortality in General Zhu Ge-Ling's troops, according to data reviewed on the website of National Toxicology Program, Department of Health and Human Services of USA [25]. Later in 1878, cyanotoxin poisoning was suspected in Australia [26]. In several US states, gastroenteritis has been suspected to be related to water blooms [27]. In China, primary liver cancer has been attributed to cyanotoxin-contaminated drinking water [28]. In a profound recent review, Svircev et al. [20] identified 42 publications that describe 33 cases of cyanotoxin poisoning in 11 countries—Australia, Brazil, Canada, China, Namibia, Portugal, Serbia, Sri Lanka, Sweden, the UK, and the USA for the period between 1960 and 2016. Although there is no definitive general conclusion in the epidemiological literature, it identifies a possible link between microcystins and cancer and other human health issues [20]. Wood [21] presents an informative table summarizing reports about acute animal and human poisonings attributed to exposure to cyanotoxins since 1800; there is an estimate of the number of affected animals and individuals in incidents of mortality and morbidity from 1900 onwards. The author identified 115 human incidents of cyanotoxin intoxications reported until the year 2010, mostly seen in the United States and Canada, followed by Europe [21]. Taking into account the great variety of cyanobacteria and their overall environmental distribution in fresh and brackish waters and the fact that more than 90 different types of cyanotoxins are produced by the blue-green algae, the various routes of cyanotoxin poisoning, as well as the variety of clinical manifestations encountered, we may expect that the above numbers are quite underestimated. In Varna region, Bulgaria, no evidences to related cases of acute poisoning to cyanotoxins have been documented according to local database [118]. Furthermore, it is not always easy to derive information about countries classified by Woods as "the rest of world," especially when information dated back centuries ago. Sometimes, data are published in the gray literature and in the local language; data available are not supported by adequate scientific information. Often clinical evidences of inflammatory response or allergic reactions are misleading for being common symptoms for other types of intoxications as well; such clinical cases remain in the group of *idiopathic* intoxications and are not reported as cases of cyanoprokaryota poisonings. Cyanobacteria content in the total mass of phytoplankton in different waters and sampling periods may vary up to 100%. Usually, in algae blooms, one species predominates and it releases various cytotoxins to the water. Some toxins have been detected even after the end of algae blooms, when cyanoprokaryota species are already in negligible concentrations [13].

Few reports describe correlation between defined clinical symptoms and/or laboratory findings and a reported contact and/or consumption of contaminated water. The most severe human intoxication with cyanotoxins occurred in Brazil in 1996, where 100 of 131 dialysis patients developed acute hepatic failure due to cyanotoxin contamination of the dialysis water applied. The death of 52 of them has been confirmed to be due to the presence on cyanotoxins in treatment water provided from a local water treatment plant [29, 30]. Another incidence, again in Brazil, associates 2000 cases of gastroenteritis and 88 deaths with blooms [31]. *Microcystis aeruginosa*–contaminated water caused pneumonia in two patients in Staffordshire, England [32]. In Australia, 140 children and 10 adults have experienced liver and kidney problems. Cylindrospermopsin is reportedly the etiological agent [33]. Giannuzzi et al. [34] report a case from Argentina in 2007. Microcystin-LR is detected in water samples, where the patient has been immersed before experiencing acute clinical symptoms. In addition, laboratory examination identified increase of markers for liver injury (ALT, AST, and GGT).

3. Cyclic peptides—toxicity and biotransformations

The cyclic pentapeptide nodularins and cyclic heptapeptide microcystins are the most widespread cyanotoxins in water blooms. MCs are produced by different cyanobacterial species (*Microcystis, Oscillatoria, Aphanocapsa, Cyanobium, Arthrospira, Limnothrix, Phormidium, Hapalosiphon, Anabaenopsis, Nostoc, and Synechocystis*). It is known that nodularins are produced only by cyanobacteria from the genus *Nodularia* (*Nodularia spumigena*) [35]. Various investigations reveal approx. 100 known variants of MCs up-to-date with the most toxic and widely distributed MC being MC-LR [36]. The maximum concentration of MC-LR is up to 1 μg/L in drinking water. This is the conditional guideline value adopted by the World Health Organization (WHO). The value is based on tolerated daily intake (TDI) 0.04 μg/kg body weight [37].

Most of the microcystins have hydrophilic structure; thus, their cell uptake should be facilitated by transporting systems, such as the organic anion transporting polypeptides (OATPs). Many OATPs are expressed in a tissue-specific way, whereas others are expressed ubiquitously [38]. A selective uptake of MCs by the cells, depending on the organ type and on the expression of different OATPs, is established in intestines, liver, muscle, and brain cells of three different catfish species [39]; the highest contents are found in liver, gonads, stomach, heart, and kidneys in Wistar rats [40]. The fact that MC accumulation is primarily in the liver is explained by the amount of OATPs present in this organ, which is why MCs are considered as hepatotoxins. More specifically, the MC-LR has been determined as a substrate for OATP1A2, OATP1B1, and OATP1B3. MCs are established to require active transport for human cell uptake, and the high expression of these OATP1B1 and OATP1B3 transporters in the liver accounts for their selective liver toxicity [41, 42]. Researches reveal that OATP1B1 and OATP1B3 expression is detected in cell lines originating from liver, colon, and pancreatic tumors [43], as well as in hepatocellular carcinoma [44]. These results account for microcystin toxicity to be examined mainly in hepatocytes *in vivo* and in cultured hepatic cells *in vitro*.

The liver of the fish species *O. bonariensis*, collected from a shallow lake in Argentina, contained 10 times higher MC-RR levels than the muscles, reports a study [45]. Another study, on mice, elucidates that 9% of the MC-LR toxin fraction is filtrated in the kidneys and eliminated through urine, thus making kidneys a possible object for MC-LR toxicity as well [46]. Pflugmacher et al. [47] determine that the first stage in the detoxification of MCs is the formation of a glutathione conjugate of MC (MC-LR-GSH) in hepatocytes, identified earlier in mice and in rat livers [48]. MC-LR-GSH is then further metabolized to a cysteine conjugate (MC-LR-Cys) for excretion via urine [49], via feces as well, as free MCs or their metabolites [50].

Chronic exposure to sublethal doses of MCs could lead to induction of oxidative stress, necrotic cell death, and liver neoplasia in animals [51] and a possible reason for that could be the depletion of GSH cell stores. A study demonstrates the bioaccumulation of microcystin-LR (MC-LR) in mammals [52]. A pig experimental model has been used because of its liver, kidney, and gastrointestinal tract function similarities to humans, as well as similarities to humans' metabolic rates [53]. Although MC-LR is not found in the serum of treated animals, free MC-LR is detected in the large intestine and kidneys, in liver as well, where the MC-LR-glutathione conjugate is in high quantity, approximately 1.1% of the applied MC-LR dose. The chemical structures of unabsorbed MCs are not modified, or few changes occur. MCs are transported to the intestine and further are excreted by feces. The other route is absorption and subsequent conjugation in the liver and rapid excretion of this compound in the bile [54]. MC-LR and its derivatives (MC-LR-GSH and MC-LR-Cys) may also enter the enterohepatic circulation and, being reabsorbed into the blood stream, may reach the brain, heart, lungs, and even testicles [55].

Animal studies mark the possible MC-LR accumulation in human hepatic tissue exposed chronically to high doses of cyanotoxins as well. Present-day study analyses daily exposure to MCs and their effects on human health; authors identify the presence of MCs in anglers' serum, most likely resulting from exposure to ingested MC from consumed fish [56]. Serum enzymes aspartate aminotransferase, alanine aminotransferase, lactate dehydrogenase, and alkaline phosphatase, which are biomarkers of hepatic function, are elevated, pointing to liver damage in the fishermen. The smaller ring structure of NODs is taken up by the liver cells more easily than MC-LR, thus probably resulting in stronger hepatocellular effects [57]. Another research provides evidence that MC-LR can be transported across the blood-brain barrier in humans [41].

3.1 Cyclic peptides—molecular toxicity mechanism in relation to carcinogenicity

Different mechanisms of cytotoxicity are observed among MC variants and nodularins in a range of *in vitro* cell culture studies on cell viability and the ability to cause apoptosis or necrosis in varying concentrations applied to different cell types. Fastner et al. [58] explicates that primary rat hepatocytes are less susceptible to MC-RR (EC_{50} 1500–4300 nM) compared to MC-LR (EC_{50} 60–200 nM). Independently of the cell culture type (primary or transfected hepatocytes), MC-RR is always less cytotoxic than MC-LR [59]. Gacsi et al. [60] have studied the effects of MC-LR on cultured Chinese hamster ovary cells (CHO-K1) in order to detect cell viability and to determine if nonviable cells go through necrosis or apoptosis. The study demonstrates that low dose of MC-LR (<10 μM) after 24 h exposure does not induce apoptosis in the cell line. The application of higher MC-LR concentrations (⩾20 μM) shows induced apoptosis in a concentration-dependent manner. The shrinkage of apoptotic cells is linked to the shortening and loss of actin filaments and microtubule depolymerization. No necrosis is observed over the concentration range tested. Piyathilaka et al. [61] evaluates the MC-LR cytotoxic and apoptotic effects on different human kidney cell lines—normal embryotic (HEK-293) and adenocarcinoma cell line (ACHN). The MTT and sulforhodamine B (SRB) cell viability assays establish that MC-LR is more cytotoxic to embryonic kidney cells compared to kidney adenocarcinoma cells after treatment with MC-LR for 24 h. In addition, morphological studies also reveal higher MC-LR toxicity to kidney cancer cells than to normal kidney cells. MC-LR does not promote cell division of human kidney adenocarcinoma cells, indicating that it cannot be a promoter of kidney cancer [61].

NODs and MCs are among the most common natural cyanotoxins. Their toxicity is mainly due to the ability to inhibit the eukaryotic protein serine/threonine phosphatase families 1 and 2A (PP1 and PP2A), which are essential for many signal transduction pathways of eukaryotic cells. This inhibition is linked to protein hyperphosphorylation, thus leading to modification of cytoskeleton and disturbances of many cellular processes: loss of cell-cell adhesion at the desmosomes [62], disruption of actin filaments [63], and altered cell signaling pathways, for example MAPKs signaling pathways that regulate cellular proliferation [55]. As potent inhibitors of protein serine/threonine phosphatase, MCs and NODs have a profound effect on cell signaling leading to the affected cell's death. Both MC-LR and NOD have inhibitory effect on protein phosphatases, independently that MC-LR binds covalently to them and NOD does not [64].

Cell signaling pathways involving MAPKs regulate cellular proliferation through phosphorylation cascades. Several types of phosphatases including the protein serine/threonine phosphatases 2A regulate the Ras-Raf-MEK-ERK cascade (PP2A). The phosphatase PP2A inhibits these pathways by dephosphorylation. The activated (phosphorylated) forms of the transcription factor ERK1/2 are translocated to the cell nucleus, thus leading to the transcription of certain proto-oncogenes [65]. Junttila et al. [66] speculate that by inhibiting PP2A, MC-LR could deregulate the ERK1/2 pathway, thus promoting cell proliferation and tumorigenesis.

NODs and MCs also play a role as potential oxidants, which could induce reactive oxygen species production, hence causing cell oxidative stress damages [67]. Many studies demonstrate that oxidative stress is involved in the liver cell toxicity due to MCs [68] and NODs [67]. Increased production of reactive oxygen species (ROS) and lipid peroxides in mouse liver because of treatment with NODs is observed [69].

MCs may increase the production of ROS by depletion of GSH due to a high rate of conjugation [8, 67]. These observations are confirmed in zebrafish [70], where MC administration leads to lipid peroxidation and a change in the antioxidant enzyme activity [71]. A study explicates MC-RR influence on gene expression of nuclear factor—erythroid 2 related factor 2 (Nrf2), a master regulator of inducible antioxidant responses, in human hepatocytes, causing mitochondria dysfunction [72]. The transcription factor Nrf2 has been identified as a key factor in the cell protection from oxidative stress and electrophilic insults [73, 74]. Many of Nrf2 target genes play essential role in maintaining cellular antioxidant responses and xenobiotic metabolism. Its constitutive activation may contribute to a malignant phenotype [75], and its elevated expression and activity have been observed in different cancer cells [76]. Nrf2 promotes the survival of tumor cells under a deleterious environment and elevates resistance to antitumor drugs [77]. These observations suggest that Nrf2 plays contrasting roles in different tumorigenesis stages and is subject to MCs' toxicity with predictable effect on further tumorigenesis.

Gan et al. have shown that MC-LR is able to enhance the stability of the Nrf2 transcription factor in the cytoplasm and its translocation to the nucleus via binding to the cytosolic regulator protein Keap1. Knockdown of Nrf2 mediated by siRNA can inhibit cell proliferation and cell cycle progression induced by MC-LR [78]. Therefore, upregulation of Nrf2 induced by MC-LR in tumor cells favors liver cancer cell growth. This study gives additional information supporting Nrf2 role in cancer tumorigenesis [78], respectively, of MC-LR. Moreover, a higher level of Nrf2 in toxin-treated rat primary hepatocytes after 48 h has been observed [79]. It is assumed that inhibition of protein phosphatases by MCs may affect the activity of DNA-dependent protein kinase (DNA-PK), an enzyme with key role in the nonhomologous terminal binding of DNA loops in the G_0-phase of the cell cycle observed in human lymphocytes [80].

Another important mechanism of genotoxicity is the impairment of DNA repair. Experimental animals exposed to sublethal low doses of MC have shown to develop tumorigenesis in coordination with the presence of dysfunctional p53 [81]. The increased formation of reactive oxygen species leads to oxidative DNA damage. A study shows that after 4 h of exposure to 0.01, 0.1, and 1 mg/mL of MC-LR DNA strand breaks were induced in dose dependent manner in human liver carcinoma cell line (HepG2 cells) [82]. Oxidized pyrimidines are repaired within a short time of exposure to MCs (8 h), while oxidized purines (mainly 8-hydroxyguanine) remain unrepaired in the DNA and accumulate [83] leading to GC-TA transversion mutations [84]. This statement has been verified *in vivo* with demonstrated elevation of 8-hydroxyguanine in male rat hepatocytes 24 h after treatment with 50 mg/

kg body weight of MC-LR [85]. In primary cultured rat liver cells exposed to NOD, the highest level of 8-oxo-2′-deoxyguanosine adducts is observed after 3 h exposure and its level decreased to control cells' levels after 24 h of exposure [85].

Many studies on MC-LR adverse effects establish its ability to change gene expression, and by these means contribute to a better understanding of MC-LR mechanisms linked to toxicity, genotoxicity, and carcinogenicity potential. Sueoka et al. [86] give the first evidence that MC-LR modulates the expression of tumor suppressor genes and oncogenes. They demonstrate that primary rat liver cells exposed to MC-LR (1 mM) for 6 h remarkably elevated the tumor necrosis factor α (TNF-α) expression, which could play the role of an endogenous tumor promoter [87]. The same study shows upregulation of early-response genes from the *jun* and *fos* gene families, proto-oncogenes, which are involved in gene regulation in response to different stimuli such as growth factors, cytokines, and viral and bacterial infections (**Table 1**).

In summary, one pathway of MC genotoxic activity is mediated by induction of ROS generation, thus leading to DNA strand breaks and at the same time significantly decreasing DNA repair system activity. The impairment of DNA repair together with DNA damage is an important factor involved in tumorigenesis. Chronic exposure to low concentrations of these cyanotoxins may increase the risk for carcinogenesis due to their potential long-term adverse effects (carcinogenic and genotoxic). For this reason, the International Agency for Research on Cancer classifies MC-LR as a possible human carcinogen [88]. **Figure 1** summarizes possible mechanisms of MR-LR genotoxicity with contribution to carcinogenesis.

Experimental model	Time/dose of exposure/method of administration	Main findings	Reference
Male Wistar rats	Single intravenous administration of MC-LR extract; 80 μg/kg body weight	The maximum MC-LR content (2.9% of the injected dose) detected 2 h after injection. Highest concentration found in kidney (0.034–0.295 μg/g dry weight); concentration in liver (0.003–0.052 μg/g dry weight).	[40]
Fish species *O. bonariensis* collected in Los Padres Lake (Argentina)	Fish residing in intoxicated water (MC-LR, -RR, -YR, and -LA total content in water: 2.8 ± 5.6 μg L^{-1})	Total content of MCs in liver (33.6 ± 37.2 μg kg^{-1}) is 10-fold higher than that in the fish muscles (3.9 ± 2.2 μg kg^{-1}).	[45]
Pigs (breed, PIC 337)	Oral administration of MC-LR in two treatment groups: 1. 0.04 μg MC-LR/kg body weight for 13 weeks 2. 2 μg toxin/kg body weight for 5 weeks	MC-LR not detected in serum; free MC-LR found in the large intestine (1.4 μg/kg dry weight) and kidney (1.9 μg/kg dry weight). The higher dosed animals accumulated MC-LR-conjugate in liver (26.4 μg/kg dry weight).	[52]
129-Trp53^{tm1Brd}N4 mice (homozygous p53 knockout B6 mice)	Intraperitoneal injection of MC-LR, 40 μg/kg body weight for 4, 24 h, and 4, 14, and 28 days	Increased proliferative response in liver after 28 days exposure time as detected by increased nuclear Ki-67 immunoreactivity and phosphohistone H3 expression.	[81]

Table 1.
Microcystins in animal studies.

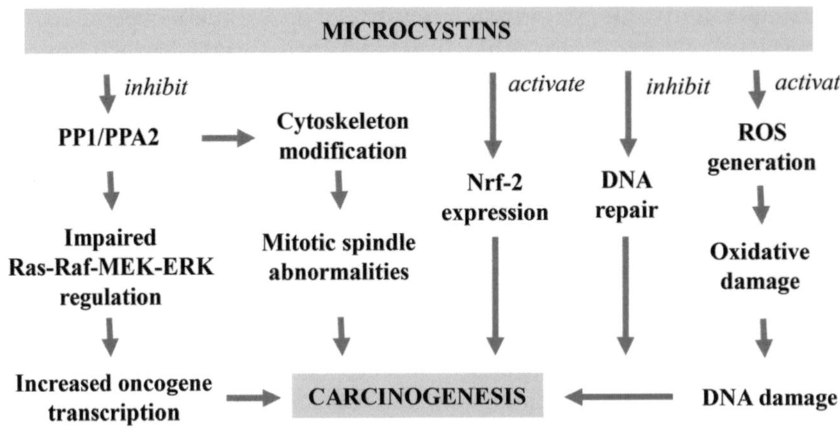

Figure 1.
Mechanisms of microcystin genotoxicity.

3.2 Cyclic peptides—potential sources of anticancer drugs

Essential for candidate molecules to be developed into useful anticancer therapeutics is their cancer selectivity. It is known that specific types of cancer can be targeted by redox-based therapies when cancer cells are assailable by increased ROS production induced by exogenous agents [89]. Thus, microcystin analogues are assumed to be selective anticancer drugs for certain types of cancer cells, specifically for those that express OATP, without causing significant toxicity to normal cells because of the differences of redox status between normal and cancer cells [90]. The development of OATP-targeting compounds based on the chemical structure of MC-LR, with unique physicochemical properties such as high water solubility, resistance to chemical hydrolysis or oxidation at near-neutral pH, and stability in pH shifts, appears to be a feasible and promising option in this direction [91]. There are studies focused on developing analogues of microcystin cyanotoxins for efficiently targeting the OATP-expressing metastatic cancers, which are resistant to conventional chemotherapy treatment [90] and many known cyanotoxins have been studied for their anticancer properties in human cell lines.

Currently, neither optimal nor targeted therapy has been developed for pancreatic cancer [92]. Overexpression of OATPs in pancreatic cancer offers an opportunity to develop effective novel cancer-targeted agents. A study demonstrates that MC-LR targeting OATP1B1 and OATP 1B3 can cause inhibition of proliferation of pancreatic cancer cells in a dose-response mode [92]. Study findings point that antiproliferative and pro-apoptotic effects are proportionally related to the expression of these transporters, thus suggesting an essential role for OATP expression in the process of MC-LR–induced cancer cell damage. Moreover, direct comparison of the inhibitory effect of MC-LR and the drug gemcitabine manifests a noticeable advantage of the toxin [92].

Monks et al. [93] have transfected cervical cancer cell line HeLa with the known OATP1B1 and OATP1B3 transporters seeking through appropriate *in vitro* models how MCs are uptaken into the cells and testing the activity of MCs against cells that express OATPs. Authors elucidate that transfected HeLa cells were 1000-fold more sensitive to MC-LR compared to the vector-transfected control cells, pointing that the expression of transporters imparts marked selectivity for MC cytotoxicity [93]. These observations suggest that MC cytotoxicity in OATP1B1- and OATP1B3-expressing HeLa cells is linked to cell-specific inhibition of PP2A and not to protein phosphatase inhibition in general.

These findings endorse the anticancer potential of MCs and raise hopes that cyanotoxins may have a promising future in cancer therapy. Challenges of potential organ-specific MC toxicity remain to be resolved by proper chemical modifications in the process of drug modulation.

4. Cylindrospermopsin—molecular mechanisms of toxicity and biotransformation

Humans are more susceptible to the exposure to cylindrospermopsin in comparison to other cyanotoxins because up to 90% of the total CYN is found outside the cyanobacterial cells [94]. Humpage et al. [95] recommend a maximum concentration of CYN in drinking water to be 1 μg/L based on tolerated daily intake, 0.03 μg/kg body weight.

CYN is generated by different freshwater cyanobacteria species, which are common worldwide, nowadays [96]. Many cyanotoxins are generally sequestered inside cyanobacteria until death, while cylindrospermopsin can be liberated in water during blooms [97].

CYN is a polycyclic uracil derivative containing guanidino and sulfate groups. The cyanobacterial toxin CYN is a tricyclic alkaloid that consists of a tricyclic guanidine moiety combined with hydroxymethyluracil. CYN has been recognized to induce cytotoxicity *in vitro* in human cell lines from liver and intestine [98]. The toxin primarily attacks the liver, but it is also a general cyanobacterial toxin that targets the spleen, kidney, heart, lungs, thymus, eyes, etc. [99].

The mechanisms of CYN toxicity and genotoxicity are not fully clarified. It is assumed that there are two types of toxic responses. It is established that CYN is more toxic in short-term (1–2 weeks) compared to long-term exposure in cell culture experiments [100]. Rapid toxicity is due to CYP450-generated metabolites [95]. The longer-term toxicity of CYN includes an irreversible inhibition of eukaryotic protein synthesis in *in vitro* experiments [98].

Many studies explore the cytotoxic effect of cylindrospermopsin and they are summarized in **Table 2**. These studies vary in type of cell culture used, time of exposure, concentrations of the CYN, and even the type of cytotoxicity test used.

Most *in vitro* experiments demonstrate that the cytotoxic effect of cylindrospermopsin is observed after long-term exposure (24–72 h). Toxicity of CYN on primary and carcinoma cell line is compared: the primary rat hepatocyte cells are more sensitive to the toxic effect of CYN, compared to KB cell line [101].

Morphological studies are more informative than cytotoxicity studies as they identify the types of cell damage. By means of microscopy, in that respect, pleomorphic nuclei, nucleolar segregation with altered nuclei, depraved Golgi apparatus, and apoptosis in human endothelial cells (HUVEC) after exposure to 0.375 μg/mL, CYN is observed [15]. The same authors also report morphological changes (mitochondrial damage, lipid degeneration, and nucleated segmentation with altered nuclei) in Caco-2 cells after exposure to a higher concentration of CYN (2.5 μg/mL). Absorption of CYN in Caco-2 cells is very limited, which explains the result [105]. Authors report that after cells being exposed to concentration of CYN 1–10 μM for 3, 10, and 24 h, the passage of CYN across the intestinal monolayer is about 2.5% after 3 h and increases slightly up to 20.5% after 24 h.

In search for possible mechanisms of CYN toxicity, it is observed that CYN significantly reduces GSH levels in rats' primary hepatocytes; a decline in the synthesis of GSH is the predominant mechanism, rather than an increased glutathione consumption [106], which could lead to increased oxidative stress. Other authors

Experimental model	Method applied	Experimental conditions	Results	Reference
Primary rat hepatocytes	MTT assay	0–10,000 ng/mL for 24, 48, 72 h exposure	The LC50 is 40 ng/mL; toxic effects are observed after 72 h.	[101]
Primary mouse hepatocytes	MTT assay	1–5 μM/mL	1–5 μM CYN induces concentration-dependent cytotoxicity in 18 h.	[102]
Primary human granulosa cells	MTT assay	0–1 μg/mL for 2, 4, 6, 24, 48, 72 h exposure	There is no effect when cells are exposed up to 1 μg/mL for short time (2–6 h). Cell viability is decreasing in a concentration-dependent way for longer time (24–72 h).	[103]
Hepatic cell lines: C3A and HepG2; colonic cell line: Caco-2	MTT assay	0.4–66 μM for 1, 2, 4, 6, 24 h exposure	The IC50 is 1.5 μM for C3A and HepG2 for 24 h exposure. The IC50 is 6.5 μM for Caco-2 for 25 h exposure.	[98]
CHO K1cells	Annexin V-FITC assay	0.1–10 μM for 12, 18, 24, 48 h exposure	Apoptosis is observed at low concentrations (1–2 μM) and short exposure (12 h). Necrosis is observed at higher concentrations (5–10 μM) and following longer exposure (24 or 48 h).	[60]
KB (human cervix carcinoma) cells	MTT assay	0–10,000 ng/mL for 24, 48, 72 h exposure	The LC50 is 200 ng/mL; toxic effects are observed after 72 h	[101]
HeLa cells	MTT assay	40, 20, 10, 5, 1, and 0.1 mg DW (lyophilized cyanobacterial biomass)/mL (cultivation medium) for 24 h of exposure	The IC50 is 0.2 ± 0.06 mg of lyophilized biomass per milliliter of culture medium.	[104]

MTT (3-(4,5-dimethylthiazol-2-yl)-2,5-diphenyltetrazolium bromide); KB (human cervix carcinoma) cells; C3A (human hepatocellular carcinoma); HepG2 (human liver hepatocellular carcinoma cell line); Caco-2 (human colorectal adenocarcinoma cell line); CHO-K1 (Chinese hamster ovary K1 cells); Annexin V-FITC (fluorescein isothiocyanate labeled annexin V); HeLa (human cervical epithelial adenocarcinoma).

Table 2.
In vitro cytotoxicity studies performed with cylindrospermopsin.

observe different and contradictory effects of CYN on the activity of gamma-glutamylcysteine synthetase (GCS)—the regulatory enzyme in GSH synthesis. In any case, reduction of GSH levels does not contribute significantly for the acute CYN toxicity *in vivo as presumed*, because no changes in the oxidative stress markers after exposure to CYN are evidenced [95].

The role of biotransformation of CYN is an important factor for understanding its toxic effect in cell lines, respectively, in various tissues. Scientific data show that toxicity and genotoxicity of CYN depend on cytochrome P450 (CYP)-mediated metabolism, as various CYP inhibitors can protect cells against toxicity, but it is not yet clear which isoforms are involved [95]. The higher activity of CYP450 in hepatocytes involved in bioactivation events is found to be important for CYN toxicity in liver cell cultures [107]. Many *in vitro* and *in vivo* studies on the toxic mechanisms of CYN prove that metabolites of the toxin produced by CYP450 are mainly responsible for its toxicity, including its genotoxicity. Thus, the activity of the cytochrome P450 enzyme system has been investigated [102], demonstrating that the inhibition of CYP450 activity by proadifen or ketoconazole in mouse hepatocytes reduces the toxicity of CYN but does not alter its effect on protein synthesis. These observations may explain lower CYN toxicity in cell lines such as human cervix carcinoma (KB cells) [101], HeLa cell types [100], and CHO-K1 cells [108] compared to primary rat hepatocytes. Another study reveals that CYP1A1 and CYP1A2 are upregulated in human peripheral blood lymphocytes after CYN exposure [109].

Due to the simultaneous presence of different cyanobacterial toxins in aquatic environment, Hercog et al. [110] investigated the genotoxic potential of MC-LR and CYN mixtures, applied on HepG2 cells. Cells are treated with different doses of CYN, a single dose of MC-LR, and several combinations. A mixture of MC-LR and CYN provokes genotoxic damages, but to a lesser extent in case of strand breaks, compared to CYN itself. Data manifest that MC-LR provoke DNA strand breaks after short-term exposure, while CYN induces DNA damage after prolonged exposure in metabolically active cells [95, 111]. These data point that CYN exhibits higher genotoxic effects compared to MC-LR in the mixture of CYN and MC-LR. The same authors disclose mRNA expression levels of certain genes after 4 and 24 h of exposition to CYN or to MC-LRs, or to a combination of both cyanotoxins. Changes in the expression levels of genes involved in the metabolism of xenobiotic, genes involved in immediate-early response/signaling, and genes involved in response to DNA damage, upon exposure to CYN/MC-LR mixture, are not different to those induced by CYN itself [110], indicating higher genotoxicity of CYN.

In summary, the main target of CYN toxic activity is the liver, and CYN metabolism plays an important part for understanding the mechanisms of its toxicity. Therefore, the activity of CYP450 enzyme system is considered a key mechanism for CYN toxicity development in hepatocyte cultures, including genotoxicity. The higher sensitivity of liver cells exposed to CYN is due to bioactivation-dependent events, research indicates [105]. One of the CYN-known mechanisms is the irreversible inhibition of protein synthesis after long-term exposure [98]. Another mechanism is via oxidative stress induced by inhibiting the regulatory enzyme in GSH synthesis [106]. CYN induces DNA damage after longer exposure in metabolically active cells [95].

4.1 Anticancer properties of cylindrospermopsin

Caco-2 cells and HepG2 are often used human cell lines for cyanotoxin effects research. A study showed that CYN is linked to a variable effect in HepG2 cell line. Cyanotoxin diminishes lipid peroxidation in cells that have not been previously induced by phenobarbital exposure for 12 h and elevates it in phenobarbital-induced cells exposed to the highest CYN concentration (10 μg/L). Lipid peroxidation increases in both cell types after 24 h exposure, only at 10 μg/L CYN [112], demonstrating that the toxicity of low concentrations of CYN (<10 μg/L) is limited in human hepatoma cells. HepG2 cells are more sensitive compared to intestinal cells, while Caco-2 cells are even less sensitive. The observation is associated with the limited CYN uptake in colon cells as described by several authors [105, 113].

Oral intake is the major route of human exposure to CYN, which makes intestine a target organ. Huguet et al. [114] examined the cellular and molecular mechanisms of cylindrospermopsin toxicity on differentiated cell line of human intestinal Caco-2 cells. This cellular monolayer provides *in vitro* model performing functional and morphological characteristics similar to those of enterocytes. Results reveal that differentiated Caco-2 cells exposed for 24 h to a subtoxic cylindrospermopsin concentration overexpress the gene products linked to DNA damage repair, including nucleosomal histone modifications [114]. Bain et al. examined the potential role of p53 tumor suppressor protein in CYN-induced gene expression in human hepatocellular carcinoma cell line [111]. Authors report that after 6 h of exposure to CYN, concentration-dependent increases in mRNA levels are observed for the p53 target genes CDKN1A, MDM2, GADD45alpha (all involved in the response to DNA damage), and BAX (involved in the apoptosis), indicating an early activation of p53 by CYN. The respective levels of mRNA for these genes remain elevated after 24 h. Data suggest that CYN can induce stress responses resulting in activation of the p53 transcription factor [111] and subsequent upregulation of DNA repair processes and activation of apoptosis.

That being said, a 72 h exposure of HepG2 cell line to CYN provokes DNA double strand breaks, providing evidence that CYN can perform as a direct genotoxin [115].

Obviously, available scientific data indicate controversial roles of CYN and its toxicity. CYN can cause severe cell damages, and it has the potential to activate DNA repair processes, which, concerning concentration and time-of-exposure–dependent activities, makes it another promising potential anticancer drug source.

5. Clinical toxicology and pharmacological aspects

Scientific paper analysis reveals some mechanisms linked to exposure to cyanotoxins and their effect on human health. Many episodes of severe poisonings have been registered after acute exposure, associated with adverse effects. Epidemiological studies reveal correlation between cyanotoxins and their toxic effects on human health [20].

Symptoms of poisoning by drinking water are much like those of gastrointestinal disturbances caused by a number of pathogenic bacteria, thus hampering differentiation of poisoning with cyanotoxins. Data for chronic exposure to low cyanobacterial toxin levels are still not well investigated.

Concerning the chemical diversity of cyanotoxins, the pathobiochemical mechanisms for cyanotoxin-associated diseases are variable [116] and the mechanism of toxicity is different. Thus, there is no universal antidote for treatment of cases of cyanobacteria intoxications. One treatment strategy is to apply chemoprotectants, especially for treatment of microcystin intoxications. However, there is less research available on cylindrospermopsin-induced toxicity treatment [99]. Commonly discussed is the application of antioxidants with vitamin E having the strongest protective effect, as oxidative stress is one of the most common pathobiochemical mechanisms of cyanobacteria intoxications. In reference to available knowledge about cellular uptake of cyanotoxins, especially microcystins, transport inhibitors are considered for potential administration in cases of cyanobacteria-related intoxications and in combination with other therapies. The antibiotic rifampin is reported as an example of such a drug approved for clinical use [117].

Due to nondefinitive manifestation of cyanotoxin poisoning, symptomatic treatment is applied, including oxygen application, aiming at respiratory distress amelioration, activated charcoal gastric lavage, forced diuresis for toxin elimination by glomerular filtration, alkalization, and hepatoprotective medication administration [118].

6. Discussion

Cyanobacterial blooms have been registered worldwide for centuries, and a correlation to associated human and animal illness has been suspected. Subsequently, it has been documented that blue-green algae produce various bioactive compounds with the common name cyanotoxins. Taking into account the wide variety of cyanobacteria, their effect on all aquatic ecosystems, and the various manifestation of cyanotoxin poisoning, it is essential to elucidate their toxicity mechanisms, as well as adequate treatment.

Most common and well-examined cyanotoxins are the ones of the microcystin family. Epidemiological studies do not provide definitive confirmation of linkage of acute or chronic exposure to cyanotoxins and human cancer development. Some animal studies demonstrate cyanotoxins' carcinogenic potential. Intraperitoneal injection of MC-LR in sublethal dose causes neoplastic nodules in mouse liver [119]. MC-LR application causes liver cancer in dose-dependent manner in rat model where protein phosphatase type 1 and type 2A activities' inhibition has been established [120]. Inhibition of serine/threonine phosphatase activity is a possible link between toxic and suspected carcinogenic potential of microcystins. Supporting evidences for this hypothesis, for example, are the findings that PP2A phosphatase inhibition by microcystins leads to disruption of MAPK signal transduction pathway [55]. This can be a possible explanation for increased proto-oncogene transcription observed [65] and promoted cell proliferation and tumorigenesis [66] in experiments with this kind of toxins. Considering research limitations of microcystin effects on humans, further investigations and evidence collection are needed to provide more robust correlation between cyanotoxin poisoning and cancer development.

CYN cancer potential has been less studied and not fully explained. It is assumed rather indirect. CYN metabolism and biotransformation with the participation of CYPs generate reactive metabolites and exhaust cellular glutathione. Thus, its toxicity and/or carcinogenic potential may be attributed to generated (geno)toxic metabolites and compromised antioxidant cellular defense.

Cellular penetration of MCs is mediated by tissue-specific OATPs. Overexpression of these transporters in certain cancer cells [92] provides an opportunity for the development of effective novel cancer-targeted agents. In support of this hypothesis, transfection of HeLa cancer cells with OATPs has been established to increase their susceptibility to MC treatment as compared to vector-transfected control cells [93]. More studies in this field are necessary to provide valuable data about MCs' application as anticancer remedies.

7. Conclusions

Cyanobacteria are proved in various habitats, such as drinking water reservoirs and recreational waters, at the basis of food chains, and thus, with a substantial impact on ecosystems and human health. Centurial observations of a correlation between water blooms and health issues in animals and humans are extended in numerous epidemiological, *in vivo* and *in vitro*, studies. Various bioactive compounds under the common name cyanotoxins are established as the reason for blooming water toxicity. Some of the toxic molecular mechanisms for certain cyanotoxins are clarified. Their bioavailability, metabolism, and biotransformation are proved as well. A possible link between cyanotoxin exposure and cancer development has been suspected and there is experimental research data in support of this hypothesis. Yet, cyanobacteria produce natural compounds with promising potential for the discovery of novel anticancer drugs. Improved alertness about cyanotoxin poisoning, its relation to water blooms, poisoning symptoms, and specific treatment is needed in view of adequate human and animal health promotion and health care. Cyanobacteria have already been in the focus of food and pharmaceutical industry and cosmetics for a long time, incorporated in different preparations and food supplements. This requires raised awareness of the population and responsible institutions about the hazards of cyanotoxin contamination regarding food, water, and health remedies.

Acknowledgements

This study was supported by the Bulgarian National Science Fund, Grant No DN13/9, 15.12.2017; project "Cyanoprokaryotes—a new potential risk factor for cancer in Bulgaria?".

Author details

Deyana Georgieva Vankova[1*], Milena Gincheva Pasheva[1], Yoana Dimitrova Kiselova-Kaneva[1], Dobri Lazarov Ivanov[2] and Diana Georgieva Ivanova[1]

1 Department of Biochemistry, Molecular Medicine and Nutrigenomics, Faculty of Pharmacy, Medical University of Varna, Varna, Bulgaria

2 Department of Biology, Faculty of Pharmacy, Medical University of Varna, Varna, Bulgaria

*Address all correspondence to: deyana.vankova@mu-varna.bg

References

[1] Awramik SM. The oldest records of photosynthesis. Photosynthesis Research. 1992;**33**:75-89

[2] Zehr JP, Waterbury JB, Turner PJ, Montoya JP, Omoregie E, Steward GF, et al. Unicellular cyanobacteria fix N2 in the subtropical North Pacific Ocean. Nature. 2001;**412**:635-638

[3] Tan LT. Bioactive natural products from marine cyanobacteria for drug discovery. Phytochemistry Reviews. 2007;**68**:954-979

[4] Meriluoto J, Blaha L, Bojadzija G, Bormans M, Brient L, Codd G, et al. Toxic cyanobacteria and cyanotoxins in European waters—Recent progress achieved through the CYANOCOST action and challenges for further research. Advances in Oceanography and Limnology. 2017;**8**(1):161-178

[5] Carmichael WW. Health effects of toxin-producing cyanobacteria: "The CyanoHABs". Human and Ecological Risk Assessment. 2001;7:1393-1407

[6] Pitois S, Jackson MH, Wood BJB. Sources of the eutrophication problems associated with toxic algae: An overview. Journal of Environmental Health. 2001;**64**:25-32

[7] Dietrich D, Hoeger S. Guidance values for microcystins in water and cyanobacterial supplement products (blue-green algal supplements): A reasonable or misguided approach? Toxicology and Applied Pharmacology. 2005;**203**:273-289

[8] Martins JC, Vasconcelos VM. Microcystin dynamics in aquatic organisms. Journal of Toxicology and Environmental Health. 2009;**12**:65-82

[9] Rodrigues MA, Reis MP, Mateus MC. Liquid chromatography/negative electrospray ionization ion trap MS2 mass spectrometry application for the determination of microcystins occurrence in southern Portugal water reservoirs. Toxicon. 2013;**74**:8-18

[10] Jia J, Chen Q, Lauridsen TL. A systematic investigation into the environmental fate of microcystins and the potential risk: Study in Lake Taihu. Toxins. 2017;**8**(6):170

[11] Liu Y, Chen W, Li D, Huang Z, Shen Y, Liu Y. Cyanobacteria/cyanotoxin contaminations and eutrophication status before Wuxi drinking water crisis in Lake Taihu. Chinese Journal of Environmental Science. 2011;**23**:575-581

[12] Peng L, Liu Y, Chen W, Liu L, Kent M, Song L. Health risks associated with consumption of microcystin-contaminated fish and shellfish in three Chinese lakes: Significance for freshwater aquacultures. Ecotoxicology and Environmental Safety. 2010;**73**:1804-1811

[13] Stoyneva-Gärtner MP, Descy JP, Latli A, Uzunov BA, Pavlova VT, Bratanova Z, et al. Assessment of cyanoprokaryote blooms and of cyanotoxins in Bulgaria in a 15-years period (2000-2015). Advances in Oceanography and Limnology. 2017;**8**(1):1-22

[14] Kaebernick M, Neilan BA. Ecological and molecular investigations of cyanotoxin production. FEMS Microbiology Ecology. 2001;**35**:1-9

[15] Gutiérrez-Praena D, Jos A, Pichardo S, Moreno IM, Cameán AM. Presence and bioaccumulation of microcystins and cylindrospermopsin in food and the effectiveness of some cooking techniques at decreasing their concentrations: A review. Food and Chemical Toxicology. 2013;**53**:139-152

[16] Messineo V, Melchiorre S, Di Corcia A, Gallo P, Bruno M. Seasonal succession of *Cylindrospermopsis raciborskii* and

Aphanizomenon ovalisporum blooms with cylindrospermopsin occurrence in the volcanic Lake Albano, Central Italy. Environmental Toxicology. 2010;**25**:18-27

[17] Saker ML, Metcalf JS, Codd GA, Vasconcelos VM. Accumulation and depuration of the cyanobacterial toxin cylindrospermopsin in the freshwater mussel Anodonta cygnea. Toxicon. 2004;**43**:185-194

[18] Cordeiro-Araújo MK, Chia MA, Bittencourt-Oliveira MC. Potential human health risk assessment of cylindrospermopsin accumulation and depuration in lettuce and arugula. Harmful Algae. 2017;**68**:217-223

[19] El-Deeb NM. Cyanobacterial toxin cylindrospermopsin: It's possible pathway from poisoning to cancer curing. Austin Biomolecules: Open Access. 2016;**1**(2):1009

[20] Svircev Z, Drobac D, Tokodi N, Mijovic B, Codd G, Meriluoto J. Toxicology of microcystins with reference to cases of human intoxications and epidemiological investigations of exposures to cyanobacteria and cyanotoxins. Archives of Toxicology. 2017;**91**:621-650

[21] Wood R. Acute animal and human poisonings from cyanotoxin exposure—A review of the literature. Environment International. 2016;**91**:276-282

[22] Backer LC, Landsberg JH, Miller M, Keel K, Canine TKT. Cyanotoxin poisonings in the United States (1920s–2012)-review of suspected and confirmed cases from three data sources. Toxins. 2013;**5**(9):1597-1628

[23] Mulvenna V, Dale K, Priestly B, Mueller U, Humpage A, Shaw G, et al. Health risk assessment for cyanobacterial toxins in seafood. International Journal of Environmental Research and Public Health. 2012;**9**(3):807-820

[24] Roy-Lachapelle A, Solliec M, Bouchard MF, Sauvé S. Detection of cyanotoxins in algae dietary supplements. Toxins. 2017;**9**(3):76-93

[25] Chorus I, Bartram J. Toxic cyanobacteria in water: A guide to their public health consequences, monitoring and Management. In: Chorus I, Bertram J, editors. World Health Organization. Suffolk, Great Britain: St Edmundsbury Press; 1999. p. 416. Available from: http://www.who.int/iris/handle/10665/42827

[26] Francis G. Poisonous Australian lake. Nature. 1878;**18**:11-12

[27] Billings W. Public health and toxic cyanobacteria. Water-associated human illness in Northeast Pennsylvania and it suspected association with blue-green algae blooms. In: Carmichael WW, editor. Handbook of The Water Environment: Algal Toxins and Health. 1st ed. NY: Plenum Press; 1981. pp. 243-255

[28] Ueno Y, Nagata S, Tsutsumi T, Hasegawa A, Watanabe M, Park H, et al. Detection of microcystins, a blue-green algal hepatotoxin, in drinking water sampled in Haimen and Fusui, endemic areas of primary liver cancer in China, by highly sensitive immunoassay. Carcinogenesis. 1996;**17**(6):1317-1321

[29] Jochimsen EM, Carmichael WW, An JS, Cardo DM, Cookson ST, Holmes CE, et al. Liver failure and death after exposure to microcystins at a hemodialysis center in Brazil. The New England Journal of Medicine. 1998;**338**:873-878

[30] Azevedo SMFO, Carmichael WW, Jochimsen EM, Rinehart KL, Lau S, Shaw GR, et al. Human intoxication by microcystins during renal dialysis treatment in Caruaru, Brazil. Journal of Toxicology. 2002;**181-182**:441-446

[31] Teixera M, Costa M, Carvalho V, Pereira M, Hage E. Gastroenteritis epidemic in the area of the Itaparica dam,

Bahia, Brazil. Bulletin of the Pan American Health Organization. 1993;**27**:244-253

[32] Turner P, Gammie A, Hollinrake K, Codd G. Pneumonia associated with contact with cyanobacteria. British Medical Journal. 1990;**300**:1440-1441

[33] Molica R, Azevedo S. Ecofisiologia de cianobactérias produtoras de cianotoxinas. Oecologia Australis. 2009;**13**:229-246

[34] Giannuzzi L, Sedan D, Echenique R, Andrinolo D. An acute case of intoxication with cyanobacteria and cyanotoxins in recreational water in Salto Grande dam Argentina. Marine Drugs. 2011;**9**:2164-2175

[35] Žegura B, Štraser A, Filipič M. Genotoxicity and potential carcinogenicity of cyanobacterial toxins—A review. Mutation Research. 2011;**727**:16-41

[36] Jaiswal KP, Yadav AS, Gothalwal R. Microcystins: An emerging biomarker and toxicity prediction in human and animal. International Journal of Biotech Trends and Technology. 2016;**17**(1):1-8

[37] WHO. Guidelines for drinking-water quality. In: Recommendations Chemical Fact Sheets. Vol. 1. Geneva, Switzerland: World Health Organization; 2004. pp. 407-408

[38] Obaidat A, Roth M, Hagenbuch B. The expression and function of organic anion transporting polypeptides in normal tissues and in cancer. Annual Review of Pharmacology and Toxicology. 2012;**52**:135-151

[39] Cazenave J, Wunderlin DA, Bistoni MA, Ame MV, Krause E, Pflugmacher S, et al. Uptake, tissue distribution and accumulation of microcystin-RR in *Corydoras paleatus*, *Jenynsia multidentata* and *Odontesthes bonariensis*. Aquatic Toxicology. 2005;**75**:178-190

[40] Wang Q, Xie P, Chen J, Liang G. Distribution of microcystins in various organs (heart, liver, intestine, gonad, brain, kidney and lung) of Wistar rat via intravenous injection. Toxicon. 2008;**52**:721-727

[41] Fischer WJ, Altheimer S, Cattori V, Meier PJ, Dietrich DR, Hagenbuch B. Organic anion transporting polypeptides expressed in liver and brain mediate uptake of microcystin. Toxicology and Applied Pharmacology. 2005;**203**:257-263

[42] Ibelings BW, Chorus I. Accumulation of cyanobacterial toxins in freshwater "seafood" and its consequences for public health: A review. Environmental Pollution. 2007;**150**:177-192

[43] Abe T, Unno M, Onogawa T, Tokui T, Kondo TN, Nakagomi R, et al. LST-2, a human liver-specific organic anion transporter, determines methotrexate sensitivity in gastrointestinal cancers. Journal of Gastroenterology. 2001;**120**:1689-1699

[44] Cui Y, Konig J, Nies AT, Pfannschmidt M, Hergt M, Franke WW, et al. Detection of the human organic anion transporters SLC21A6 (OATP2) and SLC21A8 (OATP8) in liver and hepatocellular carcinoma. Laboratory Investigation. 2003;**83**(4):527-538

[45] Amé MV, Galanti LC, Menone ML, Gerpe MS, Moreno VJ, Wunderlin DA. Microcystin-LR, -RR, -YR and -LA in water samples and fishes from a shallow lake in Argentina. Harmful Algae. 2010;**9**:66-73

[46] Robinson NA, Pace J, Matson CF, Miura GA, Lawrence WB. Tissue distribution, excretion and hepatic biotransformation of microcystin-LR in mice. The Journal of Pharmacology and Experimental Therapeutics. 1990;**256**:176-182

[47] Pflugmacher S, Wiegand C, Oberemm A, Beattie KA, Krause E,

Codd GA, et al. Identification of an enzymatically formed glutathione conjugate of the cyanobacterial hepatotoxin microcystin-LR: The first step of detoxication. Biochimica et Biophysica Acta. 1998;**1425**:527-533

[48] Kondo F, Matsumoto H, Yamada S, Ishikawa N, Ito E, Nagata S, et al. Detection and identification of metabolites of microcystins formed in vivo in mouse and rat livers. Chemical Research in Toxicology. 1996;**9**:1355-1359

[49] He J, Chen J, Xie P, Zhang D, Li G, Wu L, et al. Quantitatively evaluating detoxification of the hepatotoxic microcystins through the glutathione and cysteine pathway in the cyanobacteria-eating bighead carp. Aquatic Toxicology. 2012;**116**:61-68

[50] Li W, He J, Chen J, Xie P. Excretion pattern and dynamics of glutathione detoxification of microcystins in Sprague Dawley rat. Chemosphere. 2018;**191**:357-364

[51] Gehringer MM. Microcystin-LR and okadaic acid-induced cellular effects: A dualistic response. FEBS Letters. 2004;**557**:1-8

[52] Greer B, Meneel JP, Elliott CT. Uptake and accumulation of microcystin-LR based on exposure through drinking water: An animal model assessing the human health risk. Scientific Reports. 2018;**8**:491

[53] Swindle MM, Makin A, Herron AJ, Clubb FJJ, Frazier KS. Swine as models in biomedical research and toxicology testing. Veterinary Pathology. 2012;**49**:344-356

[54] Li W, Xie P, Chen J, He J, Guo X, Yu D, et al. Quantitative liquid chromatography-tandem mass spectrometry method for determination of microcystin-RR and its glutathione and cysteine conjugates in fish plasma and bile. Journal of Chromatography B, Analytical Technologies in the Biomedical and Life Sciences. 2014;**963**:113-118

[55] Menezes C, Elisabete Valério E, Dias E. The Kidney Vero-E6 Cell Line: A Suitable Model to Study the Toxicity of Microcystins. Vol. 2. Rijeka, Croatia: InTechOpen; 2013. pp. 29-48

[56] Chen J, Xie P, Li L, Xu J. First identification of the hepatotoxic microcystins in the serum of a chronically exposed human population together with indication of hepatocellular damage. Toxicological Sciences. 2009;**108**:81-89

[57] Ohta T, Sueoka E, Iida N, Komori A, Suganuma M, Nishiwaki R, et al. Nodularin, a potent inhibitor of protein phosphatases 1 and 2A, is a new environmental carcinogen in male F344 rat liver. Cancer Research. 1994;**54**:6402-6406

[58] Fastner J, Heinze R, Chorus I. Microcystin-content, hepatotoxicity and cytotoxicity of cyanobacteria in some German water bodies. Water Science and Technology. 1995;**32**:165-170

[59] Fischer A, Hoeger SJ, Stemmer K, Feurstein DJ, Knobeloch D, Nussler A, et al. The role of organic anion transporting polypeptides (OATPs/SLCOs) in the toxicity of different microcystin congeners in vitro: A comparison of primary human hepatocytes and OATP-transfected HEK293 cells. Toxicology and Applied Pharmacology. 2010;**245**:9-20

[60] Gacsi M, Antal O, Vasas G, Mathe C, Borbely G, Saker ML, et al. Comparative study of cyanotoxins affecting cytoskeletal and chromatin structures in CHOK1 cells. Toxicology In Vitro. 2009;**23**:710-718

[61] Piyathilaka MAPC, Pathmalal MM, Tennekoon KH, De Silva BGDNK, Samarakoon SR, Chanthirika S.

Microcystin-LR-induced cytotoxicity and apoptosis in human embryonic kidney and human kidney adenocarcinoma cell lines. Microbiologica. 2015;**161**:819-828

[62] Eriksson JE, Toivola D, Meriluoto JAO, Karaki H, Han YG, Hartshorne D. Hepatocyte deformation induced by cyanobacterial toxins reflects inhibition of protein phosphatases. Biochemical and Biophysical Research Communications. 1990;**173**:1347-1353

[63] Buratti FM, Manganelli M, Vichi S, Stefanelli M, Scardala S, Testai M, et al. Cyanotoxins: Producing organisms, occurrence, toxicity, mechanism of action and human health toxicological risk evaluation. Archives of Toxicology. 2017;**91**:1049-1130

[64] Bagu JR, Sykes BD, Craig MM, Holmes CFB. A molecular basis for different interactions of marine toxins with protein phosphatase-1. The Journal of Biological Chemistry. 1997;**272**:5087-5097

[65] Li H, Xie P, Li G, Hao L, Xiong Q. In vivo study on the effects of microcystin extracts on the expression profiles of proto-oncogenes (c-fos, c-Jun and c-myc) in liver, kidney and testis of male Wistar rats injected i.v. with toxins. Toxicon. 2009;**53**:169-175

[66] Junttila MR, Li SP, Westermarck J. Phosphatase-mediated crosstalk between MAPK signalling pathways in the regulation of cell survival. The FASEB Journal. 2008;**22**:954-965

[67] Bouaïcha N, Maatouk I. Microcystin-LR and nodularin induce intracellular glutathione alteration, reactive oxygen species production and lipid peroxidation in primary cultured rat hepatocytes. Toxicology Letters. 2004;**148**:53-63

[68] Ding WX, Shen HM, Zhu HG, Ong CN. Studies on oxidative damage induced by cyanobacteria extract in primary cultured rat hepatocytes. Environmental Research. 1998;**78**:12-18

[69] Lankoff A, Banasik A, Nowak M. Protective effect of melatonin against nodularin-induced oxidative stress in mouse liver. Archives of Toxicology. 2002;**76**:158-165

[70] Pavagadhi S, Gong Z, Hande MP, Dionysiou DD, de la Cruz AA, Balasubramanian R. Biochemical response of diverse organs in adult Danio rerio (zebrafish) exposed to sub-lethal concentrations of microcystin-LR and microcystin-RR a balneation study. Aquatic Toxicology. 2012;**109**:1-10

[71] Valério E, Vasconcelos V, Campos A. New insights on the mode of action of microcystins in animal cells—A review. Medicinal Chemistry. 2016;**16**:1032-1041

[72] Lundqvist J, Pekar H, Oskarsson A. Microcystins activate nuclear factor erythroid 2-related factor 2 (Nrf2) in human liver cells in vitro—Implications for an oxidative stress induction by microcystins. Toxicon. 2017;**126**:47-50

[73] Wild AC, Moinova HR, Mulcahy RT. Regulation of gamma-glutamylcysteine synthetase subunit gene expression by the transcription factor Nrf2. The Journal of Biological Chemistry. 1999;**274**:33627-33636

[74] Itoh K, Wakabayashi N, Katoh Y, Ishii T, Igarashi K, Engel JD, et al. Keap1 represses nuclear activation of antioxidant responsive elements by Nrf2 through binding to the amino-terminal Neh2 domain. Genes and Development. 1999;**13**:76-86

[75] Padmanabhan B, Tong KI, Ohta T, Nakamura Y, Scharlock M, Ohtsuji M, et al. Structural basis for defects of Keap1 activity provoked by its point mutations in lung cancer. Molecular Cell. 2006;**21**:689-700

[76] Singh A, Misra V, Thimmulappa RK, Lee H, Ames S, Hoque MO, et al. Dysfunctional Keap1-Nrf2 interaction in non-small-cell lung cancer. PLoS Medicine. 2006;**3**(10):1865-1876

[77] Homma S, Ishii Y, Morishima Y, Yamadori T, Matsuno Y, Haraguchi N, et al. Nrf2 enhances cell proliferation and resistance to anticancer drugs in human lung cancer. Clinical Cancer Research. 2009;**15**:3423-3432

[78] Nanqin G, Xiaoyun S, Lirong S. Activation of Nrf2 by microcystin-LR provides advantages for liver cancer cell growth. Chemical Research in Toxicology. 2010;**23**:1477-1484

[79] López-Alonso H, Rubiolo JA, Vega F, Vieytes MR, Botana LM. Protein synthesis inhibition and oxidative stress induced by cylindrospermopsin elicit apoptosis in primary rat hepatocytes. Chemical Research in Toxicology. 2013;**26**:203-212

[80] Lankoff A, Bialczyk J, Dziga D, Carmichael WW, Gradzka I, Lisowska H, et al. The repair of gamma-radiation-induced DNA damage is inhibited by microcystin-LR, the PP1 and PP2A phosphatase inhibitor. Mutagenesis. 2006;**21**:83-90

[81] Clark SP, Ryan TP, Searfoss GH, Davis MA, Hooser SB. Chronic microcystin exposure induces hepatocyte proliferation with increased expression of mitotic and cyclin-associated genes in P53-deficient mice. Toxicologic Pathology. 2008;**36**:190-203

[82] Zegura B, Sedmak B, Filipic M. Microcystin-LR induces oxidative DNA damage in human hepatoma cell line HepG2. Toxicon. 2003;**41**:41-48

[83] Zegura B, Lah TT, Filipic M. The role of reactive oxygen species in microcystin-LR-induced DNA damage. Toxicology. 2004;**200**:59-68

[84] Grollman AP, Moriya M. Mutagenesis by 8-oxoguanine: An enemy within. Trends in Genetics. 1993;**9**:246-249

[85] Maatouk I, Bouaïcha N, Plessis MJ, Périn F. Detection by 32P-postlabelling of 8-oxo-7 8-dihydro-20-deoxyguanosine in DNA as biomarker of microcystin-LR and nodularin-induced DNA damage in vitro in primary cultured rat hepatocytes and in vivo in rat liver. Mutation Research. 2004;**564**(1):9-20

[86] Sueoka E, Sueoka N, Okabe S, Kozu T, Komori A, Ohta T, et al. Expression of the tumor necrosis factor a gene and early response genes by nodularin, a liver tumor promoter, in primary cultured rat hepatocytes. Journal of Cancer Research and Clinical Oncology. 1997;**123**:413-419

[87] Komori A, Yatsunami J, Suganuma M, Okabe S, Abe S, Sakai A, et al. Tumor necrosis factor acts as a tumor promoter in BALB/3T3 cell transformation. Cancer Research. 1993;**53**:1982-1985

[88] IARC. Cyanobacterial Peptide Toxins. 2006. Available from: https://monographs.iarc.fr/wp-content/uploads/2018/06/mono94-7.pdf

[89] Wang J, Yi J. Cancer cell killing via ROS: To increase or decrease, that is the question. Cancer Biology & Therapy. 2008;**7**(12):1875-1884

[90] Sainis I, Fokas D, Vareli K, Tzakos AG, Kounnis V, Briasoulis E. Cyanobacterial cyclopeptides as lead compounds to novel targeted cancer drugs. Marine Drugs. 2010;**8**(3):629-657

[91] Zhang D, Xie P, Chen J. Effects of temperature on the stability of microcystins in muscle of fish and its consequences for food safety. Bulletin of Environmental Contamination and Toxicology. 2010;**84**:202-207

[92] Kounnis V, Chondrogiannis G, Mantzaris MD, Tzakos AG, Fokas D, Papanikolaou NA, et al. Microcystin LR shows cytotoxic activity against pancreatic cancer cells expressing the membrane OATP1B1 and OATP1B3 transporters. Anticancer Research. 2015;**35**(11):5857-5865

[93] Monks NR, Liu S, Xu Y, Yu H, Bendelow AS, Moscow JA. Potent cytotoxicity of the phosphatase inhibitor microcystin LR and microcystin analogues in OATP1B1- and OATP1B3-expressing HeLa cells. Molecular Cancer Therapeutics. 2007;**6**:587-598

[94] Rücker J, Stüken A, Nixdorf B, Fastner J, Chorus I, Wiedner C. Concentrations of particulate and dissolved cylindrospermopsin in 21 aphanizomenon-dominated temperate lakes. Toxicon. 2007;**50**:800-809

[95] Humpage AR, Fontaine F, Froscio S, Burcham P, Falconer IR. Cylindrospermopsin genotoxicity and cytotoxicity: Role of cytochrome P-450 and oxidative stress. Journal of Toxicology and Environmental Health Part A: Current Issues. 2005;**68**:739-753

[96] Kinnear S. Cylindrospermopsin: A decade of progress on bioaccumulation research. Marine Drugs. 2010;**8**:542-564

[97] Chiswell RK, Shaw GR, Eaglesham G, Smith MJ, Norris RL, Seawright AA, et al. Stability of cylindrospermopsin, the toxin from the cyanobacterium, cylindrospermopsis raciborskii: Effect of pH, temperature, and sunlight on decomposition. Environmental Toxicology. 1999;**14**:155-161

[98] Froscio SM, Fanok S, Humpage AR. Cytotoxicity screening for the cyanobacterial toxin cylindrospermopsin. Journal of Toxicology and Environmental Health Part A: Current Issues. 2009;**72**:345-349

[99] Guzmán-Guillén R, Prieto AI, Moyano R, Blanco A, Vasconcelos V, Cameán AM. Dietary l-carnitine prevents histopathological changes in tilapia (*Oreochromis niloticus*) exposed to cylindrospermopsin. Environmental Toxicology. 2017;**32**:241-254

[100] Shaw GR, Seawright AA, Moore MA, Lam PKS. Cylindrospermopsin, a cyanobacterial alkaloid: Evaluation of its toxicological activity. Therapeutic Drug Monitoring. 2000;**22**:89-92

[101] Chong MWK, Wong BSF, Lam PKS, Shaw GR, Seawright AA. Toxicity and uptake mechanism of cylindrospermopsin and lophyrotomin in primary hepatocytes. Toxicon. 2002;**40**:205-211

[102] Froscio SM, Humpage AR, Burcham PC, Falconer IR. Cylindrospermopsin-induced protein synthesis inhibition and its dissociation from acute toxicity in mouse hepatocytes. Environmental Toxicology. 2003;**18**:243-251

[103] Young FM, Micklem J, Humpage AR. Effects of blue-green algal toxin cylindrospermopsin (CYN) on human granulosa cells in vitro. Reproductive Toxicology. 2008;**25**:374-380

[104] Hrouzek P, Kapuścik A, Vacek J, Voráčová K, Paichlová J, Kosina P, et al. Cytotoxicity evaluation of large cyanobacterial strain set using selected human and murine in vitro cell models. Ecotoxicology and Environmental Safety. 2016;**124**:177-185

[105] Fernández DA, Louzao MC, Vilariño A, Fraga M, Espiña B, Vieytes MR, et al. Evaluation of the intestinal permeability and cytotoxic effects of cylindrospermopsin. Toxicon. 2014;**91**:23-34

[106] Runnegar MT, Kong S, Berndt N. Protein phosphatase inhibition and in vivo hepatotoxicity of microcystins.

American Journal of Physiology. Gastrointestinal and Liver Physiology. 1993;**265**:224-230

[107] Bazin E, Mourot A, Humpage AR, Fessard V. Genototoxicity of a freshwater cyanotoxin cylindrospermopsin, in two human cell lines: Caco-2 and HepaRG. Environmental and Molecular Mutagenesis. 2010;**51**:251-259

[108] Lankoff A, Wojcik A, Lisowska H, Bialczyk J, Dziga D, Carmichael WW. No induction of structural chromosomal aberrations in cylindrospermopsin-treated CHO-K1 cells without and with metabolic activation. Toxicon. 2007;**50**:1105-1115

[109] Straser A, Filipic M, Zegura B. Cylindrospermopsin induced transcriptional responses in human hepatoma HepG2 cells. Toxicology In Vitro : An International Journal Published in Association with BIBRA. 2013;**27**:1809-1819

[110] Hercog K, Maisanaba S, Filipic M, Jos A, Cameánn AM, Zegura B. Genotoxic potential of the binary mixture of cyanotoxins microcystin—LR and cylindrospermopsin. Chemosphere. 2017;**189**:319-329

[111] Bain P, Shae G, Patel B. Induction of P53-regulated gene expression in human cell lines exposed to the cyanobacterial toxin cylindrospermopsin. Journal of Toxicology and Environmental Health Part A: Current Issues. 2007;**70**:1687-1693

[112] Liebel S, Oliveira Ribeiro CA, Magalhaes VF, Silva C, Ramsdorf WA, Rossi SC, et al. Low concentrations of cylindrospermopsin induce increases of reactive oxygen species levels, metabolism and proliferation in human hepatoma cells (HepG2). Toxicology In Vitro. 2015;**29**:479-488

[113] Pichardo S, Cameán AM, Jos A. In vitro toxicological assessment of cylindrospermopsin: A review. Toxins. 2017;**9**(402):1-29

[114] Huguet A, Hatton A, Villot R, Quenault H, Blanchard Y, Fessard V. Modulation of chromatin remodelling induced by the freshwater cyanotoxin cylindrospermopsin in human intestinal Caco-2 cells. PLoS One. 2014;**9**(6):99-121

[115] Alja Š, Filipič M, Novak M, Žegura B. Double strand breaks and cell-cycle arrest induced by the cyanobacterial toxin cylindrospermopsin in HepG2 cells. Marine Drugs. 2013;**11**(8):3077-3090

[116] Facciponte DN, Bough MW, Seidler D, Carroll JL, Ashare A, Andrew AS, et al. Identifying aerosolized cyanobacteria in the human respiratory tract: A proposed mechanism for cyanotoxin-associated diseases. Science of the Total Environment. 2018;**645**:1003-1013

[117] Dawson RM. The toxicology of microcystins. Toxicon. 1998;**36**(7):953-962

[118] Zlateva S. Poisoning with molluscs and crustaceans. In: Kanev K, Stavrev D, editors. Handbook of Marine Toxicology. Poisoning with Sea Food and Marine Animals Incidence. 1st ed. Medical University Varna: Publishing Steno; 2018. p. 26. ISBN 978-619-221-163-0. IBSN 978-954-449-977-8

[119] Ito E, Kondo F, Terao K, Harada KI. Neoplastic nodular formation in mouse liver induced by repeated intraperitoneal injections of microcystin-LR. Toxicon. 1997;**35**(9):1453-1457

[120] Nishiwaki-Matsushima R, Oht T, Nishiwaki S, et al. Liver tumor promotion by the cyanobacterial cyclic peptide toxin microcystin-LR. Journal of Cancer Research and Clinical Oncology. 1992;**118**(6):420-424

Chapter 9

Effects of Atypical Neurotoxins on the Developing Fetal Brain

Chia-Yi Tseng

Abstract

The brain is not only a control center of the body but also a part of the way that the body can communicate with external environments. The spatial and temporal events of brain development are well-defined. These processes are sequentially regulated by intrinsic and external factors, such as gene. Disruption of these steps results in malformation and malfunction of the brain. Neurotoxin may affect our developing nervous system as a kind of endogenous and exogenous factor. For classical neurotoxins, such as heavy metals, snake venom, and bacterial toxins, the underlying toxin-mediated physiological pathways are relatively clear, and their antidotes are usually available. However, for atypical neurotoxins, such as air pollutants, food additives, and manufactural compounds, their effects on the nervous system are ordinarily extended and not easy to detect. In addition, the corresponding mechanism is too complex to define. A single and effective antidote against these atypical neurotoxins is uncommon, so prevention is better than cure with this kind of toxin. This chapter starts with the introduction of endogenous and exogenous neurotoxins, how they affect nervous system and their potential antidotes, followed by the impact of atypical neurotoxins in fetal brain development and their possible preventative or therapeutic methods.

Keywords: environmental or atypical neurotoxins, neurodevelopmental defects, neurodegenerative disorders

1. Introduction

Neurotoxins are toxic substances that destroy the nervous system. Depending on their origin, it could be divided into endogenous or exogenous neurotoxins. Endogenous is the neurotoxin produced by the human body itself, while exogenous one comes from the surrounding environment. Neurotoxins can damage neurons, nerve fibers, glias, and myelin, causing the atrophy of nerve fibers and neurons, or demyelination, which in turn affects neural circuits and functions. Ultimately, defect in nerve system affects the physiological homeostasis of human body, which results in corresponding signs and symptoms of poisoning. Macro-manifestations of neurotoxin exposure may associate a wide range of central nervous system impairments such as cognitive deficit [1], memory impairment [2], epilepsy, and dementia [3, 4].

IntechOpen

2. Classic neurotoxins and their possible mechanisms of action that damage the nervous system

2.1 Exogenous neurotoxin

Exogenous toxins are foreign synthetic by name, and common exogenous neurotoxins include metal neurotoxins (e.g., lead), microbial neurotoxins (e.g., botulinum), biotoxins (e.g., tetrodotoxin), and chemical toxoids (e.g., ethanol). Different types of toxins have their different mechanisms of action in nervous system: (1) metal neurotoxins, such as lead and aluminum, usually migrate to the brain through the blood circulation by destroying the structure of or inhibition of the blood-brain barrier (BBB) [5]. Once it penetrates the BBB and reaches the brain, it can cause damage to brain and thus the emergence of diseases such as learning disabilities [6, 7], disorders in motor coordination [8, 9], and Alzheimer's disease [10]. At present, these metal neurotoxins are still widely used in food preparation, like in the packaging factory. Furthermore, due to the environmental pollution, these substances are also widely existing in the food chain [11]. (2) Microbial neurotoxins are produced by microorganisms, mostly from bacteria, such as botulinum, tetanus toxin, and lipopolysaccharide (LPS). The main mechanism of microbial neurotoxins that disturb the nervous system is inhibiting the communication of neurons. Microbial neurotoxins prohibit the release of neurotransmitters from synaptic vesicle [12, 13], thereby terminating nerve messages, which may lead to a decrease in muscle tension [14, 15], muscle atrophy [16], and paralysis [17, 18]. If it affected the respiratory muscles, it could cause asphyxiation and death [19, 20]. (3) Bio-neurotoxins come from organisms that produce these toxins as tetrodotoxin existed inside pufferfish's skin and gastrointestinal tract, snake venom produced by snakes, and chlorotoxin produced by scorpion. Some of which reduce the permeability of the ion channels in neurons and thus decrease neuronal communication. Different bio-neurotoxins can target different ion channels. For example, the tetrodotoxin is specific to the sodium ion channel [21], while the conotoxin produced by the conch is specific to the calcium ion channel [22]. The other bio-neurotoxins may not affect ion channel but have impact on neurotransmitter gated channel, like bungarotoxin, a type of snake venom [23]. (4) Chemical neurotoxins are a class of toxins with a broader mechanism of action. For example, ethanol has been shown to induce nervous system damage and affect the body in various ways: studies show that ethanol can alter the composition of nerve cell membranes [24], inhibiting the activation of NMDA receptors [25], causing the imbalance of cellular calcium ion concentration [26], facilitating the mitochondrial dysfunction [27], and increasing the oxidative stress inside the neurons [28], and that destroy the nervous system, leading to brain atrophy, encephalitis, neurodegeneration, cognitive decline, developmental disorders, and other neurological diseases [29, 30].

2.2 Endogenous neurotoxins

Endogenous neurotoxins, such as nitric oxide and glutamate, originate in the body and usually have their typical physiological role and function in the body. When the concentration of these endogenous compounds becomes higher, it can lead to dangerous effects: (1) glutamate is the primary neurotransmitter of the nervous system, accomplishing the chemical transmission in synapses. The normal concentration of glutamate is responsible for the regular performance of neurons. One of the most critical uses in nervous system is an excitatory neurotransmitter, which is related to the long-term potentiation in memory and learning.

High concentrations of glutamate become toxic to the neurons by increasing the permeability of calcium ions. It leads to an increase in cellular calcium concentration, then over-activates the calcium-associated enzymes, and eventually results in neuronal swelling and cellular death. This phenomenon is known as excitotoxicity. Studies have linked this mechanism to many neurological disorders, such as Huntington's disease, epilepsy, and stroke [31, 32]. (2) Nitric oxide (NO) is a secondary messenger synthesized by neural nitric oxide and commonly used in neurons. It regulates synaptic plasticity of the nervous system, smooth muscle relaxation in nerve and vascular system, and neurovascular dilation [33, 34]. Abnormal concentration of NO is associated with asthma, schizophrenia, and Huntington's disease [35–37]. The neurotoxicity of NO is based on glutamate-induced excitotoxicity. NO is response to glutamate-mediated NMDA activation, which is produced by calcium-dependent signaling. An elevated rate of glutamate excitotoxicity could lead to an increase in neuronal NO level. Over-dose of NO can also increase oxidative stress, which further induces DNA damage and apoptosis [38]. Therefore, an abnormal level of NO inside the nervous system can produce significant neuronal toxic effects.

3. Common antidotes

Common antidotes, such as antioxidants and antitoxins, can effectively reduce nerve damage induced by neurotoxins: (1) Antitoxin or antiserum is an antidote that uses antibodies to neutralize specific action of the toxins. Antitoxin is produced by individual animals, plants, or bacteria that are responded to toxin exposure. Antitoxins are made in organisms and can be injected into other organisms, including humans. Its most common use in the human body is antivenom [39]. (2) Antioxidants are compounds that inhibit oxidative stress, such as glutathione or ascorbic acid (vitamin C). If neurotoxins cause oxidative stress, antioxidants can be used to reduce the toxic reactions and side effects [40, 41].

4. Neurotoxins and the developing nervous system

4.1 Brain development

Brain is the computational core of our nervous system and is a place where animals can process and coherent the stimulus gathering from outside or internal surroundings and then sending out the response. It is responsible for many higher-order functions such as coordination of movement, learning and memory, and language and speech. Therefore, a well and the fully developed brain is essential to regulate these functions. Many intrinsic and external factors are required for brain development. Intrinsic factors are like hormones or regular development-associated gene expression, and external factors are like essential nutrients. Abnormal impact on these factors results in brain malformation and malfunction. For example, abnormal expression of thyroid hormone affects cerebellar development, motor performance, and severe anxiety [42, 43]; dysfunction of cyclin-dependent kinase 5 and insulin-like growth factor-I results in neurological disorders and neurodegenerative diseases [44, 45]; iron deficiency in early life causes irreversible effect on behavioral and neural development [43, 46]; and (n-3) fatty acid plays a role in neurogenesis, neurotransmission, and protection against oxidative stress in whole life span [47].

4.2 General events during the timeline of fetal brain development

During cerebral development, brain cells go through the process that includes replication and migration. The replication of the brain cells is also called neurogenesis, which starts from the 8th week of gestation in humans and the 10th day in rodents [48]. Neurogenesis is the formation of neurons from neural stem cells near the area of lateral ventricles occurring during embryonic development and is responsible for producing all the various types of neurons of the brain. Neuronal migration mainly happens between the 12th and 24th week of gestation in humans and the 11th and 16th day in rodents [49, 50]. Neurons pass the subplate and migrate into the cortical plate along the radial glial process starting from the subventricular zone with an inside out pattern that forms six-layered neocortical laminae [51], also known as cortex. We may look at these processes in detail through rodent studies: neuronal progenitor cells (NPCs) form the earliest cortical neurons and lie inside the preplate on the 10.5th day of pregnancy, which is divided into the superficial marginal zone, the cortical plate, and the subplate. The radial glial cells (RGCs) are also generated from NPCs at around 11th to 12th day of gestation, which owns the unique morphology with their soma inside the ventricular zone, their short processes extending the apical side of ventricle, and their long processes elongating to basal lamina. Newly formed neurons use the processes of RGCs as guiding railroad to migrate from the ventricular zone toward their final destination inside the cortical plate. Early-born neurons give rise to layers I, V, and VI, and later-born neurons migrate from past layers V and VI to the other layers (layers II to IV) of the cortical plate [52]. This is also known as in-side-out migration.

Different cortical layers have different functions; for example, the neurons of the 6th layer remarkably express the T-box brain 1 (Tbr1) protein, which regulates cell migration and differentiation during embryonic development [53–55], and also is responsible for the connection between cortex and thalamus in the developed brain [56]. The cortical neurons of the 5th layer mainly express COUP-TF-interacting protein 2 (Ctip2; also known as Bcl11b), a C2H2 zinc finger transcription factor, and link the cortex with brain stem and spinal cord [57]. Special AT-rich sequence-binding protein 2 (SATB2) also known as DNA-binding protein SATB2 is highly expressed in the neurons with layers II and III, which is associated with neuronal morphogenesis [58]. In adult brain, the neurons in layers II and III mediate communication across cortical regions and with the amygdala [59, 60].

After the nerve cells migrate to the destination, they begin to develop neurites in order to form synapses, which communicate with other brain cells. Neurites are composed of axons and dendrites. Axons transmit messages, and dendrites receive them. Both of which shape neural circuits. Most of the topics discussed are dendritic patterns. Dendrites are highly branched bush-like cellular extensions that mediate the enormous majority of presynaptic and environmental inputs, which regulate neuronal communication. Dendritic patterning is critical for proper neuronal function and has served as the basis for the classification of neuronal subtypes [61, 62]. The development of dendrite is a complicated multistep process. First, neurites initiate and form a structure called lamellipodia. Axons outgrow from minor processes followed by the outgrowth of dendrites. Dendrites then start to branch and form dendritic spines. After the process of pruning, dendritic branches are fully matured, and synapses are formed [62–64]. These steps are regulated by intrinsic genetic signals and extracellular cues [64]. Disruption of these pathways results in abnormal development in dendrite patterning that sequentially affects communication between neurons, which further leads to disruption of neuronal circuitry, and finally, whole nervous system breaks down. For example, mutation in the human neural cell adhesion molecule L1 and Neuro-p24, a membranous protein, affects neurites' outgrowth and extension [65, 66]. Many well-known neurodegenerative diseases, such as Rett syndrome (RS) and autism, are genetic defects with well-defined anomalies in dendritic patterning [67, 68]. Hence, the integrity of dendrite morphology is crucial for maintaining normal function of brain circuitry and neuronal networks.

4.3 Genetic factors affect brain development

Gene is the main intrinsic factor that affects brain development, which contained highly programmed information related to neurogenesis and migration. These genetic factors include integration of reelin, Lis-1, and doublecortin [50, 69, 70]. The most studied genes are those encoding the dopamine inactivator catechol-O-methyl transferase (COMT), neurotrophin, brain-derived neurotrophic factor (BDNF), the schizophrenia candidate gene neuregulin (NRG1), and the serotonin transporter (5-HTT), for example, take neurotrophins. Neurotrophins play an essential role in mediating neuronal survival and brain development. There are four types of neurotrophins: neuronal growth factor [71], brain-derived neurotrophic factor (BDNF), neurotrophin 3 (NT-3), and neurotrophin 4/5 (NT-4/5). In their mature forms, these neurotrophins can bind as homodimers to specific tropomycin-related kinase (Trk) receptors. TrkA binds to NGF, TrkB binds to BDNF and NT-4/5, and TrkC binds to NT-3. Trk receptors are part of a group of receptor tyrosine kinases. Ligand binding results in dimerization of the receptor. The dimerized receptors phosphorylate several conserved tyrosine residues on one another [72–74]. This allows for proteins containing phosphotyrosine binding (PTB) or Src homology (SH2) domains to dock, and this docking activates intracellular signaling cascades that include Ras-Raf-Erk, PI3 kinase-Akt, PLC-γ-Ca^{2+}, NF-κB, and some protein kinase C pathways [73]. Neurotrophins exist in two states: proteolytically processed, which is the mature form and can bind the various Trk receptors, or unprocessed, which allows them to bind with high affinity to p75 neurotrophin receptor (NTR). Processed neurotrophins can still bind to p75NTR but with much lower affinity than to the Trk receptors. Binding of processed or unprocessed neurotrophins to p75 may elicit several responses including cell death [72, 73]. Recent studies also show that extracellular stimuli (NGF, BDNF, and epidermal growth factor) induced Rac activity, which is involved in neurotrophin-derived signaling and neuronal migration [75]. Deficiency in these intrinsic regulators disrupts neuronal migration and cortical laminar organization [76, 77], causing morphological abnormalities, such as schizencephaly, porencephaly, lissencephaly, macrogyria, and microgyria [78]. These lead to psychiatric and neurological disorders [69, 79, 80].

4.4 Examples of common neurotoxins on fetal brain development

The blood-brain barrier (BBB) is a crucial example of protection against toxins and other adverse compounds reaching the brain. BBB of the developing brain is not fully formed at the beginning of gestation, and therefore, fetal will be more vulnerable to the neurotoxins [81, 82]. For example, long-term exposure to nicotine during pregnancy directly affects acetylcholine systems and brain cell replication and differentiation, which consequently results in behavioral deficits of the offspring [83, 84]; prenatal, postnatal, and adolescent administration of alcohol affects gene expression (e.g. c-fos), causes abnormalities of brain structure and function, and finally disrupts brain development permanently and irreversibly [85, 86].

4.5 The impact of atypical neurotoxins on the developing brain

In the current industrialized society, atypical neurotoxins may also have hidden influence on normal brain development. The impacts of these agents on the processes of brain development are diverse and the productive time extends from prenatal to adolescent period [85]. Prenatal exposure to carbofuran, a carbamate pesticide, decreases nestin expression, histone-H3 phosphorylation, and the number of glial fibrillary acidic protein and SOX-2 co-labeled cells, which further leads to neurodegeneration and cognitive deficits in offspring [87]; Maternal application of dicholoacetonitrile (a disinfectant in our drinking water), benzyl benzoate (a antiparasitic insecticide), and trimethyltin (a stabilizer for plastics in paints) may induce oxidative stress and then result in neurodegeneration in fetal brain [88–90]; maternal infection is associated with the increased levels of proinflammatory cytokines in the amniotic fluid [91], umbilical cord plasma [92], and cerebral palsy [93, 94] as well as neurodevelopmental disorders such as schizophrenia [95] and autism spectrum disorders [96]. The findings in experimental models of maternal infection manifest the role of inflammatory response in the alteration of fetal neuronal morphology [97], astrocytosis, ventriculomegaly, changes in oligodendrocyte precursors [98], reduction of oligodendrocyte number, hypomyelination of brain [99] and a decrease of dopaminergic and serotoninergic neurons in the offspring [100], all of which are capable of leading to brain formative deficits. Indeed, maternal infection induces changes in brain developmental events, including neurogenesis, myelination, synaptogenesis as well as cell migration [101, 102]. Neuroinflammation has been reported to be highly associated with numbers of neurological and pathological diseases, such as cerebral palsy [94], schizophrenia [95], and autism spectrum disorders [96].

However, the precise molecular mechanisms of these exogenous agents that cause abnormal brain development largely remain unknown. Moreover, there are other possible harmful candidates needed to reveal. For example, monocyclic aromatic amines (MAAs) are a group of chemicals ubiquitously present in the environment. Exposure assessments indicate that most individuals experience lifelong exposure to these compounds from several sources, such as occupational exposure *via* tobacco smoke, herbicides, or hair dye, which are considerable in causing bladder cancer [103]. *In vivo* evidence has demonstrated the carcinogenic potential of most alkyl aniline compounds. For examples, 2,6-dimethylaniline (DMA) is responsible for nasal carcinogenesis [104]; Gan and colleagues indicated that 2,6-DMA, 3,5-dimethylaniline (3,5-DMA), and 3-ethylaniline (3-EA) are strongly associated with bladder cancers [105]. Currently, only 2,6-DMA is categorized as a possible human carcinogen by IARC [106]. However, the threats of other alkyl anilines cannot be neglected that 2,6-DMA, 3,5-DMA, and 3-EA can be metabolized as electrophilic intermediates, which further bind to DNA and form adducts. Skipper and colleagues report that three alkyl anilines can be metabolized as electrophilic intermediates and induce the production of DNA adducts, followed by attacking their putative targets, like bladder. Moreover, their results indicated that the adduct levels were the highest in animals given 3,5-DMA and the lowest in that given 3-EA. Furthermore, 3,5-DMA has been indicated not only to play a significant role in the etiology of bladder cancer in humans but study using *in vivo* experiments also strongly suggested that DNA adducts formed by 3,5-DMA might account for its presumptive activity [107]. A recent study additionally proves that 2,6-DMA and 3,5-DMA cause a single base-pair transition in the guanine-hypoxanthine phosphoribosyltransferase (*gpt*) gene in an *in vitro* model [108]. MMAs are activated through cytochrome P450-catalyzed oxidation of the amino group, followed by extensive esterification of *N*-hydroxylamine and heterolysis of the N—O bond to produce a reactive nitrenium ion. The ion then interacts with DNA base and forms covalent adducts [108, 109]. Furthermore, the other major product of hydroxylation, aminophenol, also has the ability to damage DNA by electrophilic attack at nucleophilic DNA bases that lead to mutagenesis and carcinogenesis. Aminophenol becomes electrophilic upon 2-electron oxidation to quinine imines, followed by Michael addition reactions as well as nucleophilic addition at the keto and imino carbon centers. Finally, DNA adducts are formed [103, 110]. Moreover, quinines react directly with proteins through thiol addition. Thioether addition products are responsible for the production of reactive oxygen species (ROS) [111, 112]. Accordingly, oxidation of alkyl anilines is generally regarded as a critical bioactivation. Indeed, studies have shown that the major metabolite of 3,5-DMA and 3,5-dimethylaminophenol (3,5-DMAP) is responsible for the ROS production, which contributes to the apoptotic cytotoxicity in mammalian cell lines [113, 114]. Furthermore, a recent *in vivo* study has shown that 3,5-DMA-induced ROS production disrupts the dendrites patterning of the cortical cells and causes the abnormal cortical layer distribution in developing fetal brain [115].

The most popular topic of air pollution, fine particular matter such as $PM_{2.5}$, has been reported to have massive impact on neurodevelopment. A study displays that $PM_{2.5}$ can enter the maternal amniotic fluid system by inhalation and directly causes the delay in brain development of the fetal rat. Besides, microarray data demonstrated that $PM_{2.5}$ mainly increases the risk of neurological diseases in the offspring, such as Alzheimer's disease, epilepsy, autism, learning and memory disorders, and emotional control disorders [116]. Up-to-date study shows that $PM_{2.5}$ increases the number of white blood cell, upregulates the inflammatory response, induces the memory impairment, and declines in dendritic branches of the hippocampi of the offspring [117].

5. Discussion and conclusion

The human brain is the most complex system in biology, and its function depends on the various connections of nerve cells or the interaction between brain regions. Besides, there is growing evidence that many mental and neurological disorders are associated with neurodevelopmental abnormalities, which, according to epidemiological statistics, include autism, attention deficit hyperactivity disorder, dyslexia, and other cognitive impairments affecting millions of children worldwide [118, 119]. During the fetal and infant periods, they are most susceptible to environmental neurotoxin, which can cause permanent brain damage during these sensitive developmental stages [82]. Classical neurotoxins, such as heavy metal neurotoxins, microbial neurotoxins, bio-neurotoxins, and chemical neurotoxins, are mentioned earlier in this chapter. As for atypical neurotoxins, such as 3,5-DMA mentioned in the previous section, their effects are not immediate and not apparent, so their damage to the nervous system is not easy to detect. Instead, once it is detected, the damage is already severe and irreversible, such as neurodegeneration or developmental disorders [120, 121]. Some of these atypical neurotoxins are hidden in the surrounding environment, and some are obvious but neglected because of slow action, such as air pollution. Because there is no immediate risk, it is often ignored in clinical or in research. Therefore, how to find an efficient antidote or effective daily health care methods against this neurotoxin, especially in current aging society, become much more critical.

Conflict of interest

The authors have declared that no competing interests exist.

Author details

Chia-Yi Tseng
Department of Biomedical Engineering, Center for Nano-Technology, Chung Yuan Christian University, Taiwan

*Address all correspondence to: cytseng@cycu.edu.tw

References

[1] Abdel-Aal RA, Assi AA, Kostandy BB. Memantine prevents aluminum-induced cognitive deficit in rats. Behavioural Brain Research. 2011;**225**(1):31-38

[2] Volpe BT et al. Loss of hippocampal CA1 pyramidal neurons correlates with memory impairment in rats with ischemic or neurotoxin lesions. Behavioral Neuroscience. 1992;**106**(3):457-464

[3] Mainardi M et al. Tetanus neurotoxin-induced epilepsy in mouse visual cortex. Epilepsia. 2012;**53**(7):e132-e136

[4] Eiser AR. Why does Finland have the highest dementia mortality rate? Environmental factors may be generalizable. Brain Research. 2017;**1671**:14-17

[5] Ronnback C, Hansson E. The importance and control of low-grade inflammation due to damage of cellular barrier systems that may lead to systemic inflammation. Frontiers in Neurology. 2019;**10**:533

[6] Zhu X et al. Perceptual training restores impaired cortical temporal processing due to lead exposure. Cerebral Cortex. 2016;**26**(1):334-345

[7] Wang M et al. Effects of carbachol on lead-induced impairment of the long-term potentiation/depotentiation in rat dentate gyrus in vivo. Food and Chemical Toxicology. 2007;**45**(3):412-418

[8] Dolinsky ZS et al. Behavioral effects of lead and *Toxocara canis* in mice. Science. 1981;**213**(4512):1142-1144

[9] Hietanen E et al. Biotransformational and neurophysiological changes in rabbits exposed to lead. Archives of Environmental Contamination and Toxicology. 1980;**9**(3):337-347

[10] Ghose AK et al. Knowledge-based, central nervous system (CNS) lead selection and lead optimization for CNS drug discovery. ACS Chemical Neuroscience. 2012;**3**(1):50-68

[11] Lee JW et al. Toxic effects of lead exposure on bioaccumulation, oxidative stress, neurotoxicity, and immune responses in fish: A review. Environmental Toxicology and Pharmacology. 2019;**68**:101-108

[12] Hassel B. Tetanus: Pathophysiology, treatment, and the possibility of using botulinum toxin against tetanus-induced rigidity and spasms. Toxins (Basel). 2013;**5**(1):73-83

[13] Poulain B. Molecular mechanism of action of tetanus toxin and botulinum neurotoxins. Pathologie Biologie. 1994;**42**(2):173-182

[14] Malgorzata P, Piotr C, Edward K. The mechanism of the beneficial effect of botulinum toxin type a used in the treatment of temporomandibular joints dysfunction. Mini Reviews in Medicinal Chemistry. 2017;**17**(5):445-450

[15] Toczyska I, Plusa T. Shiga toxin and tetanus toxin as a potential biologic weapon. Polski Merkuriusz Lekarski. 2015;**39**(231):157-161

[16] Sellin LC. The action of batulinum toxin at the neuromuscular junction. Medical Biology. 1981;**59**(1):11-20

[17] Surana S et al. The travel diaries of tetanus and botulinum neurotoxins. Toxicon. 2018;**147**:58-67

[18] Rossetto O, Pirazzini M, Montecucco C. Botulinum neurotoxins: Genetic, structural and mechanistic insights. Nature Reviews. Microbiology. 2014;**12**(8):535-549

[19] Bradford AB et al. 3,4-Diaminopyridine reverses paralysis

in botulinum neurotoxin-intoxicated diaphragms through two functionally distinct mechanisms. Toxicology and Applied Pharmacology. 2018;**341**:77-86

[20] Morton DB et al. Synaptic transmission in neurons that express the Drosophila atypical soluble guanylyl cyclases, Gyc-89Da and Gyc-89Db, is necessary for the successful completion of larval and adult ecdysis. The Journal of Experimental Biology. 2008. **211** (Pt 10):1645-1656

[21] Chulanetra M et al. Human ScFv that block sodium ion channel activity of tetrodotoxin. Toxicon. 2012;**59**(2):272-282

[22] Tisa LS, Olivera BM, Adler J. Inhibition of *Escherichia coli* chemotaxis by omega-conotoxin, a calcium ion channel blocker. Journal of Bacteriology. 1993;**175**(5):1235-1238

[23] Clarke PB. The fall and rise of neuronal alpha-bungarotoxin binding proteins. Trends in Pharmacological Sciences. 1992;**13**(11):407-413

[24] Roux A et al. Ethanol induced brain lipid changes in mice assessed by mass spectrometry. ACS Chemical Neuroscience. 2016;**7**(8):1148-1156

[25] Hermenegildo C et al. NMDA receptor antagonists prevent acute ammonia toxicity in mice. Neurochemical Research. 1996;**21**(10):1237-1244

[26] Woodward JJ. Ethanol and NMDA receptor signaling. Critical Reviews in Neurobiology. 2000;**14**(1):69-89

[27] Huang W et al. Fatty acid ethyl ester synthase inhibition ameliorates ethanol-induced Ca^{2+}-dependent mitochondrial dysfunction and acute pancreatitis. Gut. 2014;**63**(8):1313-1324

[28] Luo J. Autophagy and ethanol neurotoxicity. Autophagy. 2014;**10**(12):2099-2108

[29] Davis KM, Wu JY. Role of glutamatergic and GABAergic systems in alcoholism. Journal of Biomedical Science. 2001;**8**(1):7-19

[30] Kiecker C. The chick embryo as a model for the effects of prenatal exposure to alcohol on craniofacial development. Developmental Biology. 2016;**415**(2):314-325

[31] Savolainen KM, Loikkanen J, Naarala J. Amplification of glutamate-induced oxidative stress. Toxicology Letters. 1995;**82-83**:399-405

[32] Zadori D et al. Mitochondrial disturbances, excitotoxicity, neuroinflammation and kynurenines: Novel therapeutic strategies for neurodegenerative disorders. Journal of the Neurological Sciences. 2012;**322**(1-2):187-191

[33] Hardingham N, Dachtler J, Fox K. The role of nitric oxide in pre-synaptic plasticity and homeostasis. Frontiers in Cellular Neuroscience. 2013;**7**:190

[34] Cui X et al. Role of endothelial nitric oxide synthetase in arteriogenesis after stroke in mice. Neuroscience. 2009;**159**(2):744-750

[35] Nasyrova RF et al. Role of nitric oxide and related molecules in schizophrenia pathogenesis: Biochemical, genetic and clinical aspects. Frontiers in Physiology. 2015;**6**:139

[36] Kumar P, Kalonia H, Kumar A. Cyclosporine A attenuates 3-nitropropionic acid-induced Huntington-like symptoms in rats: Possible nitric oxide mechanism. International Journal of Toxicology. 2010;**29**(3):318-325

[37] Kim YH et al. Association of extended nitric oxide parameters with bronchial hyperresponsiveness and

bronchodilator response in children with asthma. Journal of Breath Research. 2017;**11**(4):046003

[38] Chabrier PE, Demerle-Pallardy C, Auguet M. Nitric oxide synthases: Targets for therapeutic strategies in neurological diseases. Cellular and Molecular Life Sciences. 1999;**55**(8-9):1029-1035

[39] Pucca MB et al. History of envenoming therapy and current perspectives. Frontiers in Immunology. 2019;**10**:1598

[40] Kita T et al. Protective effects of phytochemical antioxidants against neurotoxin-induced degeneration of dopaminergic neurons. Journal of Pharmacological Sciences. 2014;**124**(3):313-319

[41] Wasik A, Antkiewicz-Michaluk L. The mechanism of neuroprotective action of natural compounds. Pharmacological Reports. 2017;**69**(5):851-860

[42] Koibuchi N, Iwasaki T. Regulation of brain development by thyroid hormone and its modulation by environmental chemicals. Endocrine Journal. 2006;**53**(3):295-303

[43] Beard J. Iron deficiency alters brain development and functioning. The Journal of Nutrition. 2003;**133**(5 Suppl. 1):1468S-1472S

[44] Netchine I et al. IGF1 molecular anomalies demonstrate its critical role in fetal, postnatal growth and brain development. Best Practice & Research. Clinical Endocrinology & Metabolism. 2011;**25**(1):181-190

[45] Su SC, Tsai LH. Cyclin-dependent kinases in brain development and disease. Annual Review of Cell and Developmental Biology. 2011;**27**:465-491

[46] de Escobar GM, Obregon MJ, del Rey FE. Iodine deficiency and brain development in the first half of pregnancy. Public Health Nutrition. 2007;**10**(12A):1554-1570

[47] Innis SM. Dietary (n-3) fatty acids and brain development. The Journal of Nutrition. 2007;**137**(4):855-859

[48] Stagni F et al. Timing of therapies for down syndrome: The sooner, the better. Frontiers in Behavioral Neuroscience. 2015;**9**:265

[49] Dehay C, Kennedy H. Cell-cycle control and cortical development. Nature Reviews. Neuroscience. 2007;**8**(6):438-450

[50] Kwan KY, Sestan N, Anton ES. Transcriptional co-regulation of neuronal migration and laminar identity in the neocortex. Development. 2012;**139**(9):1535-1546

[51] Stiles J, Jernigan TL. The basics of brain development. Neuropsychology Review. 2010;**20**(4):327-348

[52] De Carlos JA, O'Leary DD. Growth and targeting of subplate axons and establishment of major cortical pathways. The Journal of Neuroscience. 1992;**12**(4):1194-1211

[53] Han W et al. TBR1 directly represses Fezf2 to control the laminar origin and development of the corticospinal tract. Proceedings of the National Academy of Sciences of the United States of America. 2011;**108**(7):3041-3046

[54] Hevner RF et al. Tbr1 regulates differentiation of the preplate and layer 6. Neuron. 2001;**29**(2):353-366

[55] McKenna WL et al. Tbr1 and Fezf2 regulate alternate corticofugal neuronal identities during neocortical development. The Journal of Neuroscience. 2011;**31**(2):549-564

[56] Lam YW, Sherman SM. Functional organization of the somatosensory cortical layer 6 feedback to the thalamus. Cerebral Cortex. 2010;**20**(1):13-24

[57] Hall JE. Guyton and Hall Textbook of Medical Physiology. Elsevier Health Sciences; 2010

[58] Zhang L et al. Satb2 is required for dendritic arborization and soma spacing in mouse cerebral cortex. Cerebral Cortex. 2012;**22**(7):1510-1519

[59] Clancy B, Darlington RB, Finlay BL. Translating developmental time across mammalian species. Neuroscience. 2001;**105**(1):7-17

[60] Bouwmeester H, Smits K, Van Ree JM. Neonatal development of projections to the basolateral amygdala from prefrontal and thalamic structures in rat. The Journal of Comparative Neurology. 2002;**450**(3):241-255

[61] MacNeil MA, Masland RH. Extreme diversity among amacrine cells: Implications for function. Neuron. 1998;**20**(5):971-982

[62] McAllister AK. Cellular and molecular mechanisms of dendrite growth. Cerebral Cortex. 2000;**10**(10):963-973

[63] Mandell JW, Banker GA. The microtubule cytoskeleton and the development of neuronal polarity. Neurobiology of Aging. 1995;**16**(3):229-237 discussion 238

[64] Urbanska M, Blazejczyk M, Jaworski J. Molecular basis of dendritic arborization. Acta Neurobiologiae Experimentalis (Wars). 2008;**68**(2):264-288

[65] Araki M et al. Developmentally regulated expression of neuro-p24 and its possible function in neurite extension. Neuroscience Research. 2002;**44**(4):379-389

[66] Michelson P et al. Missense mutations in the extracellular domain of the human neural cell adhesion molecule L1 reduce neurite outgrowth of murine cerebellar neurons. Human Mutation. 2002;**20**(6):481-482

[67] Zoghbi HY. Postnatal neurodevelopmental disorders: Meeting at the synapse? Science. 2003;**302**(5646):826-830

[68] Kaufmann WE, Moser HW. Dendritic anomalies in disorders associated with mental retardation. Cerebral Cortex. 2000;**10**(**10**):981-991

[69] Liu JS. Molecular genetics of neuronal migration disorders. Current Neurology and Neuroscience Reports. 2011;**11**(2):171-178

[70] Molyneaux BJ et al. Neuronal subtype specification in the cerebral cortex. Nature Reviews. Neuroscience. 2007;**8**(6):427-437

[71] MacKenzie AR et al. The atmospheric chemistry of trace gases and particulate matter emitted by different land uses in Borneo. Philosophical Transactions of the Royal Society of London. Series B, Biological Sciences. 2011;**366**(1582):3177-3195

[72] Chao MV. Neurotrophins and their receptors: A convergence point for many signalling pathways. Nature Reviews. Neuroscience. 2003;**4**(4):299-309

[73] Huang EJ, Reichardt LF. Trk receptors: Roles in neuronal signal transduction. Annual Review of Biochemistry. 2003;**72**:609-642

[74] Segal RA. Selectivity in neurotrophin signaling: Theme and variations. Annual Review of Neuroscience. 2003;**26**:299-330

[75] Yoshizawa M et al. Involvement of a Rac activator, P-Rex1, in neurotrophin-derived signaling and neuronal migration. The Journal of Neuroscience. 2005;**25**(17):4406-4419

[76] Tan X, Shi SH. Neocortical neurogenesis and neuronal migration. Wiley Interdisciplinary Reviews: Developmental Biology. 2013;**2**(4):443-459

[77] Douet V et al. Genetic influences on brain developmental trajectories on neuroimaging studies: From infancy to young adulthood. Brain Imaging and Behavior. 2014;**8**(2):234-250

[78] Barth PG. Disorders of neuronal migration. The Canadian Journal of Neurological Sciences. 1987;**14**(1):1-16

[79] Folsom TD, Fatemi SH. The involvement of Reelin in neurodevelopmental disorders. Neuropharmacology. 2013;**68**:122-135

[80] Gressens P. Pathogenesis of migration disorders. Current Opinion in Neurology. 2006;**19**(2):135-140

[81] Goasdoue K et al. Review: The blood-brain barrier; protecting the developing fetal brain. Placenta. 2017;**54**:111-116

[82] Sanders T et al. Neurotoxic effects and biomarkers of lead exposure: A review. Reviews on Environmental Health. 2009;**24**(1):15-45

[83] Abdel-Rahman A et al. Maternal exposure of rats to nicotine via infusion during gestation produces neurobehavioral deficits and elevated expression of glial fibrillary acidic protein in the cerebellum and CA1 subfield in the offspring at puberty. Toxicology. 2005;**209**(3):245-261

[84] Slotkin TA. Cholinergic systems in brain development and disruption by neurotoxicants: Nicotine, environmental tobacco smoke, organophosphates. Toxicology and Applied Pharmacology. 2004;**198**(2):132-151

[85] Archer T. Effects of exogenous agents on brain development: Stress, abuse and therapeutic compounds. CNS Neuroscience & Therapeutics. 2011;**17**(5):470-489

[86] Jang MH et al. Influence of maternal alcohol administration on c-Fos expression in the hippocampus of infant rats. Neuroscience Letters. 2005;**378**(1):44-48

[87] Mishra D et al. Prenatal carbofuran exposure inhibits hippocampal neurogenesis and causes learning and memory deficits in offspring. Toxicological Sciences. 2012;**127**(1):84-100

[88] Esmat A et al. Dichloroacetonitrile induces oxidative stress and developmental apoptotic imbalance in mouse fetal brain. Environmental Toxicology and Pharmacology. 2012;**33**(1):78-84

[89] Kockaya EA, Kilic A. Developmental toxicity of benzyl benzoate in rats after maternal exposure throughout pregnancy. Environmental Toxicology. 2014;**29**(1):40-53

[90] Paule MG et al. Developmental toxicology of trimethyltin in the rat. Toxicology and Applied Pharmacology. 1986;**84**(2):412-417

[91] Yoon BH et al. Fetal exposure to an intra-amniotic inflammation and the development of cerebral palsy at the age of three years. American Journal of Obstetrics and Gynecology. 2000;**182**(3):675-681

[92] Yoon BH et al. Interleukin-6 concentrations in umbilical cord plasma are elevated in neonates with

white matter lesions associated with periventricular leukomalacia. American Journal of Obstetrics and Gynecology. 1996;**174**(5):1433-1440

[93] Shatrov JG et al. Chorioamnionitis and cerebral palsy: A meta-analysis. Obstetrics & Gynecology. 2010;**116**(2 Pt 1):387-392

[94] Wu YW et al. Chorioamnionitis and cerebral palsy in term and near-term infants. JAMA. 2003;**290**(20):2677-2684

[95] Brown AS et al. Maternal exposure to respiratory infections and adult schizophrenia spectrum disorders: A prospective birth cohort study. Schizophrenia Bulletin. 2000;**26**(2):287-295

[96] Beversdorf DQ et al. Timing of prenatal stressors and autism. Journal of Autism and Developmental Disorders. 2005;**35**(4):471-478

[97] Burd I, Balakrishnan B, Kannan S. Models of fetal brain injury, intrauterine inflammation, and preterm birth. American Journal of Reproductive Immunology. 2012;**67**(4):287-294

[98] Rodts-Palenik S et al. Maternal infection-induced white matter injury is reduced by treatment with interleukin-10. American Journal of Obstetrics and Gynecology. 2004;**191**(4):1387-1392

[99] Pang Y et al. Suppression of glial activation is involved in the protection of IL-10 on maternal *E. coli* induced neonatal white matter injury. Brain Research. Developmental Brain Research. 2005;**157**(2):141-149

[100] Lin YL, Lin SY, Wang S. Prenatal lipopolysaccharide exposure increases anxiety-like behaviors and enhances stress-induced corticosterone responses in adult rats. Brain, Behavior, and Immunity. 2012;**26**(3):459-468

[101] Chao MW et al. N-acetylcysteine attenuates lipopolysaccharide-induced impairment in lamination of Ctip2- and Tbr1-expressing cortical neurons in the developing rat fetal brain. Scientific Reports. 2016;**6**:32373

[102] Boksa P. Effects of prenatal infection on brain development and behavior: A review of findings from animal models. Brain, Behavior, and Immunity. 2010;**24**(6):881-897

[103] Skipper PL et al. Monocyclic aromatic amines as potential human carcinogens: Old is new again. Carcinogenesis. 2010;**31**(1):50-58

[104] Koujitani T et al. Tumor-promoting activity of 2,6-dimethylaniline in a two-stage nasal carcinogenesis model in N-bis(2-hydroxypropyl)nitrosamine-treated rats. Cancer Letters. 1999;**142**(2):161-171

[105] Gan J et al. Alkylaniline-hemoglobin adducts and risk of non-smoking-related bladder cancer. Journal of the National Cancer Institute. 2004;**96**(19):1425-1431

[106] USNT Program. Toxicology and carcinogenesis studies of 2,6-xylidine (2,6-dimethylaniline) (CAS No. 87-62-7). Charles River CD Rats. Research Triangle Park, NC; 1990

[107] Skipper PL et al. DNA adduct formation by 2,6-dimethyl-, 3,5-dimethyl-, and 3-ethylaniline in vivo in mice. Chemical Research in Toxicology. 2006;**19**(8):1086-1090

[108] Chao MW et al. Genotoxicity of 2,6- and 3,5-dimethylaniline in cultured mammalian cells: The role of reactive oxygen species. Toxicological Sciences. 2012;**130**(1):48-59

[109] Cui L et al. Identification of adducts formed by reaction of N-acetoxy-3,5-dimethylaniline with DNA. Chemical Research in Toxicology. 2007;**20**(11):1730-1736

[110] Eyer P. Reactions of oxidatively activated arylamines with thiols: Reaction mechanisms and biologic implications. An overview. Environmental Health Perspectives. 1994;**102**(Suppl 6):123-132

[111] Slaughter DE, Hanzlik RP. Identification of epoxide- and quinone-derived bromobenzene adducts to protein sulfur nucleophiles. Chemical Research in Toxicology. 1991;**4**(3):349-359

[112] Towndrow KM et al. Stress- and growth-related gene expression are independent of chemical-induced prostaglandin E(2) synthesis in renal epithelial cells. Chemical Research in Toxicology. 2000;**13**(2):111-117

[113] Chao MW et al. Intracellular generation of ROS by 3,5-dimethylaminophenol: Persistence, cellular response, and impact of molecular toxicity. Toxicological Sciences. 2014;**141**(1):300-313

[114] Erkekoglu P et al. Antioxidants and selenocompounds inhibit 3,5-dimethylaminophenol toxicity to human urothelial cells. Arhiv za Higijenu Rada i Toksikologiju. 2019;**70**(1):18-29

[115] Chao MW et al. In vitro and In vivo analysis of the effects of 3,5-DMA and its metabolites in neural oxidative stress and neurodevelopmental toxicity. Toxicological Sciences. 2019;**168**(2):405-419

[116] Chao MW et al. Exposure to PM2.5 causes genetic changes in fetal rat cerebral cortex and hippocampus. Environmental Toxicology. 2017;**32**(4):1412-1425

[117] Tseng CY et al. The effect of *Ganoderma microsporum* immunomodulatory proteins on alleviating PM2.5-induced inflammatory responses in pregnant rats and fine particulate matter-induced neurological damage in the offsprings. Scientific Reports. 2019;**9**(1):6854

[118] Grandjean P, Landrigan PJ. Neurobehavioural effects of developmental toxicity. Lancet Neurology. 2014;**13**(3):330-338

[119] Grandjean P, Landrigan PJ. Developmental neurotoxicity of industrial chemicals. Lancet. 2006;**368**(9553):2167-2178

[120] Chinta SJ et al. Cellular senescence is induced by the environmental neurotoxin paraquat and contributes to neuropathology linked to Parkinson's disease. Cell Reports. 2018;**22**(4):930-940

[121] Spencer PS, Palmer VS, Kisby GE. Seeking environmental causes of neurodegenerative disease and envisioning primary prevention. Neurotoxicology. 2016;**56**:269-283

Chapter 10

Toxicity Potential of Cyanogenic Glycosides in Edible Plants

Kumbukani K. Nyirenda

Abstract

Cyanogenic glycosides are natural phytotoxins produced by over 2000 plant species, many of which are consumed by humans. The important food crops that contain cyanogenic glycosides include cassava (*Manihot esculenta*), sorghum (*Sorghum bicolor*), cocoyam (*Colocasia esculenta* L. and *Xanthosoma sagittifolium* L.), bamboo (*Bambusa vulgaris*), apple (*Malus domestica*), and apricot (*Prunus armeniaca*). Cyanogenic glycosides and their derivatives have amino acid-derived aglycones, which spontaneously degrade to release highly toxic hydrogen cyanide (HCN). Dietary cyanide exposure has been associated with several health challenges such as acute cyanide poisoning, growth retardation, and neurological disorders. This chapter will introduce general cyanogenesis principles, highlight major food plants with lethal cyanide levels, and provide epidemiological-based health conditions linked to cyanide intake. Furthermore, strategies for elimination of cyanogens from food crops, such as processing technologies, will be discussed. Finally, the chapter will analyze the role of cyanogenic plants in ensuring food security among resource-poor communities.

Keywords: cyanogenic glycosides, cyanogens, phytotoxins, detoxification, food safety

1. Introduction

Many plant species that are grown for food contain phytotoxins in different parts of the plant. Natural toxins are usually secondary metabolites produced by plants for defensive purposes against threats such as bacteria, fungi, insects, and predators [1]. They may also occur in food plants because of natural selection and new breeding methods that enhance protective mechanisms of the crops [2]. The most common natural toxins found in food plants include lectins in beans, glycoalkaloids in potatoes, and cyanogenic glycosides in cassava, bitter apricot seed, bamboo shoots, and flaxseeds [3]. A review of several natural toxins in food plants commonly consumed in the world, including the toxicological effects associated with the ingestion of these toxins, shows that cyanogenic glycosides are the most important and extensively studied group of phytotoxins [4].

Cyanogenic glycosides are chemical compounds that release hydrogen cyanide (HCN) and are common in certain families such as the Fabaceae, Rosaceae, Leguminosae, Linaceae, and Compositae [2]. Approximately 25 cyanogenic glycosides, which are mostly found in the edible parts of plants, have been identified [4]. The potential toxicity of cyanogenic glycosides and their derivatives largely depends on their ability to release hydrogen cyanide. Dietary cyanide exposure may result in acute poisoning and has also been associated with the etiology of several chronic diseases [5]. Therefore, the presence of cyanogenic glycosides in food and fodder presents a significant social and economic problem in many parts of the world, particularly in developing countries. In Africa, consumption of insufficiently processed cassava (*Manihot esculenta* Crantz) has been associated with cyanide poisoning, tropical ataxic neuropathy (TAN) disease, and konzo [6, 7]. In 1992, the death of three people in Nigeria was attributed to cyanide intake from cyanogenic glycosides of cassava [5], and a decade ago five Nigerians died of cyanide poison after reportedly eating a meal prepared with cassava flour.

Cyanogenic glycosides found in plants are not toxic on their own. However, when cell structures of plant are disrupted, cyanogenic glycoside will be brought together with the corresponding hydrolytic β-glucosidase enzyme. Subsequently, the glycoside degenerates to a sugar and a cyanohydrin that rapidly decomposes to hydrogen cyanide and an aldehyde or a ketone [8]. In bitter almonds and peach stones, cyanogenic glycoside, amygdalin, is converted to glucose, benzaldehyde, and toxic hydrogen cyanide. In edible plants, cyanide levels are reduced significantly during the processing to an accepted Food and Agricultural Organization (FAO)/World Health Organization (WHO) level of 10 mg HCN/kg dry weight [9]. However, when poorly processed lethal concentrations of the cyanogens may be obtained in the final edible products.

2. Cyanogenic glycosides in food plants

Cyanogenic glycosides are a structurally diverse class of secondary metabolites that are mostly used by plants as a defense against various threats such as bacteria, fungi, insects, and predators [1]. The compounds consist of α-hydroxynitrile aglycones attached to a sugar moiety (Vetter, 2000) and are widely distributed in the plant kingdom [10]. Cyanogenic glycosides are common in certain families such as the Fabaceae, Rosaceae, Leguminosae, Linaceae, and Compositae, and their constituents provide a useful tool for taxonomic identification [2]. Several important food plants are known to synthesize cyanogenic glycosides; for example, linamarin in cassava and butter bean, dhurrin in sorghum and macadamia nut, and amygdalin in almond, peach, sweet cherry, and sour cherry [2, 11].

2.1 Biosynthesis of cyanogenic glycosides

In plants, cyanogenic glycosides are derivatives of five amino acids (valine, isoleucine, leucine, phenylalanine, and tyrosine) and the non-proteinogenic amino acid, cyclopentenyl glycine. Linamarin and lotaustralin are derived from valine, isoleucine, and leucine, while dhurrin is derived from tyrosine. Amygdalin and prunasin are derived from phenylalanine [12]. The biosynthesis of various cyanogenic glycosides in different plants has been described, and the most extensively reported are dhurrin in sorghum and linamarin in cassava [10]. The generic biosynthetic pathway for the production of cyanogenic glycosides from amino acids is shown in **Figure 1**.

The first two steps of biosynthetic production of cyanogenic glycoside are catalyzed by a cytochrome P450 enzyme through two successive N-hydroxylations of the amino group of the parent amino acid. The α-hydroxynitrile (cyanohydrin) is then generated following the decarboxylation and dehydration of aldoxime and nitrile, respectively [14]. The final step that produces cyanogenic glycoside involves glycosylation of the cyanohydrin moiety, and the process is catalyzed by UDPG-glycosyltransferase [10].

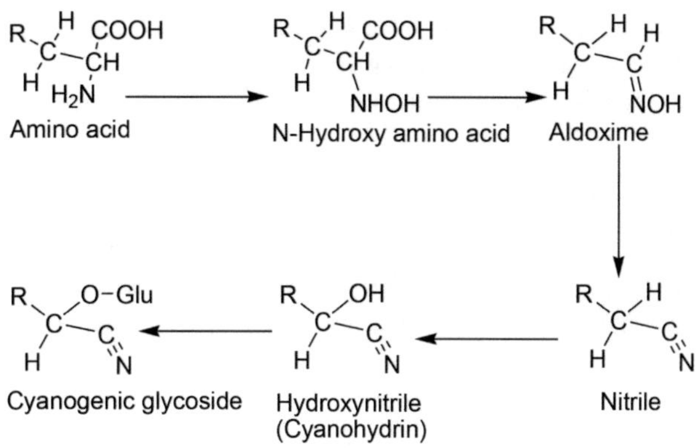

Figure 1.
The biosynthetic pathway for cyanogenic glycosides from its precursor amino acid [13].

2.2 Cyanogenesis

Cyanogenesis is the ability of some plants to synthesize cyanogenic glycosides to form hydrogen cyanide via cyanohydrin intermediate [15, 16]. The hydrolysis of the cyanogenic glycosides is accomplished by the β-glucosidase enzymes, which facilitate the cleavage of the carbohydrate moiety of the cyanogenic glycoside to yield corresponding cyanohydrins which further decompose to release hydrogen cyanide and an aldehyde or ketone [17] as illustrated in **Figure 2**. The final step that produces the toxic compound, HCN, is catalyzed by hydroxynitrile lyase enzyme, which is widespread in cyanogenic plants [16].

The cyanogenic glycosides linamarin (α-hydroxybutyronitrile-β-D-glucopyranoside) and lotaustralin (ethyl linamarin) are distributed in cassava cell vacuoles, while the enzyme linamarase is found in the cell wall [18]. The hydrolysis of linamarin in cassava starts with the disruption of the root tissue during

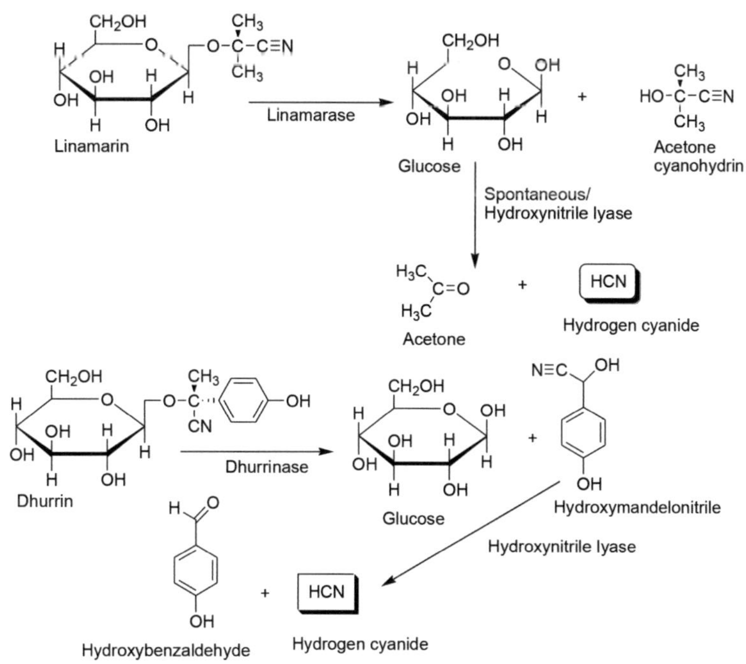

Figure 2.
Enzymatic hydrolysis of cyanogenic compounds, linamarin, and dhurrin.

processing or chewing to release the endogenous enzyme (linamarase), which catalyzes the hydrolysis of linamarin to glucose and acetone cyanohydrins. During processing factors such as reduced moisture and increased temperature facilitate the spontaneous conversion of cyanohydrins to toxic hydrogen cyanide and the corresponding ketone, acetone [19].

In sorghum, the cyanogenic glycoside dhurrin (4-hydroxymandelonitrile-β-D-glucopyranoside) and the enzyme β-glucosidase (dhurrinase) are stored in separate plant compartments. However, when the plant tissue is crushed, the enzyme and substrate dhurrin are brought in contact. The hydrolysis of dhurrin is then initiated by dhurrinase, which hydrolyzes the cyanogenic glycoside to form hydroxymandelonitrile and glucose. In acidic conditions or in the presence of hydroxynitrile lyase, the intermediate compound, hydroxymandelonitrile, further decomposes to generate hydrogen cyanide and hydroxybenzaldehyde [19] as shown in **Figure 2**. In food plants, cyanogenic glycosides are not toxic on their own. However, when cell structures of a plant are disrupted, cyanogenic glycosides will be brought together with the corresponding β-glucosidase enzyme to liberate a toxic compound, HCN.

3. Food plants with cyanogenic compounds

Cyanogenic glycosides are present in over 100 families of flowering plants, and at least 2000 plant species are known to contain this class of natural toxins. In addition to high plants, they are also found in some species of ferns, fungi, and bacteria [16]. Cyanogenic glycosides are amino acid-derived constituents of plants produced as secondary metabolites and are used as a defensive mechanism against various threats such as bacteria, fungi, insects, and other predators. There are wide variations in the levels of cyanogenic glycosides in plants due to genetic and environmental factors such as location, season, and soil types [3]. **Table 1** shows the types of cyanogenic glycosides commonly found in major edible plants.

Approximately 25 cyanogenic glycosides have been reported in different cyanogenic food plants, and **Figure 3** shows structures of examples of cyanogenic glycosides commonly found in edible plants.

3.1 Cassava

Cassava (*Manihot esculenta* Crantz) is a perennial crop that originated from South America and was introduced in Africa by the Portuguese explorers during

Species	Family	Vegetative part	Source of HCN
Cassava (*Manihot esculenta*)	Euphorbiaceae	Leaves, tuber peel, and parenchyma	Linamarin Lotaustralin
Sorghum (*Sorghum bicolor*)	Poaceae	Fruits (seeds), shoot tips, and leaves	Dhurrin
Cocoyam (*Colocasia esculenta* and *Xanthosoma sagittifolium*)	Araceae	Leaves and roots	Dhurrin
Bamboo (*Bambusa vulgaris*)	Poaceae	Stem and sprouts	Taxiphyllin
Apple (*Malus domestica*)	Rosaceae	Seeds and fruits	Amygdalin
Apricot (*Prunus armeniaca*)	Rosaceae	Kernels	Amygdalin Prunasin

Table 1.
Cyanogenic glycosides in major edible plants.

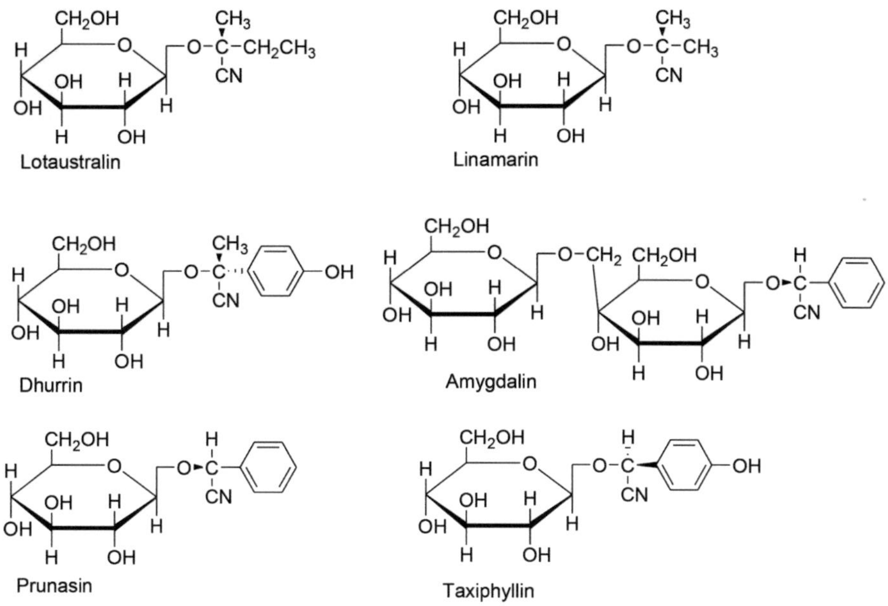

Figure 3.
Structures of cyanogenic glycosides found in major edible plants [20].

the sixteenth and seventeenth centuries. The crop is a staple food in most African communities and has economic value in Africa, South America, and Southeast Asia. The crop is widely cultivated in the tropics, and a total area of over 18 million ha is grown to cassava [21], and over half a billion of the world's population depend on cassava as their major staple [22]. Africa is the largest producer of cassava in the world and accounts for over 53% of the global production [23]. According to the Food and Agriculture Organization, cassava is ranked third, after rice and corn, as the most important source of calories in the tropics [23]. The tuberous roots of the crop have high carbohydrate content, which makes cassava a good source of calorie for over half a billion people in the world. Additionally, cassava leaves are rich in proteins, vitamin C, vitamin A, and dietary fiber. Cassava is one of the world's most important tuberous food crops, with annual global production estimated at 252 million metric tons (MT) in 2011. **Table 2** shows the production trend among the top five producing countries in the world according to the Food and Agriculture Organization statistics [23].

Country	**Annual cassava production quantity (million metric tons)**				
	2007	**2008**	**2009**	**2010**	**2011**
Nigeria	43.41	44.58	36.82	42.53	52.40
Brazil	26.54	26.70	24.40	24.50	25.45
Indonesia	19.99	21.59	22.04	23.92	24.01
Thailand	26.92	25.16	30.09	22.21	21.91
Ghana	10.22	11.35	12.23	13.50	14.24
Others	99.35	102.62	109.87	110.25	114.20
World	226.43	232.00	235.45	236.11	252.21

Table 2.
Major cassava-producing countries in the world.

Despite the nutritional and economic benefits obtained from cassava, almost all parts of the plant contain cyanogenic glycosides, which limits the potential utilization of the plant as food for human and animal consumption. Each part of the cassava plant (leaves, stem, root) contains high levels of cyanogenic glycosides, mainly linamarin and lotaustralin with the former being the most predominant cyanogen at the ratio of 9:1 [17]. The biosynthesis of the major cyanogenic glucoside in cassava, linamarin, occurs in leaves and is then transported to the tuber [24]. Cassava leaves and the cortex or peel of the roots contain large quantities of cyanogenic glycosides (900–2000 mg HCN/kg dry matter) [8], while the tuberous parenchyma has approximately 20-fold lower levels. Studies have found that cassava roots contain a total cyanide content of 10–500 mg/kg of dry matter [25] although higher contents have also been reported, particularly in bitter cultivars. All cassava varieties are known to contain cyanogenic compounds, and cyanide levels depend on factors such as variety, plant age, soil condition, fertilizer application, and environmental conditions [25].

3.2 Cocoyam

Cocoyam generally refers to two members of the Araceae family, namely, *Colocasia esculenta* (L.) Schott and *Xanthosoma sagittifolium* (L.) Schott. The plant is native to Central and South America where it has been cultivated and consumed for centuries but has since been naturalized in most tropical regions including sub-Saharan Africa [26]. Cocoyam is an important staple for most rural communities in many developing countries of Africa, Asia, and the Pacific. In sub-Saharan Africa, the most cultivated species, *Colocasia esculenta*, is extensively grown for livelihood by small-scale resource-poor farmers with minimal input.

For the last 3 decades, Africa's annual cocoyam output of about 10 MT has consistently been higher than other regions [9]. The continent's contribution to the global cocoyam output is presented in **Table 3**. The mean global production in the 2003–2012 decade was more than double the mean production obtained in the years between 1983 and 1992, which could principally be attributed to increased production in Africa. The major cocoyam-producing countries in Africa are Nigeria, Ghana, and Cameroon, which contributed about 68% of the global mean output between 2003 and 2012.

Edible cocoyam is a nutrient dense tuber crop that can be processed into flour and used to make mashed meal or porridge. The tubers can also be consumed baked or boiled. Cocoyam is rich in carbohydrates; as a result, it is an important source of

Producer	1983–1992		1993–2002		2003–2012	
	Mean[a]	%[b]	Mean	%	Mean	%
World	4.88		8.04		10.72	
Africa	2.74	56.26	5.88	73.13	8.25	76.96
China	1.20	24.62	1.40	17.47	1.61	15.04
Cameroon	0.49	10.14	0.88	10.98	1.40	13.02
Ghana	1.01	20.64	1.53	19.04	1.57	14.62
Nigeria	0.52	10.61	2.60	32.36	4.28	39.91

[a]*Mean production in million tons over 10 years.*
[b]*Percentage of contribution to global mean.*

Table 3.
Contributions of top producers to global cocoyam output in the last 3 decades [9].

calorie for millions of people in the tropical and subtropical regions [27]. In addition to carbohydrates, cocoyam contains other nutrients such as protein, vitamins, carotenoids, and minerals [28]. Apart from the nutrient composition of cocoyam tuber, antinutritional compounds such as cyanogenic glycosides have been reported in the crops albeit in lower concentrations (21.0–171.3 mg/kg dry matter) [29, 30] than other food plants.

3.3 Bamboo shoot

Fresh immature bamboo shoots are consumed as vegetable in some Asian countries, and they contain appreciable quantities of vitamin C, carbohydrates, and protein [31]. Apart from the nutritive value, bamboo shoots contain lethal concentrations of cyanogenic glycosides. The cyanogenic glycoside present in bamboo shoot is taxiphyllin, which quickly decomposes when exposed to boiling water. Cyanide contents of 1000–8000 mg HCN/kg have been reported [32]. Although cyanide content of bamboo shoot is much higher than that of cassava root, the cyanide content in bamboo shoots decreases substantially following harvesting and processing.

3.4 Sorghum

The plant sorghum [*Sorghum bicolor* (L.) Moench] belongs to the Poaceae family (tribe Andropogoneae) and is one of the most important crops in Africa, Asia, and Latin America. It is a very genetically diverse crop both in cultivated and wild species. About five sorghum's landraces are known, and the greatest variation within the sorghum genus is found in the Ethiopia-Sudan region, which is believed to be the origin of the plant. The most important global producers of sorghum are the United States of America, Nigeria, Sudan, Mexico, China, India, Ethiopia, Argentina, Burkina Faso, Brazil, and Australia [23]. Burkina Faso appears to be the world leader of sorghum production and consumption per inhabitant. There has been an increased demand for the crop in Africa over the last 50 years. Studies indicate that more than 35% of sorghum is grown directly for human consumption, while the rest is used primarily for animal feed, alcohol production, and industrial products [33]. Although sorghum is a widely grown cereal crop that resembles corn in general composition, it is an inferior crop due to the presence of cyanogenic glycosides, dhurrin and amygdalin, among other factors. The major cyanogenic glycoside in sorghum is dhurrin, and its content in shoot tips of seedlings is estimated at 30% dry weight. In young sorghum leaves, dhurrin and the enzymes responsible for its hydrolysis to hydrogen cyanide are localized in vacuoles and cytoplasm of plants, respectively. The compartmental separation of the enzyme and the substrate makes tissues free from cyanide in intact leaves. The levels of dhurrin decrease with plant age, and immature sorghum leaves contain higher concentrations of dhurrin than the mature ones [17].

3.5 Fruits and fruit kernels

Most fruits and fruit kernels contain the potentially toxic cyanogenic glycoside compound, amygdalin. The contents of amygdalin in fruit seeds vary significantly among varieties and environmental conditions [34]. The following sections will highlight two important sources of amygdalin: apple and apricot fruits.

3.5.1 Apple (Malus domestica)

Apple seeds contain appreciable amounts of amygdalin, a cyanogenic glycoside composed of cyanide and sugar. When metabolized in the digestive system, this chemical degrades into highly poisonous hydrogen cyanide. Studies have reported that amygdalin content in apple seeds ranged from 1 to 4 mg/g, while that of apple juice was reported to be between 0.001 and 0.08 mg/ml [34].

3.5.2 Apricot fruits (Prunus armeniaca)

Apricot fruits are widely cultivated in Central Asia, Africa, America, and Europe. There are two varieties of apricot kernels: bitter and sweet. Bitter apricot kernels contain a considerably high amount of the cyanogenic glycoside amygdalin and thus are unsafe for consumption. On the other hand, sweet varieties are safe for human consumption because of their low level of cyanogens [35]. The concentration of hydrogen cyanide in apricot kernels varies widely (49–4000 mg/kg), depending on whether the skin was included or not during cyanide determination. Ingestion of raw or improperly processed apricot kernels with high cyanide levels can cause serious acute problems that could lead to death [2].

4. Food processing technologies

Incidences of health conditions associated with dietary intake of cyanogens can be prevented or reduced by effective removal of cyanogenic compounds in food plants prior to consumption. Food plants are traditionally processed using various methods that vary widely depending on geographical location and ethnicity of communities [36]. The main aims of the food processing techniques are to reduce toxicity and improve palatability and storability. The main processing techniques used worldwide for most food plants include drying, boiling/cooking, soaking/wetting, fermentation, and/or a combination of the processes [8]. For example, processing techniques and stages used for production of snacks and main dishes from cassava roots are summarized in **Figure 4**.

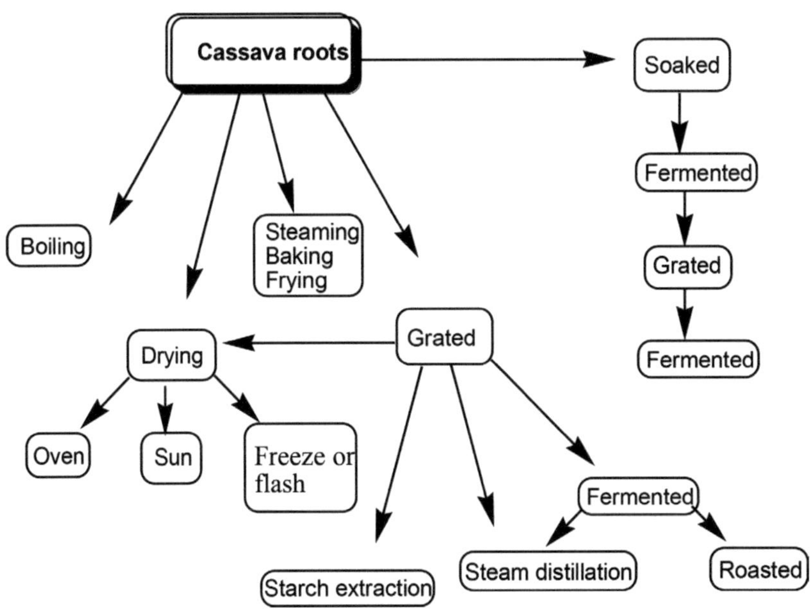

Figure 4.
Common cassava processing methods used worldwide.

4.1 Drying

Drying is one of the most appropriate processing methods for removal of cyanogenic glycosides in food plants. This is a mass transfer process which removes water from the product by evaporation and keeps the product free from microorganisms. There are several drying methods that can be employed to reduce cyanogens from food products, and they include the use of sun, oven, freeze, and superheated steam. Studies have reported that in bamboo shoots around 80% cyanogenic glycoside reduction was obtained after vacuum freeze-drying for 24 hours at −50°C. On the other hand, superheated steam drying at 120–160°C afforded significant decomposition of taxiphyllin, which causes bitterness in bamboo shoots [37], while oven-drying after grating at 60°C for 8 hours led to very high reduction of cyanogen content of up to 95% [38].

In eastern and southern Africa, cassava is traditionally processed into flour by sun drying the peeled roots followed by pounding and sieving or heap fermentation. However, because this process does not allow enough contact between linamarase and linamarin, total cyanogen content of 59 ppm of HCN equivalents has been reported in processed products, which is higher than the WHO safe level of 10 ppm [39]. The high levels of residual cyanogens can be attributed to the drying process, which restricts the contact between the endogenous enzymes linamarase and cyanogenic glucoside and promotes the retention of cyanohydrin and free cyanide in dried cassava.

4.2 Boiling/cooking

The effectiveness of boiling/cooking on cyanogen removal from various plant food products shows that the method achieves different results depending on the processing duration and part of the plant species. Several studies have reported that cooking and boiling are among the most effective practices for reducing cyanogenic compounds from food plants. These processes appear to promote the rupture of cell walls, which allow translocation of cell contents including antinutrients and toxic substances [39]. A study on bamboo plant showed that cyanogenic glycoside in the shoots of *Bambusa vulgaris* were reduced by 67.84–76.92% after boiling for 10 minutes. Boiling the shoots for an additional 10 minutes further achieved up to 87% reduction in cyanogen content [37]. Similar studies in cassava reported that the efficacy of the boiling method for cyanogen reduction is substantially improved when small-sized cassava pieces are boiled in a large volume of water [40].

However, some studies have reported that boiling can only reduce cyanogen content by 50%, and therefore, it is not an effective method for cyanide removal. The inefficiency of this processing method is attributed to the high temperatures. It is reported that at an elevated temperature of 100°C, linamarase, a heat-labile β-glycosidase, is denatured, and linamarin cannot then be hydrolyzed into cyanohydrin and subsequent HCN. A study by Cooke and Maduagwu [41] reported that bound glucosides were reduced to 45 to 50% after 25 min of boiling. Free cyanide and cyanohydrin in boiled cassava roots are found at very low concentrations.

4.3 Soaking/wetting

Like most processing methods, soaking or wetting of harvested crops helps to improve the shelf life of the food products. Additionally, processing improves the safety and quality of the products. For example, a study reported that cassava flour and to a lesser extent *gari* stored under ambient conditions retained cyanogens over long periods [25]. However, if flour is mixed with water and the resultant wet flour left in the shade for 5 hours at about 30°C to allow HCN gas to escape, the total cyanide content is reduced three to sixfold. In Africa, the wetting method is commonly practiced in villages around Uvira in South Kivu Province of the Democratic Republic of Congo (DRC) where sporadic incidences of cyanide poisoning and Konzo have been reported [42]. An improved wetting study that reduced processing time to 2 hours was found to be equally effective in removing cyanogens. However, flour samples dried at temperatures above about 80°C lead to denaturing of linamarase, and the wetting method becomes ineffective.

In Malawi, soaking of cassava roots is mostly practiced in the lakeshore areas of northern Malawi and Nkhotakota in the central region, where cassava roots are soaked peeled or unpeeled [36]. A comparative study of the two soaking methods showed that soaking of peeled roots was more effective in reducing levels of cyanogens than soaking unpeeled roots [36]. In the former case, flours of negligible cyanogen contents were obtained, and the residual cyanogen contents were below the maximum FAO/WHO limit. Soaking of unpeeled cassava roots was found to be ineffective as its products gave values above the FAO/WHO recommended limit of 10 mg HCN eq./kg dry matter. The study showed that inclusion of the peel during processing led to high retention of cyanogens in the pulp.

4.4 Fermentation

Fermentation is one of the ancient methods of food preservation and became widely accepted in many cultures due to its nutritional value and variety of sensory attributes. Fermentation enhances the nutritive value of food through biosynthesis of vitamins and essential amino acids and degradation of antinutrients [39]. In the African region, fermentation by lactic acid bacteria is one of the most practiced processing methods. Fermentation is done with grated or soaked cassava roots, which could be peeled or unpeeled [36]. The process results in a decrease in pH of the food material during processing.

In western Africa and southern America, cassava parenchyma is ground, grated, or crushed into small pieces to disrupt many plant cells and allow good contact between linamarin and linamarase. The moist mash is then left to ferment for several days, the water-soluble cyanogens is squeezed out, and the residual HCN gas is removed by roasting. This process significantly reduced the cyanogen content of the product (*gari* or *farinha*) [39].

5. Health conditions associated with cyanide exposure

Cyanide, one of the most rapidly acting poisons, exists in many forms. The most common are hydrogen cyanide and cyanide salts such as potassium cyanide, sodium cyanide, and calcium cyanide. Cyanide salts can react with acids and subsequently release HCN. In most developing countries, cyanide intake through food consumption is normally high since processed foods with residual levels of cyanogenic substances are a predominant diet among communities. However, cyanide toxicity appears to be a rare form of poisoning among the general population particularly in developed countries. Cyanide exposure occurs relatively frequently in individuals through a variety of modes including inhalation, ingestion, and dermal absorption. In food plants, ingestion of cyanogenic compounds is the most common form of cyanide exposure. The potential toxicity of cyanogenic plants is largely dependent on their ability to produce lethal concentrations of hydrogen cyanide when exposed to humans. The toxic compound, HCN, is formed following the hydrolysis of potentially toxic compounds, cyanogenic glycosides. The conversion process is initiated by the breakdown of the cyanogenic compounds upon disruption of the plant cells that occur during crushing of the edible plant material either during consumption or during processing of the food crop. The residual cyanogens in food products are the primary source of cyanide toxicity to humans when broken down in the gastrointestinal tract to form cyanide [43]. Generally, small quantities of cyanide are naturally detoxified by cellular enzymes and thiosulfates present in many tissues to form relatively harmless thiocyanate, which is excreted in the urine [44].

Human exposure to cyanide from consumption of food products with considerable amounts of cyanogenic glycosides is associated with health complications such as acute intoxications, chronic toxicity, neurological disorders, growth retardation, and goiter. The following sections will provide the epidemiological information, etiology, and prevalence of health conditions attributed to the toxic effects of cyanogenic glycosides in edible plants.

5.1 Acute toxicity

Acute cyanide poisoning occurs when the cyanide level exceeds the limit an individual can detoxify, and therefore the natural detoxification mechanisms are overwhelmed [44]. In humans, the cyanide ion (CN^-) has a strong affinity to the trivalent iron (Fe^{3+}) of the cytochrome oxidase and is readily absorbed from the intestinal and respiratory tracts [45]. A typical cherry red venous blood is seen in cases of acute cyanide poisoning because of the failure of the oxygen-saturated hemoglobin to release its oxygen at the tissues since the enzyme cytochrome oxidase is inhibited by the cyanide [44]. Thus, cyanide inhibits cytochrome oxidase preventing oxygen utilization leading to cytotoxic anoxia. This causes a decrease in the utilization of oxygen in the tissues. Additionally, increases in blood glucose and lactic acid levels and a decrease in the ATP/ADP ratio are observed, indicating a shift from aerobic to anaerobic metabolism [46].

Acute cyanide exposure mainly adversely affects the central nervous system (CNS) and the cardiovascular, endocrine, and respiratory systems. In humans, the clinical signs of acute cyanide intoxication can include rapid respiration, drop in blood pressure, dizziness, headache, stomach pains, vomiting, diarrhea, mental confusion, cyanosis with twitching, and convulsions followed by terminal coma and death. There is great variability of lethal doses reported in the literature. However, the mean lethal dose by mouth of cyanide in human adults is estimated to be in the range of 50 to 200 mg, and if untreated death is rarely delayed more than 1 hour [47].

5.2 Chronic toxicity

Persistent and prolonged exposure to low levels of cyanide is known to produce symptoms that are different from those observed in acute exposures described above. Chronic exposure to lower cyanide concentrations has been associated with several health conditions especially among cassava-eating populations. Health manifestations such as malnutrition, congenital malformations, neurological disorders, and myelopathy have been attributed to chronic cyanide toxicity [48]. Reports have also shown that goiter, the swelling of the thyroid glands, has occurred in communities where the levels of cyanogenic glycosides in cassava diets are greater than 10–50 mg/kg food [48].

5.3 Neurological effects

Although the entire human body is affected by dietary cyanide exposure, adverse effects on the central nervous system are the most prevalent because of the high metabolic demand for oxygen in neurons and its control of respiratory function. Thus, the stimulation of carotid and aortic bodies contributes to the poor functions of the central nervous system and respiratory system.

Chronic human exposure to cyanide has been studied in African regions where populations consume large amounts of cyanide-containing cassava root. Neurological findings among the affected individuals include symmetrical hyperreflexia of the upper limbs, symmetrical spastic paraparesis of the lower limbs, spastic dysarthria, diminished visual acuity, peripheral neuropathy, cerebellar signs, and deafness [6]. Cyanide intake from a cassava-dominated diet is a contributing factor in two forms of nutritional neuropathies, tropical ataxic neuropathy described from Nigeria, and epidemic spastic paraparesis described from Mozambique, Tanzania, and Zaire [49, 50].

5.3.1 Tropical ataxic neuropathy

The term tropical ataxic neuropathy refers to several neurological disorders caused by many factors including toxiconutritional agents. The syndrome, first reported in Jamaica in 1897 and named tropical ataxic neuropathy in 1959, describes several neurological symptoms effecting the mouth, eyesight, hearing, or gait. In the African population, TAN is predominantly prevalent among the elderly population of mostly older males and females. TAN is mostly attributed to cyanide intake due to constant consumption of foods derived from cassava with high levels of cyanogenic compounds [48]. Studies conducted in West Africa particularly Nigeria, Tanzania, Uganda, Kenya, the West Indies, and tropical Asia have reported that cases of TAN generally occur in older people who have consumed a monotonous cassava diet over the years.

5.3.2 Konzo

Konzo, which means "bound legs" in Yaka language of Kwango region in the Democratic Republic of Congo, was first described in 1938 by an Italian missionary doctor. It is a distinct neurological disease with selective upper motor neuron damage and is characterized by an abrupt onset of an irreversible, non-progressive and symmetrical spastic paraparesis [50]. The disease is mostly associated with high dietary cyanogen consumption from poorly processed roots of bitter cassava combined with a protein-deficient diet low in sulfur amino acids [43]. Studies have found that cassava processing methods that involve shortcuts, as practiced during times of war and famine, exacerbate the health condition among the communities. Since its first description in the DRC, Konzo epidemics have been reported from many cassava-consuming areas in rural Africa. The disease has extended beyond DRC borders, and it remains a serious health problem among African communities that subsist on cassava [48]. In sub-Saharan Africa, at least seven countries have reported the outbreaks of Konzo, and they include the Democratic Republic of Congo, Mozambique, Tanzania, Central African Republic, Angola, Cameroon, and Zambia. In most of the affected countries, the epidemics were preceded by food shortages and several weeks of exclusive consumption of poorly processed bitter cassava roots, resulting in high dietary cyanide exposure, which was confirmed by high levels of thiocyanate in serum and urine [50].

5.4 Goiter and cretinism

Goiter and cretinism are common diseases in most developing countries because of low intake of iodine (<100 μg/day) among communities. Populations that exclusively depend on cassava as a staple food have shown high incidences of endemic goiter and cretinism. Several studies have reported that populations with very low iodine intake and correspondingly high thiocyanate levels showed severe endemic goiter. The endocrine effect may be due to formation of thiocyanate, a lesser toxic metabolite of cyanide. Thiocyanate is known to block iodine uptake in the body and compete with iodide ion (I^-) as a substrate for the thyroid peroxidase, thereby decreasing the iodination of tyrosine to form iodotyrosine by the thyroid gland. Consumption of food products with residual cyanogenic glycosides even at a very low concentration can cause iodine deficiency leading to goiter [43].

5.5 Growth retardation

In humans, low birth weights among children are a common health problem especially in developing countries. Chronic exposure to cyanogenic glycosides has been reported as a major contributing factor to this health problem. Growth retardation is particularly a serious problem in populations consuming foods with inadequate proteins especially diets that are low in sulfur-containing amino acids such as methionine and cysteine. Cyanide detoxification in the human body requires sulfur donors from sulfur-containing amino acids [43], and thus, dietary exposure to cyanide has been identified as one of the contributing factors to growth retardation among children [51].

6. Cyanide detoxification

Hydrogen cyanide whether ingested directly or released from cyanogens is readily absorbed in the blood by binding to iron in hemoglobin and quickly distributed to organs such as the liver, kidney, brain, and blood tissue. However, about 80

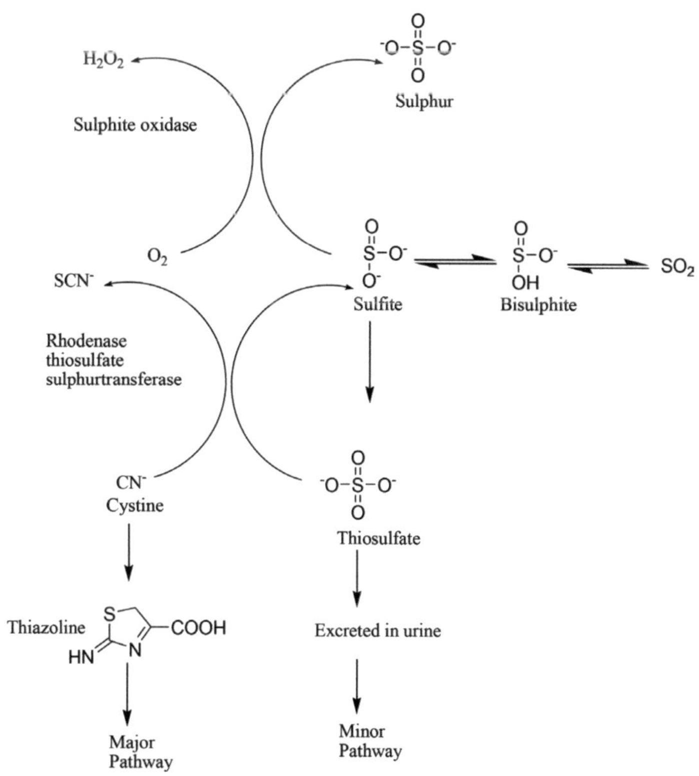

Figure 5.
Cyanide metabolism in the body [54].

percent of the absorbed cyanide is detoxified in the liver mainly by the mitochondrial enzyme rhodanese, which catalyzes the transfer of sulfur from a sulfate donor to cyanide, forming a less toxic metabolite, thiocyanate. There are two primary detoxification mechanisms of ingested cyanide in the body. The minor one involves methemoglobin in the red blood cells, which temporarily neutralize cyanide by reversible reaction [52]. The major pathway proceeds by the conversion of cyanide to a less toxic thiocyanate (SCN). This process is catalyzed by the enzyme rhodanese present in most tissues, by a reaction with sulfur [43], as shown in **Figure 5**. The two amino acids, cysteine and methionine, are the common source of sulfur [53]. The generated SCN is then slowly excreted through urine and sweat.

Other detoxification mechanisms exist and include the binding of hydroxocobalamin (vitamin B_{12}) to cyanide to form cyanocobalamin. Small quantities of cyanide along with CO_2 are eliminated through this pathway.

7. Conclusion

Cyanogenic glycosides are widely distributed in edible plants, and they play a major role in plant protection against herbivores, pathogens, and competitors. The presence of the potentially toxic compounds in food plants has also contributed to food security, particularly in the sub-Saharan African region. Most of the cyanogenic plants, such as cassava, have several agricultural advantages over other crops due to their outstanding ecological adaptation, low labor requirement, and high tolerance to extreme stress conditions such as drought and poor soils. Additionally, the cyanogenic compounds act as a deterrent against thieves and pests. However, several health disorders and diseases have been associated with consumption of food products with high quantities of residual cyanogens. Consequently, it is recommended that consumers should prepare foods properly before consumption in order to prevent adverse effects of cyanogenic glycosides in food plants. There are various traditional processing techniques that are relatively effective in removing cyanide from food plants, especially those involving grating and crushing. Generally, the efficiency of the technique largely depends on the duration of the process, material size, moisture, and temperature. In order to improve food safety, researchers have extensively studied mechanisms that accelerate cyanogenesis and cyanide volatilization during processing, which is a strategic step in detoxification of food plants. Therefore, effective processing technologies should be promoted among communities to enhance safety and organoleptic properties of products derived from cyanogenic food plants.

Conflict of interest

The author declares that there is no conflict of interest.

Author details

Kumbukani K. Nyirenda
Plant and Soil Sciences Department, University of Pretoria, Pretoria, South Africa

*Address all correspondence to: knyirenda@medcol.mw

References

[1] Wink M. Plant breeding importance of secondary metabolites for production against pathogens and herbivores. Theoretical and Applied Genetics. 1988;**75**(2):225-233

[2] Vetter J. Plant cyanogenic glycosides. Toxicon [Internet]. 2000;**38**(1):11-36. DOI: 10.1016/S0041-0101(99)00128-2

[3] Onojah PK, Odin EM. Cyanogenic glycoside in food plants. The International Journal of Innovation in Science and Mathematics [Internet]. 2015;**3**(4):2347-9051. Available from: https://www.ijism.org/administrator/components/com_jresearch/files/publications/IJISM_402_Final.pdf

[4] Bolarinwa IF, Oke MO, Olaniyan SA, Ajala AS. A review of cyanogenic glycosides in edible plants. In: Soloneski S, Larramendy ML, editors. Toxicology—New Aspects to This Scientific Conundrum. Rijeka, Croatia: Intech; 2016

[5] Monago CC, Akhidue V. Cyanide poisoning. Journal of Applied Sciences and Environmental Management. 2002;**6**(1):22-25

[6] Tylleskär T, Rosling H, Banea M, Bikangi N, Cooke RD, Poulter NH. Cassava cyanogens and konzo, an upper motor neuron disease found in Africa. Lancet. 1992;**339**(8787):208-211

[7] Mlingi N, Poulter NH, Rosling H. An outbreak of acute intoxications from consumption of insufficiently processed cassava in Tanzania. Nutrition Research. 1992;**12**(6):677-687

[8] Cardoso A, Mirone E, Ernest M, Massza F, Cliff J, Haque R, et al. Modification of nutritional quality of cassava through plant nutrition. Journal of Food Composition and Analysis. 2005;**18**:451-461

[9] FAO/WHO. WHO Food Additive Series: 65. Safety evaluation of certain food additives and contaminants. Prepared by the 74th Meeting of the Joint FAO/WHO Expert Committee on Food Additives (JECFA). Geneva; 2012

[10] Jones PR, Møller BL, Høj PB. The UDP-glucose:p-hydroxymandelonitrile-O-glucosyltransferase that catalyzes the last step in synthesis of the cyanogenic glucoside dhurrin in Sorghum bicolor. Isolation, cloning, heterologous expression, and substrate specificity. The Journal of Biological Chemistry. 1999;**274**(50):35483-35491

[11] Jones DA. Why are so many food plants cyanogenic? Phytochemistry. 1998;**47**(2):155-162

[12] Francisco IA, Pinotti MHP. Cyanogenic glycosides in plants. Brazilian Archives of Biology and Technology. 2000;**43**(5):487-492

[13] Ganjewala D, Kumar S, Devi SA, Ambika K. Advances in cyanogenic glycosides biosynthesis and analyses in plants: A review. Acta Biologica Szegediensis. 2010;**54**(1):1-14

[14] Bak S, Kahn RA, Nielsen HL, Møller BL, Halkier BA. Cloning of three A-type cytochromes P450, CYP71E1, CYP98, and CYP99 from *Sorghum bicolor* (L.) Moench by a PCR approach and identification by expression in Escherichia coli of CYP71E1 as a multifunctional cytochrome P450 in the biosynthesis of the cyanogen. Plant Molecular Biology. 1998;**36**(3):393-405

[15] Harborne JB. Recent advances in chemical ecology. Natural Product Reports. 1986;**3**:323-344

[16] Harborne JB. Plant toxins and their effects on animals. In: Introduction to Ecological Biochemistry. London: Academic Press; 1993. pp. 71-103

[17] Poulton JE. Cyanogenesis in plants. Plant Physiology. 1990;**94**(2):401-405

[18] Gruhnert C, Biehl B, Selmar D. Compartmentation of cyanogenic glucosides and their degrading enzymes. Planta. 1994;**195**(1):36-42

[19] McMahon JM, White WLB, Sayre RT. Cyanogenesis in cassava (*Manihot esculenta* Crantz). Journal of Experimental Botany. 2005;**46**(288): 731-741

[20] JECFA. Cyanogenic glycosides. In: Toxicological evaluation of certain food additives and naturally occurring toxicants. 39th Meeting of the Joint FAO/WHO Expert Committee on Food Additive (WHO Food Additives Series 30). Geneva; 1993

[21] Baguma Y, Sun C, Borén M, Olsson H, Rosenqvist S, Mutisya J, et al. Sugar-mediated semidian oscillation of gene expression in the cassava storage root regulates starch synthesis. Plant Signaling & Behavior. 2008;**3**(7):439-445

[22] Aryee FNA, Oduro I, Ellis WO, Afuakwa JJ. The physicochemical properties of flour samples from the roots of 31 varieties of cassava. Food Control. 2006;**17**(11):916-922

[23] FAO. FAOSTAT [Internet]. Rome; 2015. Available from: faostat.fao.org/site/339/default.aspx

[24] Wheatley C, Chuzel G. Cassava: The nature of the tuber and use as a raw material. In: Macrae R, Robinson RK, Sadler M, editors. Encyclopedia of Food Science, Food Technology and Nutrition. San Diego, California: Academic Press; 1993. pp. 964-970

[25] Chiwona-Karltun L, Afoakwa EO, Nyirenda D, Mwansa CN, Kongor EJ, Brimer L. Varietal diversity and processing effects on the biochemical composition, cyanogenic glucoside potential (HCNp) and appearance of cassava flours from South-Eastern African region. The International Food Research Journal [Internet]. 2015;**22**(3):973-980. Available from: www.ifrj.upm.edu.my

[26] Onwueme IC. Tropical Root and Tuber Crops—Production, Perspectives and Future Prospects. Rome: FAO; 1994. ISBN: 92-5-103461-3

[27] Nail H. Understanding the production of the major tropical/subtropical root crops: cassava, potatoes, yams and cocoyams. In: Technical Paper, China; 2010. pp. 17-35

[28] FAO. Roots, Tubers, Plantain and Bananas in Human Nutrition. Rome: FAO; 1991. ISBN: 92-5-103138-X

[29] Olajide R, Akinsoyinu AO, Babayemi OJ, Omojola AB, Abu AO, Afolabi KD. Effect of processing on energy values, nutrient and anti-nutrient components of wild cocoyam [*Colocasia esculenta* (L.) Schott] corm. Pakistan Journal of Nutrition. 2011;**10**(1):29-34

[30] Igbadul BD, Amoye J, Twadue I. Effect of fermentation on the proximate composition , antinutritional factors and functional properties of cocoyam (*Colocasia esculenta*) flour. African Journal of. Microbiology Research [Internet]. 2014;**8**(3):67-74. Available from: 10.1016/j.foodchem.2013.01.059%5Cnhttp://www.davidpublishing.com/davidpublishing/Upfile/12/1/2014/2014120172701049.pdf%5Cnhttp://academicjournals.org/journal/AJMR/article-abstract/07E643346419%5Cnhttp://academicjournals.org/journal/AJMR/

[31] Bhargava A, Kumbhare V, Srivastava A, Sahai A. Bamboo parts and seeds for additional source of nutrition. Journal of Food Science and Technology. 1996;**33**(2):145-146

[32] Ferreira VL, Yotsuyanagi K, Carvalho CR. Elimination of cyanogenic compounds from bamboo shoots *Dendrocalamus giganteus* Munro. Tropical Science. 1995;**35**(4):342-346

[33] Awika JM, Rooney LW. Sorghum phytochemicals and their potential impact on human health. Methods in Molecular Biology. 1931;**2019**:121-140

[34] Bolarinwa IF, Orfila C, Morgan MRA. Amygdalin content of seeds, kernels and food products commercially-available in the UK. Food Chemistry. 2014;**152**:133-139

[35] Bolarinwa IF, Orfila C, Morgan MRA. Determination of amygdalin in apple seeds, fresh apples and processed apple juices. Food Chemistry. 2015;**170**:437-442

[36] Kalenga Saka JD, Nyirenda KK. Effect of two ethnic processing technologies on reduction and composition of total and non-glucosidic cyanogens in cassava. Food Chemistry. 2012;**130**(3):605-609

[37] Rawat K, Nirmala C, Bisht MS. Processing techniques for reduction of cyanogenic glycosides from bamboo shoots. In: 10th World Bamboo Congress, Korea 2015. 2015

[38] Lambri M, Fumi MD. Food technologies and developing countries: A processing method for making edible the highly toxic cassava roots. Italian Journal of Agronomy. 2014;**9**(2):79-83

[39] Montagnac JA, Davis CR, Tanumihardjo SA. Nutritional value of cassava for use as a staple food and recent advances for improvement. Comprehensive Reviews in Food Science and Food Safety. 2009;**8**(3):181-194

[40] Oke OL. Eliminating Cyanogens from cassava through processing: Technology and tradition. Acta Horticulturae. 1994;**375**(375):163-174

[41] Cooke RD, Maduagwu EN. The effects of simple processing on the cyanide content of cassava chips. International Journal of Food Science and Technology. 1978;**13**(4):299-306

[42] Bradbury JH. Simple wetting method to reduce cyanogen content of cassava flour. Journal of Food Composition and Analysis. 2006;**19**(4):388-393

[43] Rosling H. Measuring effects in humans of dietary cyanide exposure from cassava. Acta Horticulturae. 1994;**375**(375):271-284

[44] Salkowski AA, Penney DG. Cyanide poisoning in animals and humans: A review. Veterinary and Human Toxicology. 1994;**36**(5):455-466

[45] Way JL. Cyanide intoxication and its mechanism of antagonism. Annual Review of Pharmacology and Toxicology. 1984;**24**(1):451-481

[46] WHO. Toxicological evaluation of certain food additives and naturally occurring toxicants. WHO Food Additive Series: 30. Geneva, Switzerland: World Health Organization; 1993

[47] Gosselin R, Hodge H, Smith R, Gleason MN. Clinical Toxicology of Commercial Products, Annals of Internal Medicine. 4th ed. Vol. 85. Baltimore: Williams and Wilkins; 1976. 554 p

[48] FSANZ. Final assessment report proposal P257. Advice on the preparation of cassava and bamboo shoots. Canberra; 2004

[49] Osuntokun BO. Cassava diet, chronic cyanide intoxication and neuropathy in the Nigerian Africans. World Review of Nutrition and Dietetics. 1981;**36**:141-173

[50] Tylleskar T, Banea M, Bikangi N, Fresco L, Persson LA, Rosling H. Epidemiological evidence from Zaire

for a dietary etiology of konzo, an upper motor neuron disease. Bulletin of the World Health Organization. 1991;**69**(5):581-589

[51] Banea-Mayambu JP, Tylleskär T, Tylleskär K, Gebre-Medhin M, Rosling H. Dietary cyanide from insufficiently processed cassava and growth retardation in children in the Democratic Republic of Congo (formerly Zaire). Annals of Tropical Paediatrics. 2000;**20**(1):34-40

[52] Lundquist P, Rosling H, Sorbo B. Determination of cyanide in whole blood, erythrocytes, and plasma. Clinical Chemistry. 1985;**31**(4):591-595

[53] Diasolua D, Kuo Y, Lambein F. Cassava cyanogens and free amino acids in raw and cooked leaves. Food and Chemical Toxicology. 2003;**41**(8):1193-1197

[54] Omaye ST. Food and Nutritional Toxicology. Boca Raton, USA: CRC Press LLC; 2004

Chapter 11

Intoxication by Harmel

Djafer Rachid

Abstract

Herbal medicine has taken a prominent place in the North African skincare system because of the increased installation of herbalists and healers, but unfortunately most of these do not have the required level to practice this medicine. The Harmel (*Peganum harmala* L.) belongs to the family Zygophyllaceae, which has 24 genera and 240 species. It is a herbaceous plant, perennial, glabrous, and bushy, from a height of 30–100 cm, with a thick rhizome, its strong, unpleasant odor reminiscent of that of the Rue (*Ruta graveolens*). The Harmel is a toxic plant widespread in North Africa which has an important place in traditional medicine in several indications. It is used as a sedative, antitussive, antipyretic, antirheumatic, and antihelminthic, and to treat some skin diseases. Harmel is ingested with a glass of water or mixed with honey or pounded with olive oil. The intoxications are mainly due to overdose; the absorption of a quantity of seed greater than a teaspoon causes hallucinations and vomiting. In France, Harmel as well as its compounds (Harmine, Harmaline, Harmol, and harmalol) have been classified among the astonishing substances. The clinical manifestations described in the literature include: digestive disorders, bradycardia; neurological disorders paralysis, central nervous system depression; renal disorders; and in severe cases, dyspnoea and hypothermia and hypotension.

Keywords: intoxication, Harmel, toxic plant, botanical study, toxicological analysis

1. Introduction

North Africa has one of the oldest and richest traditions associated with the use of medicinal plants where they are very important to people in many places.

In recent years, there has been a significant increase in phytotherapy, which has led to several studies on traditional herbal treatments that have identified problems of toxicity or interaction that may cause therapeutic failures or accidents.

The aim of our work is to make a complete toxicological study of Harmel, which is a plant widely used in traditional medicine in the Maghreb countries, but given its richness in toxic alkaloids of type β-carboline, it causes many accidents and intoxications in humans and animals.

2. Botanical study

2.1 Botanical description

Peganum harmala L. belongs to the Zygophyllaceae family, which has 24 genera and 240 species. It is a herbaceous plant, which is perennial, hairless, bushy, and from a height 30–100 cm tall, with thick rhizome, and it has a strong, unpleasant smell reminiscent of that of the Rue and its bitter taste repels the animals [1–3].

The erect, very rowing stems disappear in winter. They have alternate leaves, divided into narrow strips that remain green for part of the dry season.

The solitary flowers with five elliptic, solitary petals are large (25–30 mm) and yellowish-white green (**Figure 1**). They are formed by small white flowers at the axils of the branches and a globose fruit containing several flattened seeds [3, 4].

The fruits are small spherical capsules with three chambers from 6 to 10 mm in diameter that stand straight on its stem and depressed at the top. Capsules contain more than 50 small triangular seeds [5].

The seeds, dark brown in color, are small and angular and have a diameter of 3–4 mm × 2 mm (**Figure 2**) [1].

The outer seed coats are cross-linked and have a bitter taste, with a particular smell, because they contain a red pigment called "Turkey red" and a

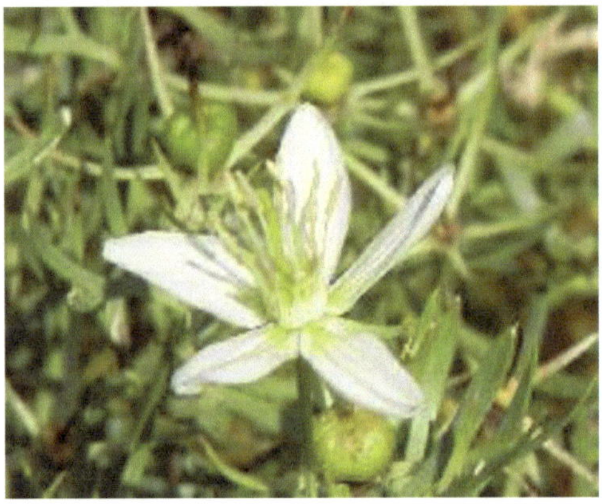

Figure 1.
Harmel flower [4].

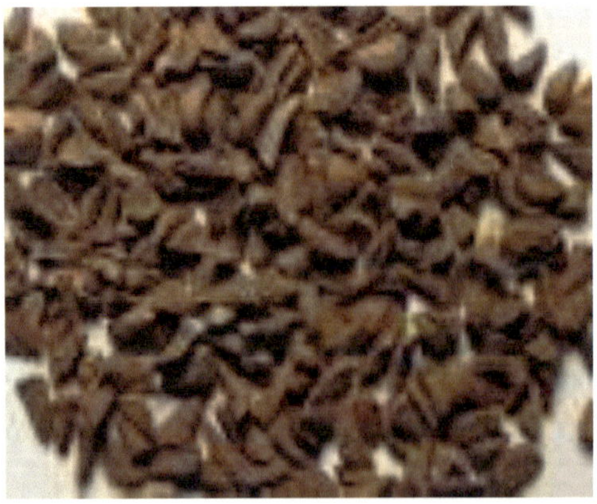

Figure 2.
Harmel seeds [4].

fluorescent compound. The harvest is done in summer because the seeds are rich in alkaloids [6].

2.2 Botanical classification

Branch: Spermatophytes
Sub-branch: Angiosperms
Class: Dicotyledonous
Subclass: Rosidae
Order: Sapindales
Family: Zygophyllaceae
Genre: *Peganum*
Species: *Peganum harmala* L. [3]

2.3 Appellations

Arabic name: Harmel
English name: Harmel, syrian rue, African rue, wild rue
French name: Harmel, rue syrienne, rue africaine
Spanich name: armalà, harmagà

3. Geographic distribution

Harmel is a plant that grows spontaneously throughout the world, generally in the Mediterranean area, especially in the quite dry areas in Europe (Spain, Russia, and Hungary); in North Africa in the steppe and semi-arid regions (Eastern Morocco, Northern Sahara and Algerian highlands, Tunisia, Libya steppes, and deserts of Egypt); and in Asia, it is widespread in the steppes of Iran, Pakistan, Turkestan to Tibet, and Siberia [7].

4. Chemical composition

Harmel contains the following chemical compounds:

- Amino acids: phenylalanine, valine, histidine, glutamic acid
- Flavonoids: coumarin, tannins, sterols.
- Alkaloids (toxic principles): Harmane, harmine, harmaline, harmol [8, 9].

The alkaloids are more concentrated in the seeds than in the other parts of the plant (3–4%): the leaf (0.52%) and the root or the stem (0.36%).

Their content increases in summer due to the maturity of the seed [10].

Roots contain 2% harmine and 1.4% harmol.

- Harmalin or Harmidine (3,4-dihydroharmine) or (7-methoxy-1-methyl-4,9-dihydro-3H-β-carboline) is of a general formula $C_{13}H_{14}N_2O$. It is the main alkaloid of *Peganum harmala* and the first that was isolated by Göbel from seeds and roots. This compound is slightly soluble in water and alcohol, and quite soluble in hot alcohol and dilute acids. Harmalin is almost twice more toxic than harmine. It forms the 2/3 total toxic alkaloids of the seed [8].

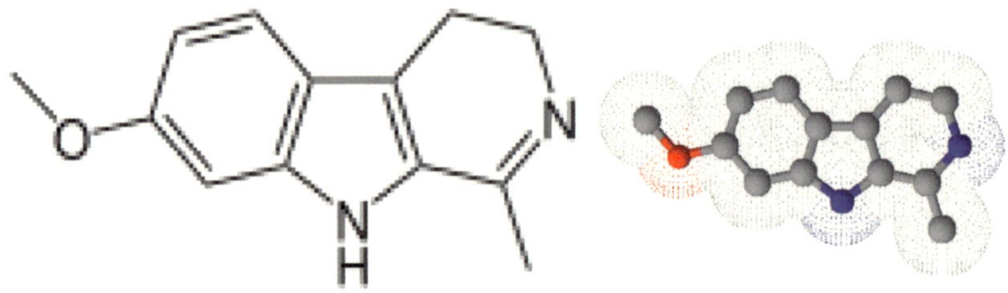

Harmalin

- Harmane (1-methyl-9-pyrido [3,4-b]indole) is of a general formula $C_{12}H_{10}N_2$. This alkaloid is crystallized in several organic solvents as colorless prisms. It is readily soluble in methanol, acetone, chloroform, or ether, but moderately soluble in hot water [8].

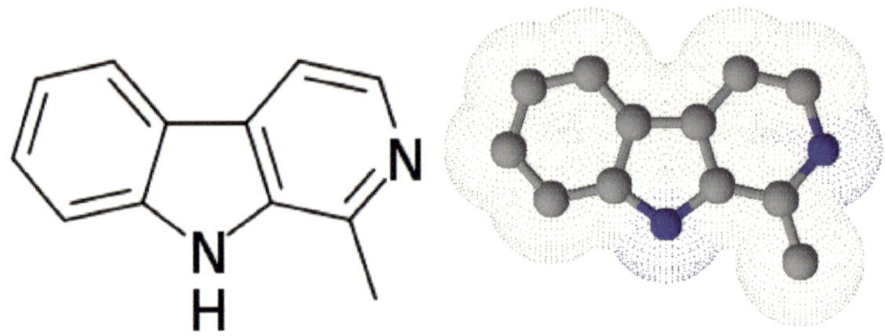

Harmane

- Harmine or Banisterin (7-methoxy-1-methyl-9-pyrido[3,4-b]indole) is of a general formula $C_{13}H_{12}N_2O$. It is slightly soluble in water, alcohol or ether.

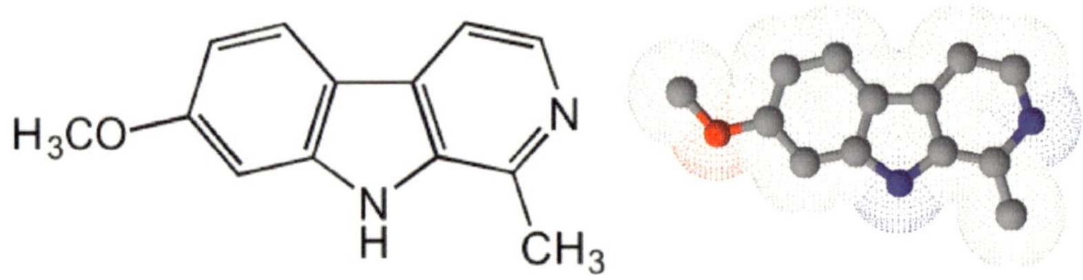

Harmine

- Harmalol (1-methyl-4,9-dihydro-3H-β-carbolin-7-ol) is of a general formula $C_{12}H_{12}N_2O$. It is an unstable alkaloid when exposed to air. It is crystallized in water as tri-hydrate. It is soluble in hot water, acetone, or chloroform, but poorly soluble in benzene [8].

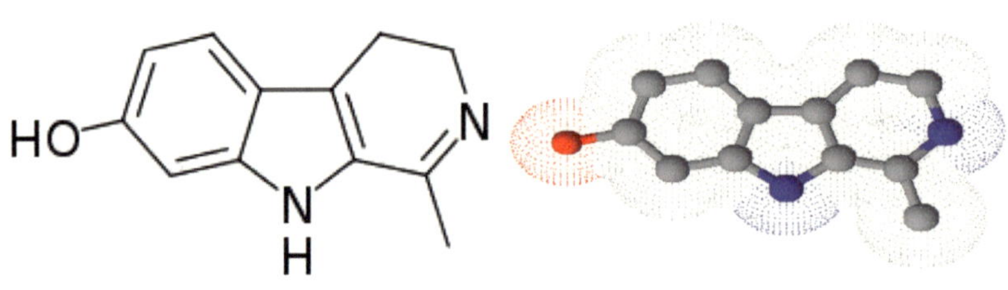

Harmalol

DOI: http://dx.doi.org/10.5772/intechopen.92936

- Other β-carbolines isolated from the plant *Peganum harmala* are: Harmalicidine and tetrahydroharmine.

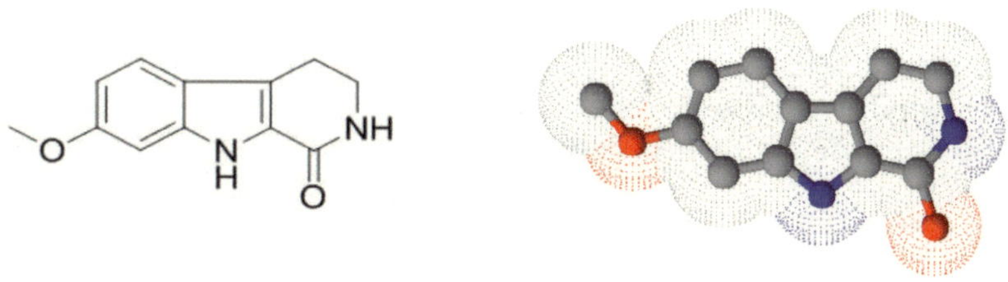

Harmalicidine

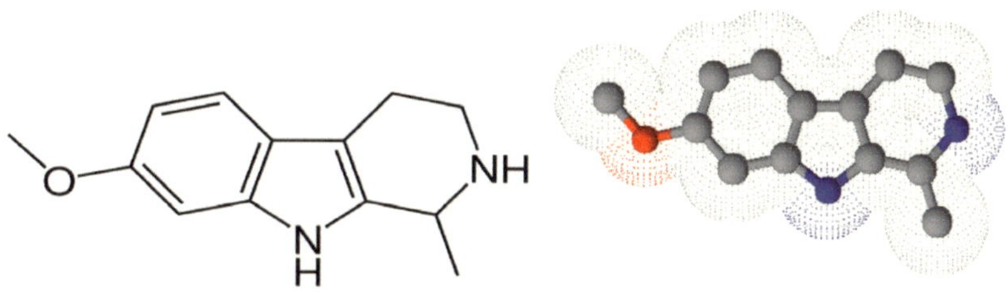

Tétrahydroharmine

5. Traditional use of the plant

Peganum harmala L. is considered one of the most famous medicinal plants in traditional medicine to treat several disorders.

- General disorders: hypnotic, antipyretic, analgesic, and antitussive.
- Gynecologic disorders: emmenagogue and abortifacient agent [11, 12].
- Digestive disorders: colic and hemorrhoids.
- Skin disorders: antiseptic and healing, dermatosis (eczema) and burning and blepharitis, and alopecia.
- Infectious disorders: neonatal tetanus, anthelmintic, antimalarial, and mumps.
- To treat certain nervous system disorders such as Parkinson's disease [13], in psychiatric conditions such as nervousness and insomnia in adults and children [7].
- Other diseases such as diabetes, high blood pressure, poisoning, snake venom, and rheumatism [11, 14].
- External use: the fresh plant either chopped and used in poultices, or after extraction of the juice for the composition of a liniment based on sheep fat, or use the dry plant or the seeds in the form of fumigations (to treat depression and insomnia in children) [7].

Seed oils obtained by decoction of the seeds in olive oil are very effective (rheumatic diseases). The dried plants, or the seeds, are sprayed and sieved to give the powder of the Harmel and also the decoction of roots.

- Internal use: seeds—a tea spoon, about 2.5 g, swallowed directly with a glass of water or mixed with honey or crushed with olive oil, fresh plant chopped and boiled in oil, or dry leaves in decoction.

6. Pharmacodynamics

6.1 Cardiovascular effects

In vivo studies have shown that different extracts of *Peganum harmala* where its main active alkaloids, harmine, harmalin, harman, and harmalol, have different cardiovascular effects, such as bradycardia, decreased blood pressure, peak aortic flow and contractile strength of the heart and vasodilator, and antigenic inhibitory effects [15].

6.2 Effects on the nervous system

Many in vitro and in vivo studies have indicated that alkaloids of *Peganum harmala* act on both the central and peripheral nervous system by inducing effects such as analgesia, hallucination, excitation, and antidepressant effect [16]. In addition, *Peganum harmala* β-carbolines have been shown to interact with dopamine, GABA, 5-hydroxytryptamine, benzodiazepines, and imidazoline at the level of their receptors present in the nervous system and in this way inducing their numerous psychotic pharmacological effects [17, 18].

6.3 Antibacterial, antifungal, insecticide, and antiparasitic

Different studies have shown different pharmacological effects such as antiparasitic effect, antifungal, antibacterial [18], and insecticides effects [19] of alkaloids derived from *Peganum harmala* seeds.

6.4 Effects on the immune system

Peganum harmala β-carbolines have been shown to have immunomodulatory effects in several studies [20]. Extracts of this plant have a significant anti-inflammatory effect via the inhibition of prostaglandin (mediator of inflammation).

6.5 Antidiabetic effects

Harmine is the main alkaloid of *Peganum harmala* that is involved in the antidiabetic effect. One study showed that this compound regulates the expression of the receptor Peroxysomes Gamma Proliferator-Activated (PPARγ), the main regulator of adipogenesis and the molecular target of antidiabetic drugs, by inhibition of the signaling pathway [21]. Studies have indicated that harmel extract has no activity on insulin secretion, as this hypoglycemic activity is associated with the pancreas. It affects the use and/or absorption of glucose [22].

6.6 Anticancer effects

In vitro studies have demonstrated a decrease in cell viability of cancer cells from various brain, colon, breast, lung, liver, esophagus, and stomach tissues following harmine treatment. Several researchers have shown the cytotoxicity of different *Peganum harmala* extracts in tumor cell lines in vitro and in vivo [23].

7. Toxicokinetic

7.1 Absorption

The main way of administration is the oral way by ingestion of preparation based on seeds or all parts of the plant.

After ingestion, the alkaloids are well absorbed by the gastrointestinal tract. The dermal way is used as a poultice and ointments where the seeds are mixed with olive oil which will increase the penetration of alkaloids by the skin.

Inhalation of alkaloids by fumigation is possible because this practice is used for the therapeutic or prophylaxis of magic [14, 24].

7.2 Distribution

Alkaloids cross the blood-brain barrier to the central nervous system. They distribute throughout the body (heart, liver, kidneys, and lungs).

7.3 Metabolism

- Phase I: alkaloids undergo hepatic O-demethylation by cytochrome P450 2D6, giving harmol and harmalol.

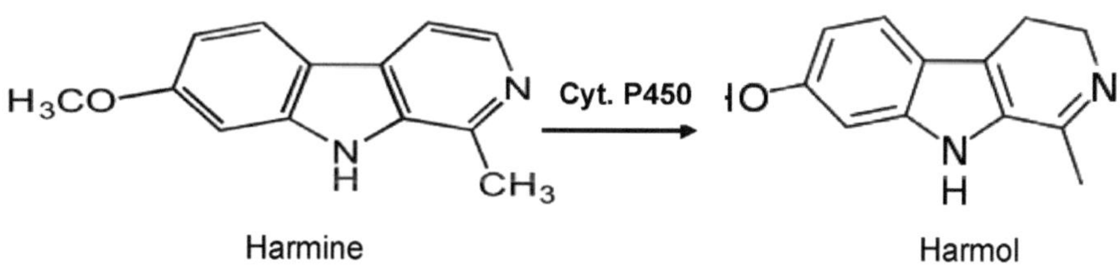

- Phase II: the metabolites of the oxidation phase will undergo glycuro- and sulfoconjugation processes.

- Phase III: β-carbolines alkaloids are excreted by bile and urine in conjugated form (glucuronates and sulfates); excretion of unchanged harmine should account only about 0.6% of a dose [25].

8. Mechanism of toxic action

Harmine reversibly inhibits monoamine oxidase A (MAO-A) and thus increases the central levels of amines such as noradrenaline (NA) and serotonin (5-HT) at the brain level which may explain the antidepressant effect of the plant.

Harmine is neurotoxic in vivo. Indeed, it has been shown that this injection is accompanied by tetany, convulsion movements or tremors, and these effects fade several minutes after injection [26].

All β-carbolines have in common an indole nucleus with a structural analogy to the serotonin molecule known for its important role in the functioning of the central nervous system. Harmalin and harmine are serotonin antagonists. It is likely that the hallucinogenic and behavioral modifying activity of these substances is related to this indolic structure [15].

Harmine and harmalin would exert a central anticholinergic action but at high doses can cause seizures and digestive manifestations, while harmane exerts an inhibitory action of the central dopaminergic system, inducing high-dose sedation and REM sleep disturbances [27–29].

The use of this plant for abortive purposes or to activate the term work is known. This abortive activity of harmel is due to these derivatives of quinazoline, which cause the contraction of the uterine muscle via induction of prostaglandin secretion [29].

9. Plants toxicity

9.1 In animals

Intoxication in animals is expressed by excitability, trembling, muscular rigidity, staggering gait, and jerky breathing. The animal is in an interrupted narcotic state with a short period of excitement. After a few hours, there is onset of dyspnea and mydriasis, hypothermia, and urinary disorders with abortion in case of gestation [24, 30].

- The aqueous seed extract has a myorelaxant effect on smooth rabbit and guinea pig muscles in vitro. These studies suggest that this extract has antispasmodic, antihistamine, and anti-adrenergic effects.

The laboratory animal studies have shown the following results [8]:

- Harmane: DL 50 in mice is 50 mg/kg intraperitoneally.
- Harmine: DL 50 in mice is 38 mg/kg intravenously.
- Harmalin: lethal dose in rats is 120 mg/kg subcutaneously.

9.2 In humans

Clinical observations of acute intoxications by Harmel showed that Harmalin, at a dose of 4 mg/kg, would produce psycho-mimetic effects in humans [16].

Ingestion: 10–30 min after the ingestion of a teaspoon of seeds (2.5 g) appears the following clinical signs:

- Euphoria or intoxication, violent headache, and tingling extremities.
- Hypoacusia and amaurosis neurosensory disorders and visual hallucinations (flame vision).

Then, abdominal pain is accompanied by bilious vomiting.

Four hours after ingestion the patient presents:

- Obnubilation.

- Sharp and symmetrical osteotendinous reflexes.

Seven hours after absorption, we note:

- Intense asthenia.

- Diffuse abdominal pain.

- Persistence of headaches.

These phases can change favorably in a few hours.

In severe cases, paralysis, CNS depression, dyspnea and hypothermia, and low blood pressure occur.

Inhalation: 5 min after fumigation inhalation appears intoxication and visual hallucinations.

10. Diagnosis of acute harmel intoxication

The diagnosis is based on the history and/or the appearance of nausea, vomiting, and hallucinations.

Vomiting, spontaneous or induced, and gastric washing fluids are kept in clean pots that must be kept and sent to the laboratory to identify the plant with certainty by searching for debris and alkaloids.

Send plant leaf, fruit, and seed samples used in the laboratory for plant identification.

10.1 Botanical identification

From gastric washing and/or from vomiting, recover debris (leaves, seeds, etc.). See the botanical description section and extract to search for alkaloids.

10.2 Toxicological analysis

Extract by chloroform in an alkaline medium to extract the alkaloids after drying under nitrogen, collect the residue by methanol and pass to the ultraviolet spectrophotometer [31] the maximum absorption in methanol:

- Harmane 234, 287 and 347 nm.

- Harmine 241, 301 and 336 nm.

- Harmaline 218, 260 and 376 nm.

Perform thin-layer chromatography with GF254 Silica Gel as stationary phase and elute with the mobile phase (ammonia 1.5 and methanol 100), use iodoplatinate developer reagent, and calculate alkaloid Rfs:

- Harmane 0.70.

- Harmine 0.68.
- Harmaline 0.38.

11. Treatment of acute intoxication

There is no antidotic treatment for Harmel intoxication. In the event of a coma, the symptomatic treatment must be instituted as a matter of urgency in order to maintain the vital functions [32].

11.1 Evacuator and scrubber treatment

Emergency gastric washing is used to remove parts of the plant that are not yet absorbed, and administration of activated charcoal is used to trap the rest of the plant. Induce osmotic diuresis is used in order to increase the renal elimination of alkaloids by perfusing hypertonic fluids (10% mannitol, 10% glucose serum). We need to monitor hemodynamic parameters.

11.2 Symptomatic treatment

Hospitalization in intensive care of the intoxicated provides an early respiratory resuscitation by tracheal intubation and mechanical ventilation in case of coma. Cautious warming in case of hypothermia (cover the patient and then give him a hot drink) and administration of diazepam are performed to treat seizures.

12. Conclusion

The injudicious taking of *Peganum harmala* causes clinical manifestations of intoxication; digestive disorders—bradycardia; neurological disorders—euphoria, hallucinations, generalized tremors, and even convulsive seizures; kidney disorders—uremia and anuria; and in severe cases, paralysis, central nervous system depression, dyspnea, as well as arterial hypotension.

Cases of poisoning by medicinal plants are very frequent and poorly known by the health services because the majority of victims do not come to the hospital for consultation. Today, African legislation is needed to regulate this profession of herbalists and herbalists.

Author details

Djafer Rachid
Department of Toxicology, Faculty of Medicine, University of Annaba, Algeria

*Address all correspondence to: djafertox@yahoo.fr

References

[1] Chopra IC, Abral BK, Handa KL. Les plantes médicinales des régions arides considérées surtout du point de vue botanique. UNESCO; 1960. p. 48

[2] Quezel P, Santa S. Nouvelle flore de l'Algérie et des régions désertiques méridionales. CNRS. 1963;**2**:59

[3] Ozenda P. Flore du Sahara. CNRS. 2004:312-322

[4] Weckesser W. First record of *Peganum harmala* (Zygophyllaceae) in Val Verde County, Texas, and subsequent eradication treatment. Phytoneuron. 27 September 2013;**71**:1-5. ISSN: 2153 733X

[5] Moloudizargari M, Mikaili P, Aghajanshakeri S, Asghari MH, Shayegh J. Pharmacological and therapeutic effects of *Peganum harmala* and its main alkaloids. Pharmacognosy Reviews. 2013;7(14):199

[6] Yahya M. A phytochemical studies of the plants used in traditional medicine of Saudi Arabia. Fitoterapia. 1986;**3**(52):179-182

[7] Hammiche V, Merad R, Azzouz M. Plantes toxiques à usage médicinal du partour méditerranéen. Saint Etienne: Springer; 2013

[8] Mahmoudian M, Jalipour H, Dardashti PS. Toxicity of *Peganum harmala*: Review and a case report. Iranian Journal of Pharmacology and Therapeutics. 2002;**1**:1-4

[9] Lamchouri F, Settaf A, Cherrah Y, El Hamidi M, Tligui N, Lyoussi B, et al. Experimental toxicity of *Peganum harmala* seeds. Annales Pharmaceutiques Françaises. 2002;**60**:123-129

[10] Ben Salah N, Amamou M, Jerbi Z, Ben Salah F, Yacoub M. One case of overdose with *Peganum harmala*. Journal de Toxicologie Clinique et Expérimentale. 1986;**6**:319-322

[11] Bellakhdar J. La pharmacopée marocaine traditionnelle: Médecine arabe ancienne et savoirs populaires. Paris: Ibis Press; 1997. p. 764

[12] Sincich F. Bedouin traditional medicine in the syrian steppe. Rome: FAO; 2002. pp. 114-115

[13] Leporatti ML, Ghedira K. Comparative analysis of medicinal plants used in traditional medicine in Italy and Tunisia. Journal of Ethnobiology and Ethnomedicine. 2009;**5**(31)

[14] Hammiche V, Merad R. *Peganum harmala* L. Poisons Information Monograph 402. International Programme on Chemical Safety; 1991. Available from: http://www.inchem.org/documents/pims/plant/pim402fr.htm

[15] Aarons DH, Victor Rossi G, Orzechowski RF. Cardiovascular actions of three harmala alkaloids: Harmine, harmaline, and harmalol. Journal of Pharmaceutical Sciences. 1977;**66**(9):1244-1248

[16] Frison G, Favretto D, Zancanaro F, Fazzin G, Ferrara SD. A case of β-carboline alkaloid intoxication following ingestion of *Peganum harmala* seed extract. Forensic Science International. 2008;**179**:37-43

[17] Pennes HH, Hoch PH. Psychomimetics, clinical and theoretical considerations: Harmine, Win-2299 and naline. The American Journal of Psychiatry. 1957;**113**:887-892

[18] Nenaah G. Antibacterial and antifungal activities of (beta)-carboline alkaloids of *Peganum harmala* (L.) seeds and their combination effects. Fitoterapia. 2010;**81**:779-782

[19] Rharrabe K, Bakri A, Ghailani N, Sayah F. Bioinsecticidal effect of harmaline on *Plodia interpunctella* development. 2013;**89**:137-145

[20] Farzin D, Mansouri N. Antidepressant-like effect of harmane and other β-carbolines in the mouse forced swim test. European Neuropsychopharmacology. 2006;**16**:324-328

[21] Waki H, Park KW, Mitro N, Pei L, Damoiseaux R, Wilpitz DC, et al. Smallmolecule harmine is an antidiabetic cell-type-specific regulator of PPARγ expression. Cell Metabolism. 2007;**5**(5):357-370

[22] Asgarpanah J, Ramezanloo F. Chemistry, pharmacology and medicinal properties of *Peganum harmala* L. African Journal of Pharmacy and Pharmacology. 2012;**6**(22):1573-1580

[23] Khlifi D, Sghaier RM, Amouri S, Laouini D. Composition and anti-oxidant, anti-cancer and anti-inflammatory activities of *Artemisia herba-alba*, *Ruta chapensis* and *Peganum harmala* L. Food and Chemical Toxicology. 2013;**55**:202-208

[24] Tahri N, Rhalem R, Soulaymani A, Achour S, Rhalem N, Khattabi A. *Peganum harmala* L. poisoning in Morocco: About 200 cases. Thérapie. 2011;**67**(1):53-58

[25] Slotkin TA, Di Stefano AWY. Blood levels and urinary excretion of harmine and its metabolites in man and rats. The Journal of Pharmacology and Experimental Therapeutics. 1970;**173**:26-30

[26] Meinguet C, Wouters J. Les dérivés de l'harmine, nouvelles molecules aux propriétés anti cancéreuse: De la conception aux études in vivo. Chimie Nouvelle. 2015;**120**:26-30

[27] Glennon RA, Dukat M, Grella B, Hong S, Contantino L, Teider M, et al. Binding of βcarolines and related agents at serotonin (5-HT2 and 5-HT1A), dopamine (D2) and benzodiazepine receptors. Drug and Alcohol Dependence. 2000;**60**:121-132

[28] Achour S, Saadi H, Turcant A, Banani A, Mokhtari A, Soulaymani A, et al. Intoxication au *Peganum harmala* L. et grossesse: Deux observations marocaines. Médecine et Santé Tropicales. 2012;**22**:84-86

[29] Zutshi U, Rao PG, Soni A, Gupta OP, Atal CK. Absorption and distribution of vasicine a novel uterotonic. Planta Medica. 1980;**40**:373-377

[30] El Bahri L, Chemli R. *Peganum harmala* L.: A poisonous plant of North Africa. Veterinary and Human Toxicology. 1991;**33**:276-277

[31] EGC C. Isolation and Identification of Drugs in Pharmaceuticals Body Fluids and Post-Mortem Material. Vol. 1. London: The Pharmaceutical Press; 1974. p. 358

[32] Djafer R, Akil Dahdouh S, Boukachabia R, Megueddem M. A case of intoxication caused by the injudicious use of harmel (*Peganum harmala* L.). Phytothérapie. 2017;**15**:288-289

Section 4

Interaction in Clinics

Chapter 12

Interaction between Pyridostigmine Bromide and Oxidative Stress

Verônica Farina Azzolin, Fernanda Barbisan, Ivo Emilio da Cruz Jung, Cibele Ferreira Teixeira, Euler Esteves Ribeiro, Raquel de Souza Praia and Ivana Beatrice Mânica da Cruz

Abstract

In this chapter the following topics will be addressed: (1) actions of the cholinergic system in the nervous system, commenting on acetylcholine metabolism and acetylcholinesterase metabolism; (2) acetylcholinesterase inhibitors as subtitle in this topic: pharmacological characterization of pyridostigmine bromide, mechanism of action, and therapeutic effect of the drug; (3) use of pyridostigmine bromide in Persian Gulf War; and (4) potential effect of pyridostigmine bromide in oxidative stress, addressing as subtitle the influence of pyridostigmine bromide on the superoxide-hydrogen peroxide imbalance model. Studies indicate that the interaction between pyridostigmine bromide and stressors could trigger genotoxicity, the mechanism associated with the induction of oxidative stress that leads to this side effect of this drug; however, this discussion needs to be better elucidated and may be more discussed as there is interaction between the pyridostigmine bromide and an endogenous oxidative imbalance caused by it or even by the possible interaction of this with genetic variations present in the antioxidant metabolism.

Keywords: acetylcholinesterase inhibitor, oxidative stress, neurotoxicity, superoxide dismutase 2, neuromuscular junction

1. Introduction

Pyridostigmine bromide (PB) is a reversible acetylcholinesterase (AChE) inhibitor and the first line of choice for the treatment of symptoms associated with myasthenia gravis (MG) and other neuromuscular junction disorder prophylactic treatment in the Persian Gulf War, for prevention of post-traumatic stress and heat and pesticide exposure. However, evidence suggests that PB may be associated with Gulf War illness, characterized by the presence of fatigue, headaches, cognitive dysfunction, and respiratory, gastrointestinal, and musculoskeletal disorders [1–4]. However studies in animal models showed that if used without any association did not cause extensive cytotoxicity and genotoxicity to these animals. But the association of these drugs with other chemical or even physical agents caused cellular apoptosis and genotoxicity in animals. These studies would suggest that this toxicity caused in association was due to oxidative stress [5, 6].

2. Actions of the cholinergic system in the nervous system

Within the neurotransmitters acting on the body's nervous system is the so-called cholinergic system associated with the release of the acetylcholine (ACh) molecule in the synaptic cleft [7–10]. ACh is considered to be one of the major chemical neurotransmitters of the peripheral nervous system being released by all preganglionic, parasympathetic, and some sympathetic postganglionic fibers, as well as by motor neurons that project to the skeletal muscles. It was the researcher Otto Loewi who discovered this molecule when he observed in his study the release of a biochemical substance by the parasympathetic nerve endings, which he called ACh [8, 11].

In cholinergic synapses, cholinesterases are present, which consist of a class of enzymes that catalyze the hydrolysis of ACh in acetic acid and choline in the synaptic cleft, and thus allow the cholinergic neuron to return to its resting state after activation. The most common cholinesterases present in the synaptic cleft are butyrylcholinesterase (BuChE) and AChE [12].

Although they are evolutionarily similar, these enzymes differ in their distribution in tissues, their kinetic properties, and the specificity of their substrates. AChE is found most abundantly in the central nervous system (CNS), in the skeletal muscles, and in the erythrocyte membrane, while BuChE is mostly found in blood plasma and is therefore also known as plasma cholinesterase [13].

Acetylcholinesterase and BuChE exhibit structural similarities, with their amino acids having approximately 50% homology. The other 50% heterogeneity among amino acids is responsible for the selectivity differences of both the substrates and the inhibitors of these enzymes. AChE preferentially hydrolyzes ACh, whereas BuChE is less selective and acts by hydrolyzing both ACh and butyrylcholine (BuCh) in comparable amounts [14].

In general, AChE is an enzyme that acts by hydrolyzing ACh in precursor molecules by rapidly closing the signaling of this molecule in the post-synaptic neuron or target tissue. Thus, AChE is a target enzyme in the treatment of various diseases, since anticholinesterase drugs act via their inhibition (**Figure 1**) [7–10].

Acetylcholine plays a crucial role in controlling numerous physiological processes in all divisions of the nervous system. However, it is also involved in various neurological and muscular dysfunctions. The apparently antagonistic action of ACh occurs due to the existence of different cholinergic receptors, which are present according to each type of target tissue. The knowledge of the various forms of ACh activity allowed the identification of causal mechanisms of several neuromorbidities associated with neuromotor plaque disorders, mainly related to changes in cholinergic receptors.

This knowledge, in turn, led to the development or understanding of the performance of drugs related to the control of symptoms of neurological diseases through differential modulation of the cholinergic system [7, 8, 10]. Among the morbidities with etiophysiopathology associated with changes in cholinergic response, MG and other forms of myasthenic syndromes are prominent. In these diseases, AChE inhibitors are used to control clinical symptoms [16]. In addition to its role in MG, more recent studies indicate that ACh could be a key molecule in the progression and control of symptoms of other neurodegenerative diseases, such as Alzheimer's disease and other types of dementia [17, 18]. Because of its very specific physiological action, drugs associated with modulation of cholinergic neurons have also

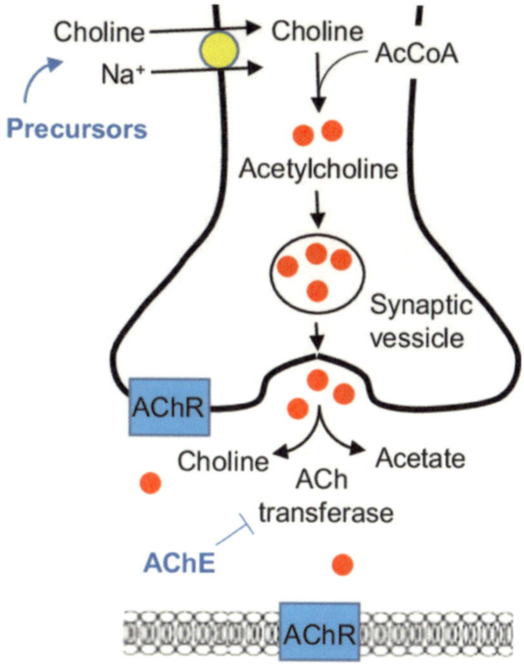

Figure 1.
Synthesis, storage, release, and degradation pathways of acetylcholine. Source: adapted Rang et al. [15]. AChR, acetylcholine receptor; ACh, acetylcholine; AChE, acetylcholinesterase.

been prophylactically used to prevent populations subject to exposure to molecules potentially used in biological warfare, such as sarin gas [19]. For this reason, studies involving pharmacology related to the cholinergic system are considered clinical and epidemiologically relevant, in addition to their action in MG.

2.1 Acetylcholinesterase inhibitors

Acetylcholinesterase inhibitory drugs are termed anticholinesterases, and these are therapeutically used to reverse the neuromuscular blockade promoted by depolarizing myorelaxants, in the treatment of neurological diseases such as MG and myasthenic syndrome, in smooth muscle atony, in strabismus, and in the treatment of symptoms of Alzheimer's disease, among others. An anticholinesterase drug delays the degradation of ACh, so the neurotransmitter spends more time in the synaptic cleft, thus intensifying cholinergic transmission, as can be observed in **Figure 2** [20–22].

Physostigmine, an alkaloid obtained from *Physostigma venenosum* L., was the first AChE inhibitor to be discovered. Thus, its cholinergic effects have been known for many years, and as early as 1923, the molecular structure of the active substance was elucidated. In 1929 Stedman demonstrated that the cholinomimetic effects of physostigmine were due to the reversible inhibition of AChE [24]. Although it is old, this drug is still in use and is currently used in the treatment of glaucoma and in cases of overdose by anticholinergic compounds, such as atropine, and tricyclic antidepressants such as amitriptyline [25]. Other drugs with inhibitory action of AChE have been developed, such as neostigmine and PB, which are simplified analog of physostigmine [20].

There are two classes of AChE inhibitors, based on their mechanism of action, and may be reversible or irreversible depending on the type of action with the active site of the drug. Reversible agents are still present in two groups: short-acting and intermediate-acting agents [26].

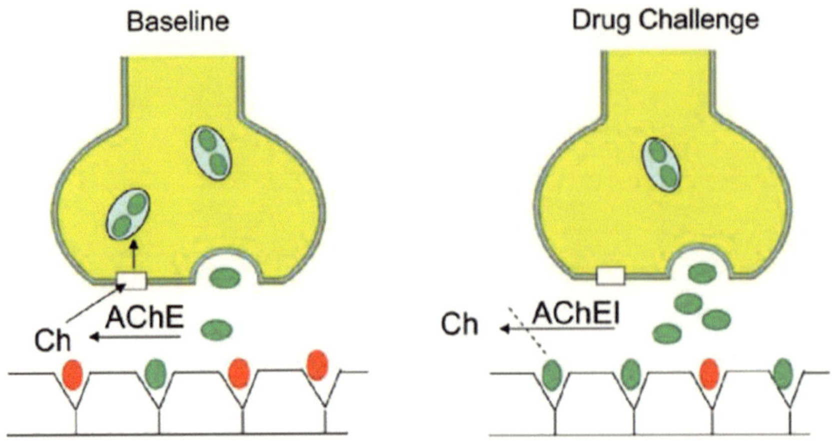

Figure 2.
Cholinergic synapse in the absence and in the presence of an AChE inhibitor. Source: adapted Araújo et al. [23]. AChE, acetylcholinesterase; ch, choline.

Edrophonium, a quaternary ammonium compound that binds only to the anionic site of the enzyme, is one of the short-acting reversible anticholinesterases. The ionic bond formed is easily reversed, and the action of the drug is brief. It is mainly used as a diagnostic purpose, since the improvement of muscle strength observed with the use of an anticholinesterase is a characteristic of MG, but it does not occur when muscle weakness results from other causes [27]. In contrast, the anticholinesterases of intermediate duration include neostigmine, PB, and physostigmine that are composed of quaternary ammonium of clinical importance [26].

In chemical terms, all of these drugs are carbamoyl esters, once acetyl esters, and have basic groups that bind to the anionic site. The transfer of the carbamyl group to the hydroxyl group of the serine from the esterase site occurs in the same way as with ACh, but the carbamylated enzyme undergoes hydrolysis much more slowly, taking minutes instead of microseconds. The anticholinesterase drugs are therefore hydrolyzed, but at an insignificant rate when compared to ACh, and the slow recovery of the carbamylated enzyme indicates that the action of these drugs is quite prolonged [12].

Irreversible anticholinesterases are compounds that have a pentavalent phosphorus containing a leaving group, such as fluoride, or an organic group. Upon binding the enzyme, this group is released, leaving the hydroxyl group of the serine of the enzyme phosphorylated. Most of these organophosphorus compounds have been developed to be used as a chemical weapon in the form of toxic gases, and as a pesticide, but also for clinical use. They interact only with the esterase site of the enzyme and do not have a cationic group. Ecotiopate is an exception, since it has a quaternary nitrogen group that also binds to the anionic site [12].

When AChE is in inactive phosphorylated form, this molecule is generally very stable. With drugs such as diflos, there is no appreciable hydrolysis, and the recovery of enzymatic activity depends on the synthesis of new molecules of the enzyme, a process that can take weeks. With other drugs like the ecotiopate, slow hydrolysis takes place in the course of a few days, so that its action is not strictly irreversible. The diflos and the parathion are apolar substances volatile with high lipid solubility, quickly absorbed through the mucous membranes and even through the integral skin and the cuticle of the insects. The use of these agents as a chemical weapon or as an insecticide is based on this property. The absence of a quaternary group that confirms specificity indicates that most of these drugs block other serine hydrolases, although their pharmacological effects stem mainly from inhibition of AChE [26].

Acetylcholinesterase inhibitors affect both peripheral, autonomic cholinergic synapses and CNS synapses. It is also important to note that some organophosphorus compounds are capable of producing a severe form of neurotoxicity leading to irreversible changes in the cholinergic system, especially triggering effects on autonomic cholinergic synapses. These implications mainly reflect increased ACh activity in parasympathetic postganglionic synapses (increased secretions of salivary, lacrimal, bronchial, and gastrointestinal glands, increased peristaltic activity, bronchodilation, bradycardia, hypotension, pupillary constriction, fixation of vision accommodation for near, drop in intraocular pressure). Larger doses are able to stimulate, and subsequently block, autonomic ganglia, producing complex autonomic effects. Blockade when it occurs consists of depolarization blockade and is associated with accumulation of ACh in plasma and in organic liquids. Neostigmine and PB tend to affect neuromuscular transmission more than the autonomic system, while physostigmine and organophosphates show the opposite pattern. The reason for this disparity is not clear, but therapeutic use takes advantage of this partial selectivity [26].

The main effect of these drugs is under neuromuscular junction; they increase the force of the contraction of a muscle stimulated by means of its motor nerve, thanks to the repetitive discharge in the muscular fiber associated with a prolongation of the action potential. Normally, ACh is hydrolyzed so quickly that each stimulus initiates only one action potential in the muscle fiber. However, when AChE is inhibited, there is a short series of action potential in the muscle fiber and, as a consequence, a greater tension. Much more important, however, is the effect produced when the transmission is blocked by a non-depolarizing blocking agent such as pancuronium. In this case, the addition of an anticholinesterase drug can dramatically restore transmission. When a large number of receptors are blocked, most ACh molecules will normally find AChE molecules and will be destroyed by them before reaching a vacant receptor. The inhibition of AChE gives ACh molecules a greater chance of finding a vacant receptor before being destroyed and as a consequence increases the action potential such that it reaches the threshold. Transmission does not occur in MG because there are very few ACh receptors, and in this case inhibition of AChE improves transmission [12].

Acetylcholinesterase inhibitors rarely fully induce symptom relief in myasthenic patients and do not affect disease progression; however, they may be sufficiently effective for proper management in certain patients with mild or purely ocular nonprogressive disease [28]. It is also important to note that people with MG are susceptible to presenting the so-called myasthenic crisis that involves weakness in respiratory muscles, upper airway muscles, or a combination of both muscle groups. Both inspiratory and expiratory respiratory muscles may be affected, manifesting as dyspnea. Respiratory dysfunction may also manifest as upper airway obstruction if bulbar or upper airway muscle weakness occurs. Signs of bulbar weakness include dysphagia, nasal regurgitation, nasal quality of speech, staccato speech, weakness of the mandible (closure of the mandible weaker than the opening of the mandible), bifacial paresis, and weakness of the tongue. Weakness of the upper airways can lead to failure by oropharyngeal collapse or tongue obstruction by increasing the work of already fatigued respiratory muscles. In epidemiological terms, it is estimated that 2/3 of myasthenic patients who present with myasthenic crisis need to be intubated and receive mechanical ventilation [29].

On the other hand, patients who ingest excess AChE inhibitors like PB may precipitate a cholinergic crisis characterized as muscarinic and nicotinic toxicity. Symptoms include increased sweating, lacrimation, salivation and pulmonary secretions, nausea, vomiting, diarrhea, bradycardia, and fasciculations. Although the cholinergic crisis is an important consideration in the evaluation of the patient in a myasthenic crisis, it is quite uncommon in these patients. In the case of suspected cholinergic crisis, AChE inhibitors should be significantly reduced or discontinued [29].

In Ref. [30], the author described in his work that the natural course of MG, using only anticholinesterase drugs, with no other type of treatment, showed remission of symptoms in 20% of the patients and mortality in 25%. However, various therapies that involve thymectomy, immunosuppression, infection control, and others positively affect the natural history of the disease. Still in that decade, this author concluded that the mortality in patients with MG is practically zero and the great majority of the patients have normal life, thanks to the improvement in the assistive technology related to the management of myasthenic crisis.

2.2 Use of pyridostigmine bromide in Persian gulf war

The use of chemical warfare agents is one of the greatest threats in the world today. Chemical warfare is based on the use of substances with toxic properties that are capable of killing, for mass destruction, and causing severe damage to the environment. The most prominent and dangerous chemical warfare agents are neurotoxic organophosphates which, due to their high toxicity, are sufficient in small amounts to cause seizures and death [31].

One of the biggest reasons for the use of chemical weapons in war and terrorist actions is that this war strategy ends up being cheaper than conventional weapons such as bombs, projectiles, and explosives. For example, to kill all people in an area of 1 km^2, the use of chemical weapons can cost approximately 40% less than if traditional weapons were used. The other reason is that chemical weapons, in addition to causing death quickly and efficiently, also cause psychological problems to those who can survive intoxication, thus being more worrisome than other weapons of war [32].

The agents of chemical warfare were used several times in wars since antiquity, although being agents is not well defined nor very efficient. Already several more effective toxic agents received major importance in 1915, when the German army sent gases like chlorine and mustard against French troops during the First World War, causing countless losses in the enemy army. From that date the development of neurotoxic agents was more intense for several armies. Before World War II, the German army began the development of the first neurotoxic organophosphates as chemical warfare agents, especially tabun, sarin, and soman. Nevertheless, these agents, as well as mustard gas and other toxic substances, were not used during World War II. In the 1950s, the neurotoxic organophosphates of the V family were developed, which are more toxic and persistent in the environment, being that the first, called VX, was developed in England. Later similar compounds were created, especially in the former Soviet Union [32].

One of the first countries to use neurotoxic organophosphates was Iraq, under Saddam Hussein's command in the war against Iran between 1980 and 1988, leading to hundreds of deaths of Iranians [33]. In 1994, sarin was used in Japan against civilians in a terrorist attack that resulted in the death of 7 people and 200 intoxications [34, 35]. On the other hand, poisoning of American soldiers by sarin occurred during the Gulf War in 1991 [33]. Recently, chemical weapons were used in Syria, killing about 1300 people, especially civilians and children, making it one of the worst chemical weapon use events in the world.

Organophosphate, pesticides, carbamates, chemical agents such as sarin, and the drug PB all belong to a class of chemicals that inactivate the circulation of cholinesterase enzymes such as AChE, BuChE, paraoxonase, and neurotoxic esterase resulting in interference with the breakdown of ACh neurotransmitter among other effects [36, 37]. Exposures lead to increased ACh in the brain and peripheral nerve endings, with overestimation resulting from cholinergic nerve receptors [38] and subsequent reduction of ACh available, as well as altered gene expression and late cognitive effects [39]. At high exposure doses, AChE inhibitors may be toxic or fatal and at lower doses may lead to long-term health effects [40], one of its mechanisms being oxidative stress [37]. The main symptoms secondary to AChE inhibition in people with deficiency in central and peripheral cholinergic function are similar to those reported by Gulf War illness soldiers, such as skeletal muscle fatigue, cognitive deficit, and gastrointestinal, sleep, and temperature regulation problems [1, 41].

Exposures to toxic agents in the Gulf War were considered contributors to numerous long-term health problems. Post-war effects include pesticide effects, uranium munitions, air contaminants from fires in Kuwait oil wells, and chemical nerve agents. PB was then used as a prophylactic measure against possible exposure to these nerve agents, and to other risks, such as psychologically stressful conditions and heat. A military who underwent several exposures in different combinations presented synergic effects that have not yet been determined in this population [4].

Gulf War illness is considered a chronic multi-symptom condition that affected 25–32% of soldiers who operated in the Gulf War. It is clinically characterized by the presence of fatigue; headaches; cognitive, respiratory, and musculoskeletal dysfunction; and gastrointestinal disorders [1–4]. Inflammation and increased oxidative stress associated with mitochondrial dysfunction may negatively affect cognitive function and mood, either directly or indirectly, through the reduction of hippocampal neurogenesis [42–44]. Therefore, chronic inflammation and oxidative stress are likely to be among the leading causes of Gulf War illness brain dysfunction.

Studies were conducted to identify possible causal factors, and evidence has suggested that PB may be associated with etiopathogenesis of Gulf War illness. One of the first studies carried out by [45] described the development of three syndromes associated with PB use: (1) impaired cognition, (2) confusion-ataxia, and (3) neuropathy. However, complementary investigations have also suggested that the use of PB without any other chemical or physical stressor in neuronal cells of animals does not cause great damages, such as decreased viability and increased cellular apoptosis [8, 46]. Thus, it appears that the interaction of PB with other endogenous or exogenous factors is what would trigger the Gulf War illness.

2.3 Potential effect of pyridostigmine bromide in oxidative stress

Considering the results of epidemiological and in animal experiments, the data described so far reinforce the hypothesis that the interaction between PB and other drugs, such as organophosphates, or perhaps other stress factors, could contribute to the rupture of homeostasis neural, via amplification of oxidative stress and of chronic inflammatory conditions that would trigger systemic neural dysfunctions associated with Gulf War illness [42–44, 47–49].

In recent decades the role of reactive species in pathophysiological processes related to oxidative stress has been intensively investigated. The reactive species are molecules that contain one or more unpaired electrons in the last electron layer [50]. These reactive molecules are generally unstable and originate from oxygen, nitrogen, or sulfur [51]. When the generation of reactive species exceeds the antioxidant capacity of the organism, an imbalance occurs in the cellular redox state, promoting oxidative stress and subsequent oxidative damage [52].

Mitochondria are the main site of reactive oxygen species (ROS) production [53]. Much of the energy produced in the body is generated through oxidative phosphorylation. Therefore, paradoxically, a fundamental process for the development of the life of eukaryotes (oxidative phosphorylation) is also one of the main responsible for the production of ROS. These species are also produced by other electron transfer reactions between different redox reactive agents, such as those involved in defense mechanisms against pathogens, for example, the case of nicotinamide adenine dinucleotide phosphate oxidase (NADPH oxidase) [54].

The production of ROS in various metabolic processes plays an important role in the functioning of the organism. They are dose dependent, and some types of ROS when in low concentrations are considered important signaling molecules responsible for the transport of electrons in the respiratory chain [54]. ROS have a deleterious effect on the body when there is an excessive increase in its production or when there is a decrease in antioxidant agents. The three main types of ROS are superoxide anion ($O_2^{\bullet-}$), hydrogen peroxide (H_2O_2), and hydroxyl radical ($OH^{\bullet}$).

Among the ROS, the $O_2^{\bullet-}$ radical is the most common, abundant, and quite diffusible both inside and between cells in vivo, the first ROS being formed by the reduction of oxygen by a single electron during oxidative phosphorylation that occurs in the mitochondria [52]. It is a poorly reactive ROS and has no ability to penetrate lipid membranes, thus acting only in the compartment where it is produced [55]. H_2O_2 is not a free radical, but an intermediate metabolite of oxygen, which in uncontrolled amounts becomes extremely deleterious, because it participates as an intermediate in the reaction that produces the $OH^{\bullet}$ radical. H_2O_2 has long life and is able to cross biological membranes. The $OH^{\bullet}$ radical is considered the most reactive ROS in biological systems, being capable of causing more damage than any other ROS. It is formed from H_2O_2, in a reaction catalyzed by transition metal ions (Fe^{2+} or Cu^{+}), called the Fenton reaction. This $OH^{\bullet}$ radical can also initiate the oxidation of the polyunsaturated fatty acids of the cell membranes (lipoperoxidation) [55–57].

However, in order to maintain the balance in the ROS generation, there is the antioxidant system, but when the ROS are in excess and the antioxidant system cannot keep the balance, processes of damage to the organism can occur, and this situation of imbalance is denominated oxidative stress [58].

The antioxidant system has the function of inhibiting the oxidative damages caused by excess reactive species. These are divided into enzymatic or endogenous antioxidants and nonenzymatic or exogenous antioxidants, the latter being mainly acquired by the diet [59].

Nonenzymatic antioxidants include ascorbic acid (vitamin C), which inhibits the action of oxidized low-density lipoprotein (LDL) and protects against the action of ROS; phenolic acids; resveratrol; catechins; β-carotene (vitamin A), which protects against lipid peroxidation and damage to DNA; α-tocopherol (vitamin E); copper (Cu); zinc (Zn); and others. As for enzymatic antioxidants, we have superoxide dismutase (SOD), which facilitates the conversion of the radical $O_2^{\bullet-}$ into H_2O_2; catalase (CAT), which converts H_2O_2 to O_2 and H_2O; and glutathione peroxidase (GPx), which has the capacity to reduce H_2O_2 to H_2O [60].

Oxidative stress is involved in several non-transmissible chronic diseases, such as atherosclerosis, hypertension, neurodegenerative diseases, cancer, and type II diabetes mellitus. In the latter, for example, excess reactive species have a detrimental influence on glucose uptake by muscle and adipose tissues, as well as decreasing insulin secretion, neuronal death, and apoptosis of various cells [61–64].

2.3.1 Influence of pyridostigmine bromide on the superoxide-hydrogen peroxide imbalance model

A large body of evidence suggests that oxidative stress is associated with cell aging, dysfunctions, and diseases [65]. However, it was long believed that ROS were largely responsible for these deleterious processes. For this reason, about 20 years ago, studies were begun to investigate the beneficial health effects of supplementing large amounts of antioxidants. The results, surprisingly, were not good. In some studies, higher morbidity loads were reported in subjects supplemented with high-dose vitamin than in the placebo group. The explanation for this apparent paradox soon emerged: many ROS, in low concentrations, were actually signaling molecules of various cellular functions. Among these, nitric oxide (NO) and H_2O_2 stand out, so the neutralization of these molecules by antioxidants influenced the cellular homeostasis processes [66].

It was hypothesized that maintenance of redox balance was a relevant aspect to avoid non-transmissible chronic morbidities or to decrease the side effects related to the ingestion of some drugs [67]. This hypothesis was tested and corroborated by genetic studies involving the imbalance of the endogenous antioxidant system. This is the case of the point polymorphism observed in the SOD2 enzyme gene called Val16Ala-SOD2 [68].

The enzyme SOD2 is synthesized from a nuclear gene located on chromosome 6, subregion 6q25, which codes for a homotetramer which binds to a manganese ion per subunit. This protein structure synthesized in the rough endoplasmic reticulum is still enzymatically inactive and has a peptide sequence known as the mitochondrial target sequence (MTS) that directs SOD2 into the mitochondria. As it passes through the pores of the inner mitochondrial membrane, the MTS peptide segment is cleaved by lysosomes, and the mature protein aggregates into an active form, making it a functional SOD2 enzyme [69, 70].

Previous studies have identified a single nucleotide polymorphism (SNP) in the MTS region of the SOD2 gene, in which a thiamine (T) is replaced by a cytosine (C) in exon 2, nucleotide 47. Substitution affects the codon 16, which encodes for amino acid 9, mutating a valine (GTT) in an alanine (GCT), and hence the polymorphism is called Val16Ala-SOD2 [69]. Therefore, this polymorphism is associated with the presence of two alleles alanine (A) and valine (V) and three possible genotypes: AA, AV, and VV. In phenotypic terms, the Ala-SOD2 variant generates a protein with α-helix structure, thus being easily imported into the mitochondria. The Val-SOD2 variant, on the other hand, generates a protein with a partial β-lamina structure, which causes the inactive SOD2 protein to be partially retained in the pores of the mitochondrial inner membrane, as it is being imported into the mitochondria. In the presence of the two alleles that form the heterozygous genotype, the Ala-/Val-SOD2 protein presents helical structure [70, 71].

In vitro investigations have demonstrated that Ala-SOD2 is capable of generating SOD2 homotetramer with 30–40% greater enzymatic activity than the matrix processed with Val-SOD2 precursor [70]. Despite the increased efficiency of SOD2 produced from the A allele, many epidemiological studies have described association between this genetic variant and various types of cancer [72] including prostate [73], breast [74], and lung [75] cancer.

It is believed that this phenomenon occurs due to the higher efficiency of SOD2 that, if not accompanied by an increase in the levels of GPX and CAT, or of nonenzymatic antioxidant compounds stored in the cell, ends up generating excess H_2O_2 that can react with transition metals via the Fenton reaction originating the strongly mutagenic $OH^{\bullet}$ radical.

On the other hand, previous investigations related to the Val-SOD2 allele suggest that this allele and/or the VV genotype would increase the risk of some chronic non-transmissible diseases and also differential response to xenobiotic agents [68]. In fact, the VV genotype has a lower enzymatic efficiency of SOD2 and thus potentially leads to the basal accumulation of higher concentrations of the radical anion $O_2^{\bullet-}$ within the mitochondria. This ROS is poorly permeable to membranes, and highly reactive in the presence of NO, which leads to the production of peroxynitrite ($ONOO^-$). In turn, this molecule has great affinity with lipids, thus causing an extensive oxidation of cell membranes, a phenomenon known as lipid peroxidation or lipid peroxidation. In addition, the excess of the radical anion $O_2^{\bullet-}$ can lead to the production of other ROS that contribute to establish oxidative stress states [76].

Thus, the VV-SOD2 genotype has been associated with endothelial dysfunction, elevated oxidized LDL levels [77], the presence of microvascular complications associated with diabetes including retinopathies and nephropathies [78], elevated levels of inflammatory cytokines [79, 80], increased risk of developing obesity [81], hypercholesterolemia [82], and association between dyslipidemia and stroke [83]. Although AA genotype increases the risk of breast cancer, in certain populations, VV genotype appears to amplify tumor aggressiveness as it increases the potential for breast cancer metastasis [84, 85].

In addition, in vitro investigations have also shown that Val16Ala-SOD2 polymorphism differentially affects the toxicity of lymphocytes exposed to ultraviolet radiation [86], to the methylmercury heavy metal [87], and the pharmacological response of hypercholesterolemic patients to rosuvastatin [88]. This polymorphism also altered the antioxidant response of peripheral blood mononuclear cells (PBMCs) exposed to resveratrol [89] and to seleno-L-methionine [90].

Due to the importance of this genetic polymorphism for human health, an experimental pharmacological model was developed by [91], for prostate cancer,

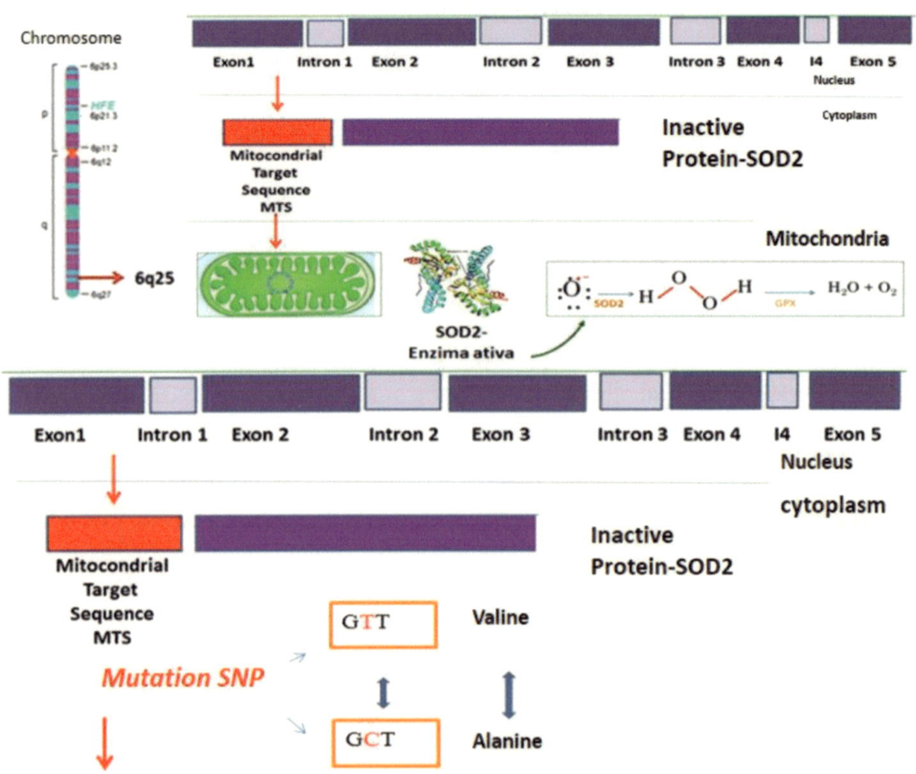

Figure 3.
This figure summarizes the Val16Ala-SOD2 polymorphism. This protein has a small peptide region known as the mitochondrial target sequence (MTS) that directs SOD2 protein into the mitochondria. Within this organelle, the enzyme SOD2 finally becomes active. This polymorphism causes a thymine to be exchanged for a cytosine at codon 16. This exchange leads to the substitution of the amino acid valine by the amino acid alanine. Thus, there are three possible genotypes related to this polymorphism: AA, VV, and AV. Source: adapted Barbisan et al. [93].

and by [92], for colorectal cancer, showing in tumor cells the difference in treatment by superoxide-hydrogen peroxide (S-HP) imbalance.

In this S-HP pharmacological imbalance model, two molecules, paraquat and porphyrin, were used. Paraquat is an $O_2^{\bullet -}$ anion generator, whose higher levels of this molecule are observed in VV-like cells. On the other hand, porphyrin is a molecule that acts similar to SOD2 (SOD2-like), thus causing an increase in H_2O_2 levels, as observed in cells with the genotype AA-like [91, 92], simulating in vitro the two genotypes of the polymorphism. A schematic summary of this genetic polymorphism is illustrated in **Figure 3**.

In summary, considering that PB seems to interact with other exogenous pro-oxidant agents, triggering symptoms recognized in Gulf War illness, the hypothesis of interaction between this drug and the Val16Ala-SOD2 polymorphism cannot be ruled out.

3. Discussion

Pyridostigmine bromide was used to treat changes in neuromuscular junction [21, 20] and was also used prophylactically in GWI for stress prevention and against chemical and physical agents, which soldiers were exposed to during the war [49]. However, this drug was associated with several adverse effects detected during and after the war in soldiers who prophylactically ingested 30 mg/3 times a day of this drug. Among these effects, the main ones were skeletal muscle fatigue, headache, attention deficit, cognition problems, gastrointestinal disorders, and sleep and temperature regulation problems, among other autonomic alterations [1, 2, 4].

These results suggested that BP could have a relevant cytotoxic effect on humans. However, previous animal cell studies have suggested that isolated exposure to CP would not cause extensive damage including decreased cell viability and cellular apoptosis [8, 46]. However, other studies have shown that when animals were treated with CP associated with other chemical molecules that were potentially used in biological warfare or in the prophylaxis of other diseases or even parasitic diseases, such as permethrin, used to prevent infestation by head lice, results were quite different. These results then indicated the interaction of BP with chemical agents or even physical factors such as intense physical activity and psychological stress such as oxidative stress and inflammation [6].

Considering that most of the agents in which BP interacts are factors that increase oxidative stress and body inflammation, an open question concerns the potential occurrence of interaction between BP and oxidative imbalances associated with individuals' genetic characteristics, as is the case of the Val16Ala-SOD2 polymorphism. This question is quite pertinent since, so far, doubts remain about the efficacy and safety of the use of BP as a drug and also about the fact that it was pointed as the cause of GWI disease.

So two studies were very important that showed that pyridostigmine bromide affected in vitro cytogenotoxicity and AChE enzyme activity of SHSY-5Y neural cells, in a concentration-dependent manner, showing decreased cell viability, increased oxidative stress, and apoptosis mainly when they were exposed to the highest concentration tested at 80 ng/mL. However, over a longer period of exposure, there was an increase in cell proliferation rate, suggesting that the oxidative effects triggered by CP exposure may be transient and reversible in these neural cells [94]. However, when exposed to different Val16Ala-SOD2 genotypes, the cytogenotoxicity and efficacy in inhibiting AChE induced by CP exposure were directly modulated by the Val16Ala-SOD2 polymorphism that alters the basal oxidative state of human peripheral blood polymorphonuclear cells. In this case, cells with higher basal production of H2O2 had higher cytotoxic sensitivity to CP, while cells with higher basal production of O^{2-} anion showed higher resistance to inhibition of AChE enzyme. These results suggest a potential pharmacogenetic effect of S-HP imbalance on BP efficacy and safety [95].

These results found in the literature suggest that the efficacy and toxicity to CP are influenced by the interaction with oxidative imbalance by Val16Ala-SOD2 polymorphism, indicating potential toxicogenetic and pharmacogenetic effects of this drug. The data presented here may potentially contribute to elucidate the interaction between BP and oxidative stress-inducing agents and may also be relevant to the clinical and epidemiological field related to the use of AChE inhibitors as therapeutic agents [94, 95].

4. Conclusion

Studies indicate that the interaction between pyridostigmine bromide and stressors could trigger genotoxicity, the mechanism associated with the induction of oxidative stress that leads to this side effect of this drug; however, this discussion needs to be better elucidated and may be more discussed as there is interaction between the pyridostigmine bromide and an endogenous oxidative imbalance caused by it or even by the possible interaction of this with genetic variations present in the antioxidant metabolism.

This chapter was developed to show studies related to the toxicity of pyridostigmine bromide and its influence with oxidative stress, as we conclude that:

Results suggested that the exposure of neural cells to PB without other chemical and physical stressors does not cause extensive toxicity that could explain the clinical symptoms observed in GWI.

Study demonstrated that PB can transiently modulate redox metabolism in cells. However, factors that increase HP levels, such as the AA-SOD2 genotype, may affect PB efficiency and efficacy by inducing AChE inhibition and oxidative stress. Data from these in vitro studies may be useful for complementing population studies investigating PB or other AChE inhibitors.

Our results suggest that the efficacy and toxicity to CP are influenced by the toxicogenetic and pharmacogenetic interactions of this drug. The results presented here may potentially contribute to elucidate the interaction between CP and oxidative stress-inducing agents and may also be relevant to the clinical and epidemiological field related to the use of AChE inhibitors as therapeutic agents.

Conflict of interest

The authors declare no conflict of interest.

Author details

Verônica Farina Azzolin[1*], Fernanda Barbisan[2], Ivo Emilio da Cruz Jung[2], Cibele Ferreira Teixeira[2], Euler Esteves Ribeiro[1], Raquel de Souza Praia[1] and Ivana Beatrice Mânica da Cruz[2]

1 Open University Foundation of the Third Age, Manaus, Amazonas, Brazil

2 Federal University of Santa Maria, Santa Maria, Rio Grande do Sul, Brazil

*Address all correspondence to: ivana.ufsm@gmail.com

References

[1] Golomb BA. Acetylcholinesterase inhibitors and gulf war illnesses. Proceedings of the National Academy of Sciences of the United States of America. 2008;**105**:4295-4300. DOI: 10.1073/pnas.0711986105

[2] Janulewicz PA, Krengel MH, Maule A, White RF, Cirillo J, Sisson E, et al. Neuropsychological characteristics of gulf war illness: A meta-analysis. PLoS One. 2017;**12**:e0177121. DOI: 10.1371/journal.pone.0177121

[3] Odegard TN, Cooper CM, Farris EA, Arduengo J, Bartlett J, Haley R. Memory impairment exhibited by veterans with gulf war illness. Neurocase. 2013;**19**:316-327. DOI: 10.1080/13554794.2012.667126

[4] White RF, Steele L, O'Callaghan JP, Sullivan K, Binns JH, Golomb BA, et al. Recent research on gulf war illness and other health problems in veterans of the 1991 gulf war: Effects of toxicant exposures during deployment. Cortex. 2016;**74**:449-475. DOI: 10.1016/j.cortex.2015.08.022

[5] Abu-Qare AW, Abou-Donia MB. Combined exposure to sarin and pyridostigmine bromide increased levels of rat urinary 3-nitrotyrosine and 8-hydroxy-2′-deoxyguanosine, biomarkers of oxidative stress. Toxicology Letters. 2001;**123**:51-58. DOI: 10.1016/S0378-4274(01)00380-0

[6] Abou-Donia MB, Suliman HB, Khan WA, Abdel-Rahman AA. Testicular germ-cell apoptosis in stressed rats following combined exposure to pyridostigmine bromide, N,N-diethyl m-toluamide (DEET), and permethrin. Journal of Toxicology and Environmental Health. Part A. 2003;**66**:57-73. DOI: 10.1080/15287390306463

[7] Pohanka M. Alpha7 nicotinic acetylcholine receptor is a target in pharmacology and toxicology. International Journal of Molecular Sciences. 2012;**13**:2219-2238. DOI: 10.3390/ijms13022219

[8] Pohanka M. Cholinesterases, a target of pharmacology and toxicology. Biomedical Papers of the Medical Faculty of the University Palacky, Olomouc, Czech Republic. 2011;**155**:219-229. DOI: 10.5507/bp.2011.036

[9] Sofuoglu M, Mooney M. Cholinergic functioning in stimulant addiction: Implications for medications development. CNS Drugs. 2009;**23**:939-952. DOI: 10.2165/11310920-000000000-00000

[10] Ventura ALM, Abreu PA, Freitas RCC, Sathler PC, Loureiro N, Castro HC. Cholinergic system: Revisiting receptors, regulation and the relationship with Alzheimer disease, schizophrenia, epilepsy and smoking. Archives of Clinical Psychiatry. 2010;**37**:74-80. DOI: 10.1590/S0101-60832010000200007

[11] Bartolini A, Di Cesare ML, Ghelardini C. Analgesic and antineuropathic drugs acting through central cholinergic mechanisms. Recent Patents on CNS Drug Discovery. 2011;**6**:119-140. DOI: 10.2174/157488911795933901

[12] Čolović MB, Krstić DZ, Lazarević-Pašti TD, Bondžić AM, Vasić VM. Acetylcholinesterase inhibitors: Pharmacology and toxicology. Current Neuropharmacology. 2013;**11**:315-335. DOI: 10.2174/1570159X11311030006

[13] Müller TC, Rocha JB, Morsch VM, Neis RT, Schetinger MR. Antidepressants inhibit human acetylcholinesterase and butyrylcholinesterase activity. Biochimica et Biophysica Acta.

2002;**1587**:92-98. DOI: 10.1016/s0925-4439(02)00071-6

[14] Pezzementi L, Nachon F, Chatonnet A. Evolution of acetylcholinesterase and butyrylcholinesterase in the vertebrates: An atypical butyrylcholinesterase from the Medaka Oryzias latipes. PLoS One. 2011;**6**:e17396. DOI: 10.1371/journal.pone.0017396

[15] Rang HP, Dale MM, Ritter JM. Farmacologia. 4th ed. Rio de Janeiro: Guanabara Koogan; 2001. 703 p

[16] Paiva JT. The Use of Anticholinesterasic Employees in Myasthenia Gravis [Monography]. São João Del Rei: Federal University of São João Del-Rei; 2013

[17] Hepnarova V, Korabecny J, Matouskova L, Jost P, Muckova L, Hrabinova M, et al. The concept of hybrid molecules of tacrine and benzyl quinolone carboxylic acid (BQCA) as multifunctional agents for Alzheimer's disease. European Journal of Medicinal Chemistry. 2018;**150**:292-306. DOI: 10.1016/j.ejmech.2018.02.083

[18] Knight R, Khondoker M, Magill N, Stewart R, Landau S. A systematic review and meta-analysis of the effectiveness of acetylcholinesterase inhibitors and memantine in treating the cognitive symptoms of dementia. Dementia and Geriatric Cognitive Disorders. 2018;**45**:131-151. DOI: 10.1159/000486546

[19] Rao AN, Patil A, Brodnik ZD, Qiang L, España RA, Sullivan KA, et al. Pharmacologically increasing microtubule acetylation corrects stress-exacerbated effects of organophosphates on neurons. Traffic. 2017;**18**:433-441. DOI: 10.1111/tra.12489

[20] Silva P. Farmacologia. 6th ed. Rio de Janeiro: Guanabara Koogan; 2002

[21] Inouye K, Oliveira GH. Critical evaluation of current pharmacological treatment for Alzheimer's disease. Infarma—Pharmaceutical Sciences. 2004;**15**:80-84

[22] Hardman JG, Limbird LE, Gilman AG, editors. Goodman & Gilman—As bases Farmacológicas da Terapêutica. 10th ed. Rio de Janeiro: McGraw-Hill; 2005. 1647 p

[23] Araújo CRM, Santos VLA, Gonsalves AA. Acetylcholinesterase—AChE: A pharmacological interesting enzyme. Revista Virtual de Química. 2016;**8**:1818-1834. DOI: 10.21577/1984-6835.20160122

[24] Lemke TL, Williams DA, Roche VF, Zito SW, editors. Foye's Principles of Medicinal Chemistry. 6th ed. Philadelphia: Lippincott Williams & Wilkins; 2008. 1381 p

[25] Cataldo Neto A, Gauer GJC, Furtado NR. Psiquiatria Para Estudantes de Medicina. 2nd ed. Edipucrs: Porto Alegre; 2013. 692 p

[26] Rang HP, Dale MM, Ritter JM, Flower RJ, Henderson G. Rang & Dale—Farmacologia. 7th ed. Rio de Janeiro: Elsevier; 2011. 808 p

[27] Marrs TC. Organophosphate poisoning. Pharmacology & Therapeutics. 1993;**58**:51-66

[28] Meriggioli MN, Sanders DB. Autoimmune myasthenia gravis: Emerging clinical and biological heterogeneity. Lancet Neurology. 2009;**8**:475-490. DOI: 10.1016/S1474-4422(09)70063-8

[29] Wendell LC, Levine JM. Myasthenic crisis. Neurohospitalist. 2011;**1**:16-22. DOI: 10.1177/1941875210382918

[30] Oosterhuis HJ. The natural course of myasthenia gravis: A long term follow up study. Journal of Neurology,

Neurosurgery, and Psychiatry. 1989;**52**:1121-1127. DOI: 10.1136/jnnp.52.10.1121

[31] Silva FC, Cardeal ZL, De Carvalho CR. Determination of organophosphorus pesticides in water using SPME-GC-MS. Química Nova. 1999;**22**:197-200

[32] Silva GR, Borges I Jr, Figueroa-Villar JD, De Castro AT. Chemical defense: History, warfare agent classification and action of neurotoxic agents. Química Nova. 2012;**35**:2083-2091

[33] Holstege CP, Kirk M, Sidell FR. Chemical warfare: Nerve agent poisoning. Critical Care Clinics. 1997;**13**:923-942. DOI: 10.1016/S0749-0704(05)70374-2

[34] Morita H, Yanagisawa N, Nakajima T, Shimizu M, Hirabayashi H, Okudera H, et al. Sarin poisoning in Matsumoto, Japan. Lancet. 1995;**346**:290-293. DOI: 10.1016/s0140-6736(95)92170-2

[35] Okumura T, Takasu N, Ishimatsu S, Miyanoki S, Mitsuhashi A, Kumada K, et al. Report on 640 victims of the Tokyo subway sarin attack. Annals of Emergency Medicine. 1996;**28**:129-135. DOI: 10.1016/s0196-0644(96)70052-5

[36] Gordon JJ, Inns RH, Johnson MK, Leadbeater L, Maidment MP, Upshall DG, et al. The delayed neuropathic effects of nerve agents and some other organophosphorus compounds. Archives of Toxicology. 1983;**52**:71-82

[37] Soltaninejad K, Abdollahi M. Current opinion on the science of organophosphate pesticides and toxic stress: A systematic review. Medical Science Monitor. 2009;**15**:RA75-RA90

[38] Terry AV Jr. Functional consequences of repeated organophosphate exposure: Potential non-cholinergic mechanisms. Pharmacology & Therapeutics. 2012;**134**:355-365. DOI: 10.1016/j.pharmthera.2012.03.001

[39] Kaufer D, Friedman A, Seidman S, Soreq H. Acute stress facilitates long-lasting changes in cholinergic gene expression. Nature. 1998;**393**:373-377. DOI: 10.1038/30741

[40] Sanborn M, Kerr KJ, Sanin LH, Cole DC, Bassil KL, Vakil C. Non-cancer health effects of pesticides: Systematic review and implications for family doctors. Canadian Family Physician. 2007;**53**:1712-1720

[41] Khan F, Kennedy G, Spence VA, Newton DJ, Belch JJ. Peripheral cholinergic function in humans with chronic fatigue syndrome, gulf war syndrome and with illness following organophosphate exposure. Clinical Science. 2004;**106**:183-189. DOI: 10.1042/CS20030246

[42] Jenrow KA, Brown SL, Lapanowski K, Naei H, Kolozsvary A, Kim JH. Selective inhibition of microglia-mediated neuroinflammation mitigates radiation-induced cognitive impairment. Radiation Research. 2013;**179**:549-556. DOI: 10.1667/RR3026.1

[43] Kohman RA, Rhodes JS. Neurogenesis, inflammation and behavior. Brain, Behavior, and Immunity. 2013;**27**:22-32. DOI: 10.1016/j.bbi.2012.09.003

[44] Parihar VK, Hattiangady B, Kuruba R, Shuai B, Shetty AK. Predictable chronic mild stress improves mood, hippocampal neurogenesis and memory. Molecular Psychiatry. 2011;**16**:171-183. DOI: 10.1038/mp.2009.130

[45] Haley RW, Kurt TL. Self-reported exposure to neurotoxic chemical

combinations in the Gulf War. A cross-sectional epidemiologic study. Journal of the American Medical Association. 1997;**277**:231-237. DOI: 10.1001/jama.1997.03540270057027

[46] Berríos VO, Boukli NM, Rodriguez JW, Negraes PD, Schwindt TT, Trujillo CA, et al. Paraoxon and pyridostigmine interfere with neural stem cell differentiation. Neurochemical Research. 2015;**40**:2091-2101. DOI: 10.1007/s11064-015-1548-7

[47] Carreras I, Aytan N, Mellott T, Choi JK, Lehar M, Crabtree L, et al. Corrigendum to "anxiety, neuroinflammation, cholinergic and GABAergic abnormalities are early markers of gulf war illness in a mouse model of the disease" [2018;**1681**:34-43]. Brain Research. 2018;**1688**:113-115. DOI: 10.1016/j.brainres.2018.03.005

[48] Kodali M, Hattiangady B, Shetty GA, Bates A, Shuai B, Shetty AK. Curcumin treatment leads to better cognitive and mood function in a model of gulf war illness with enhanced neurogenesis, and alleviation of inflammation and mitochondrial dysfunction in the hippocampus. Brain, Behavior, and Immunity. 2018;**69**:499-514. DOI: 10.1016/j.bbi.2018.01.009

[49] Sullivan K, Krengel M, Bradford W, Stone C, Thompson TA, Heeren T, et al. Neuropsychological functioning in military pesticide applicators from the Gulf War: Effects on information processing speed, attention and visual memory. Neurotoxicology and Teratology. 2018;**65**:1-13. DOI: 10.1016/j.ntt.2017.11.002

[50] Valko M, Rhodes CJ, Moncol J, Izakovic M, Mazur M. Free radicals, metals and antioxidants in oxidative stress-induced cancer. Chemico-Biological Interactions. 2006;**160**:1-40. DOI: 10.1016/j.cbi.2005.12.009

[51] Panasenko OM, Gorudko IV, Sokolov AV. Hypochlorous acid as a precursor of free radicals in living systems. Biochemistry (Mosc). 2013;**78**:1466-1489. DOI: 10.1134/S0006297913130075

[52] Halliwell B. Biochemistry of oxidative stress. Biochemical Society Transactions. 2007;**35**:1147-1150. DOI: 10.1042/BST0351147

[53] Barja G. Mitochondrial oxygen consumption and reactive oxygen species production are independently modulated: Implications for aging studies. Rejuvenation Research. 2007;**10**:215-224. DOI: 10.1089/rej.2006.0516

[54] Dowling DK, Simmons LW. Reactive oxygen species as universal constraints in life-history evolution. Proceedings of the Biological Sciences. 2009;**276**:1737-1745. DOI: 10.1098/rspb.2008.1791

[55] Nordberg J, Arnér ES. Reactive oxygen species, antioxidants, and the mammalian thioredoxin system. Free Radical Biology & Medicine. 2001;**31**:1287-1312

[56] Ferreira ALA, Matsubara LS. Free radicals: Concepts, associated diseases, defense system and oxidative stress. Revista da Associação Médica Brasileira. 1997;**43**:61-68

[57] Maia MS. Sperm viability and reactive oxygen species (ROS) generation in ram semen cryopreserved in extenders supplemented with sodium lauryl ulfate (OEP), Trolox-C and catalase [thesis]. Botucatu: Faculdade de Medicina Veterinária e Zootecnia, Universidade Estadual Paulista; 2006

[58] Obayan AOE. Oxidative stress: natural history and modulation in surgery and trauma patients [hesis]. Saskatoon: University of Saskatchewan; 2004

[59] Koury JC, Donangelo CM. Zinc, oxidative stress and physical activity.

Brazilian Journal of Nutrition. 2003;**16**:433-441

[60] Vincent HK, Innes KE, Vincent KR. Oxidative stress and potential interventions to reduce oxidative stress in overweight and obesity. Diabetes, Obesity & Metabolism. 2007;**9**:813-839. DOI: 10.1111/j.1463-1326.2007.00692.x

[61] Rudich A, Tirosh A, Potashnik R, Hemi R, Kanety H, Bashan N. Prolonged oxidative stress impairs insulin-induced GLUT4 translocation in 3T3-L1 adipocytes. Diabetes. 1998;**47**:1562-1569. DOI: 10.2337/diabetes.47.10.1562

[62] Brownlee M. Biochemistry and molecular cell biology of diabetic complications. Nature. 2001;**414**:813-820. DOI: 10.1038/414813a

[63] Maddux BA, See W, Lawrence JC Jr, Goldfine AL, Goldfine ID, Evans JL. Protection against oxidative stress-induced insulin resistance in rat L6 muscle cells by micromolar concentrations of alpha-lipoic acid. Diabetes. 2001;**50**:404-410. DOI: 10.2337/diabetes.50.2.404

[64] Green K, Brand MD, Murphy MP. Prevention of mitochondrial oxidative damage as a therapeutic strategy in diabetes. Diabetes. 2004;**53**:S110-S118. DOI: 10.2337/diabetes.53.2007.s110

[65] Leite LEA, Resende TL, Nogueira GM, da Cruz IBM, Schneider RH, Gottlieb MGV. Aging, oxidative stress and sarcopenia: A systemic approach. Revista Brasileira de Geriatria e Gerontologia. 2012;**15**:365-380

[66] Wallace DC. Mitochondrial diseases in man and mouse. Science. 1999;**283**:1482-1488. DOI: 10.1126/science.283.5407.1482

[67] Dusse LMS, Vieira LM, Carvalho MG. Nitric oxide revision. Jornal Brasileiro de Patologia e Medicina Laboratorial. 2003;**39**:343-350

[68] Bresciani G, Cruz IB, de Paz JA, Cuevas MJ, González-Gallego J. The MnSOD Ala16Val SNP: Relevance to human diseases and interaction with environmental factors. Free Radical Research. 2013;**47**:781-792. DOI: 10.3109/10715762.2013.836275

[69] Zelko IN, Mariani TJ, Folz RJ. Superoxide dismutase multigene family: A comparison of the CuZn-SOD (SOD1), Mn-SOD (SOD2), and EC-SOD (SOD3) gene structures, evolution, and expression. Free Radical Biology & Medicine. 2002;**33**:337-349

[70] Sutton A, Khoury H, Prip-Buus C, Cepanec C, Pessayre D, Degoul F. The Ala16Val genetic dimorphism modulates the import of human manganese superoxide dismutase into rat liver mitochondria. Pharmacogenetics. 2003;**13**:145-157. DOI: 10.1097/01.fpc.0000054067.64000.8f

[71] Bag A, Bag N. Target sequence polymorphism of human manganese superoxide dismutase gene and its association with cancer risk: A review. Cancer Epidemiology, Biomarkers & Prevention. 2008;**17**:3298-3305. DOI: 10.1158/1055-9965.EPI-08-0235

[72] Kang SW. Superoxide dismutase 2 gene and cancer risk: Evidence from an updated meta-analysis. International Journal of Clinical and Experimental Medicine. 2015;**8**:14647-14655

[73] Taufer M, Peres A, de Andrade VM, de Oliveira G, Sá G, do Canto ME, et al. Is the Val16Ala manganese superoxide dismutase polymorphism associated with the aging process? Journals of Gerontology Series A-Biological Sciences and Medical Sciences. 2005;**60**:432-438. DOI: 10.1093/gerona/60.4.432

[74] Bica CG, de Moura da Silva LL, Toscani NV, da Cruz IB, Sá G, Graudenz MS, et al. MnSOD gene polymorphism association with steroid-dependent cancer. Pathology Oncology Research. 2009;**15**:19-24. DOI: 10.1007/s12253-008-9064-6

[75] Zejnilovic J, Akev N, Yilmaz H, Isbir T. Association between manganese superoxide dismutase polymorphism and risk of lung cancer. Cancer Genetics and Cytogenetics. 2009;**189**:1-4. DOI: 10.1016/j.cancergencyto.2008.06.017

[76] Bresciani G, da Cruz IB, González-Gallego J. Manganese superoxide dismutase and oxidative stress modulation. Advances in Clinical Chemistry. 2015;**68**:87-130. DOI: 10.1016/bs.acc.2014.11.001

[77] Gottlieb MG, Schwanke CH, Santos AF, Jobim PF, Müssel DP, da Cruz IB. Association among oxidized LDL levels, MnSOD, apolipoprotein E polymorphisms, and cardiovascular risk factors in a South Brazilian region population. Genetics and Molecular Research. 2005;**4**:691-703

[78] Tian C, Liu T, Fang S, Du X, Jia C. Association of C47T polymorphism in SOD2 gene with coronary artery disease: A case-control study and a meta-analysis. Molecular Biology Reports. 2012;**39**:5269-5276. DOI: 10.1007/s11033-011-1324-y

[79] Montano MA, da Cruz IB, Duarte MM, da Krewer C, da Rocha MI, Mânica-Cattani MF, et al. Inflammatory cytokines in vitro production are associated with Ala16Val superoxide dismutase gene polymorphism of peripheral blood mononuclear cells. Cytokine. 2012;**60**:30-33. DOI: 10.1016/j.cyto.2012.05.022

[80] Barbisan F, Azzolin VF, Ribeiro EE, Duarte MMMF, da Cruz IBM. The in vitro influence of a genetic superoxide-hydrogen peroxide imbalance on immunosenescence. Rejuvenation Research. 2017;**20**:334-345. DOI: 10.1089/rej.2016.1892

[81] Montano MA, Barrio Lera JP, Gottlieb MG, Schwanke CH, da Rocha MI, Manica-Cattani MF, et al. Association between manganese superoxide dismutase (MnSOD) gene polymorphism and elderly obesity. Molecular and Cellular Biochemistry. 2009;**328**:33-40. DOI: 10.1007/s11010-009-0071-z

[82] Duarte MM, Moresco RN, Duarte T, Santi A, Bagatini MD, da Cruz IB, et al. Oxidative stress in hypercholesterolemia and its association with Ala16Val superoxide dismutase gene polymorphism. Clinical Biochemistry. 2010;**43**:1118-1123. DOI: 10.1016/j.clinbiochem.2010.07.002

[83] Flores AE, Pascotini ET, Kegler A, Gabbi P, Bochi GV, Barbisan F, et al. ALA16VAL-MnSOD gene polymorphism and stroke: Association with dyslipidemia and glucose levels. Gene. 2017;**627**:57-62. DOI: 10.1016/j.gene.2017.05.055

[84] Bica CG, da Silva LL, Toscani NV, Zettler CG, Gottlieb MG, Alexandre CO, et al. Polymorphism (ALA16VAL) correlates with regional lymph node status in breast cancer. Cancer Genetics and Cytogenetics. 2010;**196**:153-158. DOI: 10.1016/j.cancergencyto.2009.09.011

[85] Wang C, Liu Y, Zhou J, Ye L, Chen N, Zhu M, et al. There is no relationship between SOD2 Val-16Ala polymorphism and breast cancer risk or survival. Molecular and Clinical Oncology. 2017;**7**:579-590. DOI: 10.3892/mco.2017.1376

[86] Montagner GFS, Sagrillo M, Machado MM, Almeida RC, Mostardeiro CP, Duarte MM, et al.

Toxicological effects of ultraviolet radiation on lymphocyte cells with different manganese superoxide dismutase Ala16Val polymorphism genotypes. Toxicology In Vitro. 2010;**24**:1410-1416. DOI: 10.1016/j.tiv.2010.04.010

[87] Algarve TD, Barbisan F, Ribeiro EE, Duarte MM, Mânica-Cattani MF, Mostardeiro CP, et al. In vitro effects of Ala16Val manganese superoxide dismutase gene polymorphism on human white blood cells exposed to methylmercury. Genetics and Molecular Research. 2013;**12**:5134-5144. DOI: 10.4238/2013.October.29.7

[88] Duarte T, da Cruz IB, Barbisan F, Capelleto D, Moresco RN, Duarte MM. The effects of rosuvastatin on lipid-lowering, inflammatory, antioxidant and fibrinolytics blood biomarkers are influenced by Val16Ala superoxide dismutase manganese-dependent gene polymorphism. The Pharmacogenomics Journal. 2016;**16**:501-506. DOI: 10.1038/tpj.2015.91

[89] Capeleto D, Barbisan F, Azzolin V, Dornelles EB, Rogalski F, Teixeira CF, et al. The anti-inflammatory effects of resveratrol on human peripheral blood mononuclear cells are influenced by a superoxide dismutase 2 gene polymorphism. Biogerontology 2015;16:621-630. DOI: 10.1007/s10522-015-9561-4

[90] Schott KL, Assmann CE, Barbisan F, Azzolin VF, Bonadiman B, Duarte MMMF, et al. Superoxide-hydrogen peroxide genetic imbalance modulates differentially the oxidative metabolism on human peripheral blood mononuclear cells exposed to seleno-L-methionine. Chemico-Biological Interactions. 2017;**273**:18-27. DOI: 10.1016/j.cbi.2017.05.007

[91] Berto MD, Bica CG, de Sá GP, Barbisan F, Azzolin VF, Rogalski F, et al. The effect of superoxide anion and hydrogen peroxide imbalance on prostate cancer: An integrative in vivo and in vitro analysis. Medical Oncology. 2015;**32**:251. DOI: 10.1007/s12032-015-0700-1

[92] Azzolin VF, Cadoná FC, Machado AK, Berto MD, Barbisan F, Dornelles EB, et al. Superoxide-hydrogen peroxide imbalance interferes with colorectal cancer cells viability, proliferation and oxaliplatin response. Toxicology In Vitro. 2016;**32**:8-15. DOI: 10.1016/j.tiv.2015.12.001

[93] Barbisan F, Motta JR, Trott A, Azzolin V, Dornelles EB, Marcon M, et al. Methotrexate-related response on human peripheral blood mononuclear cells may be modulated by the Ala16Val-SOD2 gene polymorphism. PLoS One. 2014;**9**:e107299. DOI: 10.1371/journal.pone.0107299

[94] Azzolin VF, Barbisan F, Lenz LS, Teixeira CF, Fortuna M, Duarte T, et al. Effects of pyridostigmine bromide on SH-SY5Y cells: An in vitro neuroblastoma neurotoxicity model. Mutation Research—Genetic Toxicology and Environmental Mutagenesis. 2017;**823**:1-10. DOI. DOI: 10.1016/j.mrgentox.2017.08.003

[95] Azzolin VF, Barbisan F, Teixeira CF, Pillar D, Mastella MH, Duarte T, et al. The Val16Ala-SOD2 polymorphism affects cyto-genotoxicity of pyridostigmine bromide on human peripheral blood mononuclear cells. Toxicology in Vitro. 2019;**60**:237-244. DOI: 10.1016/j.tiv.2019.06.004

Chapter 13

The Clinical Importance of Herb-Drug Interactions and Toxicological Risks of Plants and Herbal Products

Cigdem Kahraman, Zekiye Ceren Arituluk and Iffet Irem Tatli Cankaya

Abstract

Approximately 70% of the world's population has been using medicinal herbs as a complementary or alternative medicine that has grown tremendously in both developed and developing countries over the past 20 years (World Health Organization Drugs Strategy 2002–2005). This increase in consumer demand for medicinal plants continues, although scientific data are rare to create safety and efficacy profiles. Its popularity is also related to easy availability, cost-effectiveness leading to better purchasing power, and various factors that perceive that they are generally safe. Herbs are often administered simultaneously with therapeutic drugs for the treatment of major ailments, and herb-drug interactions (HDIs) increase their potential. The main routes proposed for HDIs include cytochrome P450 (CYP450)-mediated inhibition or induction and transport and flow proteins. In our review, we highlighted herbal medicines used for the treatment of various diseases with pharmacokinetic, pharmacodynamic analysis and case reports together with their adverse effects and herb-drug interactions. Therefore, this review can be used as a quick reference database for physicians and healthcare professionals involved in therapy, aiming to maximize clinical outcomes by reducing the negative and toxic effects of plants along with avoiding herb-drug interactions.

Keywords: herbs/plants, herbal products, natural products, drugs, interactions, toxicity

1. Introduction

Herbal products are considered the best choice as complementary medicine in western countries, especially in the United States and Europe. Annual sales of dietary herbal supplements in the United States increase 6.8% year over year. In addition, China and India are the top export countries, while Hong Kong, Japan, the United States, and Germany are the leading importers. The Confederation of Indian Industry (CII) presented that the market size of the Ayurvedic industry in the country is $ 4.4 billion, and the total market size of the Indian health industry is $ 11.8 billion. There has been an increase in demand for "complementary" medicines, including those of plant origin. In addition, there is a significant increase in the self-administration of herbal medicines among the public. In the context of the

IntechOpen

growing demand and use of herbal medicines for patients and the public, and the subsequent interests of the regulatory authorities, comprehensive research on the safety and effectiveness of herbal products, including the possibility of interactions when simultaneous application is required, should be encouraged. This is because all herbal medicines and dietary supplements are a complex mixture containing multiple active phyto-components that increase the possibility of herb-drug interaction (HDI). Most people who consume herbal products and supplements do not show this to their pharmacist or doctor, thereby increasing the likelihood of HDI being identified and resolved over time. However, data from recent studies show that there is potential for serious interaction between some commonly used herbs/herbal products and commonly used standard medications [1].

In our review, we highlighted herbal medicines used for the treatment of various diseases with their adverse effects and herb-drug interactions, and stated recommendations for proper use of plants that might prevent possible risks for future incidents.

2. Toxicological risks of plants and herbal products

General risks associated with herbs and/or herbal products include:

- Misidentification without assigning with Latin names. Possible causes of misidentification include contamination of cultivated plants with weeds, and resembling plants mistaken for herbs collected in the wild.

- Contamination with harmful substances such as heavy metals, polycyclic aromatic hydrocarbons, dioxins, as well as natural toxins or microorganisms.

- Interaction with other drugs, such as antagonism or synergism, and medical tests that potentially lead to misdiagnosis.

- Adulteration with other medicinal drugs.

- Intrinsic toxicity caused by the presence of natural toxins, such as aristolochic acids [2].

2.1 Nephrotoxicity

The drug or toxin that causes kidney damage when exposed to a certain level cannot pass the excess urine, and the waste product is what is called nephrotoxicity. In this case, there is an increase in blood electrolytes, such as potassium and magnesium. This situation begins temporarily but can be serious if it is not detected before. Blood urea nitrogen (BUN) test and creatinine levels in the blood are two simple tests called as kidney function tests used to detect the nephrotoxicity. For healthy individuals, the normal levels of BUN and creatinine are between 10–25 mg/dl and 0.7–1.4 mg/dl, respectively. The following factors may increase these values:

a. Dehydration.

b. Obstruction of blood flow to or from kidney caused by a tumor, stone, or irregular heart rhythms.

c. Nephritis or urinary tract infection.

d. The aftermath of diseases such as diabetic neuropathy, congestive heart failure, and enlarged prostate gland in man.

e. Gastrointestinal bleeding.

f. Prolonged hypotension.

g. Protein-rich diets.

h. Radiocontrast dye injected intravenously to improve visibility.

i. Drug toxicity with some chemotherapeutics (carboplatin, carmustine, cisplatin, methotrexate, and mitomycin) and biological therapeutic agents (interleukin-2 and interferon-alpha), antibiotics (amphotericin B, gentamicin, and vancomycin), NSAIDs (ibuprofen), diuretics (furosemide), and ACE inhibitors (captopril, benazepril, and enalapril).

j. Nephrotoxicity after taking herbal medicine.

The cause of nephrotoxicity after taking herbal medicine may be the addition of toxins during careless preparation, addition of adulterants, heavy metals, and some pharmaceutical products intentionally reducing costs or increasing effectiveness [3].

About 50 plants were related to kidney damage case reports published in PubMed in the last 50+ years (from 1966 to May 2016). Herbs include *Aristolochia fangchi* Y.C.Wu ex L.D.Chow & S.M.Hwang, *Artemisia herba-alba* Asso, *Callilepis laureola* DC., *Cupressus funebris* Endl., *Ephedra sinica* Stapf, *Hypericum perforatum* L., *Taxus celebica* (Warb.) H.L.Li, *Tribulus terrestris* L., and *Tripterygium wilfordii* Hook.f. *Aristolochia* species containing aristolochic acid, *Aristolochia fangchi*, had the highest number of publications (not actual cases) [4].

2.2 Hepatotoxicity

Hepatotoxicity ("Hepar" means liver and "Toxicon" means poison in ancient Greek) implies liver damage caused by medication, chemical, herbal, or dietary supplements. Stomach pain, vomiting, nausea, chance in urine and stool color, rash, jaundice, frequent tiredness, weakness, fatigue, and fever are the main symptoms of the damage. Some liver function tests performed on blood samples allow detecting hepatotoxicity in the laboratory. These tests include alanine transaminase test (normal range 7–55 U/l), alkaline phosphatase test (normal range 45–115 U/l), albumin test (normal range 3.5–5.0 g/dl), aspartate transaminase test (normal range 8–48 U/l), and bilirubin test (normal range 0.1–1.2 mg/dl). Increased ALT, ALP, AST, and bilirubin and decreased albumin levels demonstrate hepatotoxicity. The levels of ALP also increase during pregnancy [3].

The causes of liver damage are both hepatocellular and extracellular mechanisms such as hepatocyte disruption, transport protein disruption, T-cell activation, hepatocyte apoptosis, disruption of mitochondria, injury of bile duct, drug toxicity, and drug interaction [3].

Drug toxicity mechanisms: drugs are the main cause of hepatotoxicity. About 900 drugs, toxins, and herbs have been reported for hepatotoxicity. There are two types of drug reactions: the first is the reaction that directly affects the liver, called internal drug reactions; and the other is the reaction that mediates the immune response, called idiosyncratic drug reactions. In the first category, the drug itself or its metabolite produces a dose-dependent injury, such as paracetamol and carbon tetrachloride. In the second category, hypersensitivity reactions, for example, phenytoin reaction, cause an immunoallergic or metabolic idiosyncratic reaction due to fever, rash, eosinophilia and indirect drug reaction for a short time. The second reaction type response rate is variable, for example, halothane [3].

Drug interaction mechanisms: when some drugs are taken at the same time, they react together and cause liver damage. For example, the combination of tylenol with INH, histamine, laniazide, and nydrazide can be hepatotoxic [3].

When hepatotoxicity caused by herbal drug intake is discussed, case rates are often reported. The severity of toxicity varies greatly between mild hepatitis and acute liver failure. The scoring system for allopathic drugs can be evaluated, but not suitable for herbal medicines and needs validation. Many Ayurvedic and Chinese herbal medicines are reported to cause hepatotoxicity. The main hepatotoxic herbs are *Cimicifuga racemosa* (L.) Nutt., *Larrea tridentata (*Sessé & Moc. ex DC.) Coville, *Scutellaria baicalensis* Georgi, *Scutellaria lateriflora* L., *Teucrium chamaedrys* L., etc. [3].

2.3 Cardiotoxicity

Cardiotoxicity is a term used for damage to the heart or change heart functions. It is a condition where there is a change in the electrophysiological function of the heart or damage to the heart muscle, weakening the heart and causing poor blood circulation. This can be detected by symptoms such as dry, unproductive cough; inflammation in the ankles, hands, feet, and neck vessels; irregular heartbeat; tachycardia; cardiomegaly; weakness; dizziness; etc. [3].

Herbal drugs that have a direct effect on the heart include medicine prepared from plants such as *Aconitum napellus* L., *Atropa belladonna* L., *Catharanthus roseus* (L.) G.Don, *Digitalis purpurea* L., *Ephedra distachya* L., *Glycyrrhiza glabra* L., *Mandragora officinarum* L., etc. [3].

2.3.1 Potential precautions of plants on hypertension

Herbal products are widely used in the general population and many are encouraged for the natural treatment of hypertension. Patients with hypertension often prefer to use these products in addition to or instead of pharmacological antihypertensive agents. Due to the frequent use of herbal products, both consumers and healthcare providers should be aware of the major issues surrounding these products and factors affecting both effectiveness and damages (**Table 1**) [5].

Herbal/natural products for evidence of benefit	Herbs/herbal products for evidence of harm	Causes
Coenzyme Q10	*Ephedra* spec. (Ephedra)	Cardiac effects, hypertension, palpitations, tachycardia, stroke, seizures
Fish oil	*Citrus × aurantium* L. (Bitter orange)	Blood pressure increases occur in healthy people
Allium sativum L. (Garlic)	*Eleutherococcus senticosus* (Rupr. & Maxim.) Maxim. (Siberian Ginseng)	Hypertension, tachycardia, palpitations
Vitamin C	*Glycyhrriza glabra* (Licorice)	Mineralocorticoid excess syndrome, subsequent hypertension

Table 1.
Herbal/natural products in hypertension for their benefits and disadvantages.

DOI: http://dx.doi.org/10.5772/intechopen.92040

2.4 Neurotoxicity

The physical brain damage occurred by exposure to neurotoxin is stated as neurotoxicity. Neurotoxin is a substance that causes changes in the nervous system activity by disrupting or killing neurons. Neurotoxicity symptoms are generally emotional disorders, visual impairment, extremity failing, sexual dysfunction, headache, and behavioral alteration. *Atropa belladonna*, *Brugmansia* species, *Catharanthus roseus*, *Cannabis sativa* L., *Conium maculatum* L., *Coscinium fenestratum* (Goetgh.) Colebr., *Datura stramonium* L., *Hyoscyamus niger* L., and *Papaver somniferum* L. are the common medicinal herbs that have potential neurotoxic effects [3].

2.4.1 Psychiatric and neurological adverse effects

Psychiatric and neurological patients often try herbal medicines assuming they are safe. Numerous case reports include various adverse events such as cerebral arteritis, cerebral edema, delirium, coma, confusion, encephalopathy, hallucinations, intracerebral hemorrhage and other cerebrovascular accidents, movement disorders, mood disorders, muscle weakness, paresthesia, and seizures. Some deaths have been recorded. Misuse is caused by toxicity of herbal ingredients, contamination and adulteration, and herb-drug interactions [6] (**Table 2**).

Herbs	Adverse effects	Potential drug interactions
Panax ginseng C.A.Mey.	Insomnia, vaginal bleeding, mastalgia, mania	Phenelzine, hypoglycemic drugs
Valeriana officinalis L. (Valerian)	Headache, GI symptoms, hangover	Other CNS depressants
Datura stramonium (Jimson weed)*	Ataxia, blurred vision, disorientation, other cholinergic signs	Other anti-cholinergic agents
Glycyrrhiza glabra (Licorice)	Mineral corticoid effects	Antihypertensives, corticosteroids, digoxin
Passiflora incarnata L. (Passionflower)	Nausea, drowsiness, ventricular tachycardia	Other CNS depressants
Mentha pulegium L. (Pennyroyale)	GI symptoms and cramps, confusion, hallucination, liver failure	Inhibitors of cytochrome P-450 system
Piper methysticum G.Forst. (Kava)*	GI symptoms, restlessness, allergies, hepatitis	Other CNS depressants
Ephedra sinica (Ma Huang)*	Anxiety, confusion, insomnia, psychosis	Other CNS-stimulants, beta-blockers, MAO-inhibitors, phenothiazines, theophylline
Ginkgo biloba L.	GI symptoms, allergies, headache, dizziness, bleeding	Anticoagulants
Tripterygium wilfordii (Thunder God Vine)*	Dryness of mouth, nausea, GI symptoms, leukopenia	Not known
Eucalyptus sp.	Cyanosis, delirium, GI symptoms	Not known
Hypericum perforatum (St. John's wort)	GI symptoms, allergies, fatigue, anxiety	Serotonin reuptake inhibitors, hepatic enzyme inducer
Aconitum sp. (Aconite)*	Acidosis, bradycardia, diarrhea, hypokalemia	Antiarrhythmics, antihypertensives

**Although we know the unconscious use of plants or their products, some of the plants given in the table are potent plants that are undesirable to be used in phytotherapy, but they are generally used in Traditional Chinese Medicine.*

Table 2.
Herbal remedies implicated in causing neurological adverse effects [6].

2.5 Skin toxicity

Cutaneous toxicity is a term used for a pronounced negative effect such as skin irritation, inflammation, or rashes of the epidermal growth factor receptor caused by exposure to a plant, chemical, or environmental factor. Skin consisting of a layer of dead cells and several layers of living cells is the largest organ and a defensive barrier of the body. When irritant influences into the skin, the living cells react due to cause inflammation or dermatitis. Inflammation consists of four parts including redness, pain, heat, and swelling. Skin toxicity can be detected easily as the reaction is observed immediately. The most common sources of skin toxicity are food and cosmetics, and others are medicated lotions, balms, creams, inhalers, and essential oils. Various herbal ingredients are available in all the cosmetics and medicinal products mentioned above. Types of skin sensitization reactions include:

Primary irritant dermatitis: it is a direct irritation of the skin, such as redness, itching, pain, blusters, peeling, or open wounds. Primary irritant dermatitis may be caused by plants such as, *Asclepias syriaca* L., *Cannabis sativa*, *Dieffenbachia amoena* Bull., *Digitalis purpurea*, *Ficus carica* L., *Hevea brasiliensis* (Willd. ex A.Juss.) Müll. Arg., *Narcissus pseudonarcissus* L., *Primula veris* L., *Ranunculus acris* L., *Ricinus communis* L., *Tulipa gesneriana* L., etc. Common foods such as *Agaricus bisporus* L., *Apium graveolens* L., *Brassica rapa* L., *Cucumis sativus* L., *Daucus carota* L., *Pastinaca sativa* L., *Petroselinum crispum* (Mill.) Fuss, and *Solanum lycopersicum* L. can also cause primary irritant dermatitis.

Allergic contact dermatitis: it is a real allergic response and varies from person to person. *Toxicodendron diversilobum* (Torr. & A.Gray) Greena and *Toxicodendron rydbergii* (Small ex Rydb.) Greene, *Allium cepa* L., *Allium sativum, Anacardium occidentale* L., *Apium graveolens, Cedrus deodara* (Roxb. ex D.Don) G.Don, *Dendranthema grandiflorum* (Ramat.) Kitam., *Hedera helix* L., *Marchantiophyta* species, *Narcissus pseudonarcissus*, *Primula vulgaris* Huds., *Pinus sabiniana* Douglas, *Toxicodendron vernix* (L.) Kuntze, and *Tulipa gesneriana* are the most common plants that produce allergic contact dermatitis.

Photosensitization dermatitis: it is a cutaneous toxic response caused by exposure to sunlight when a photosensitizer (sunlight sensitive compound) is present in the body and can be detected by sunburn-like reactions in pigment-free areas. Plants such as *Agave lechuguilla* Torr., *Bassia scoparia* (L.) A.J.Scott, *Hypericum* species (St John's wort), *Lantana camara* L., *Tetradymia* species, and *Tribulus terrestris* cause photosensitive dermatitis [3].

There is another type of phototoxic photosensitization caused by contact with some plants. Such a reaction occurs when a photoactive chemical produced by plants touches the skin, and is absorbed and activated by sunlight. Intensity varies depending on time and exposure amount. *Anethum graveolens* L., *Apium graveolens* L., *Brassica oleracea* L., *Citrus aurantiifolia* (Christm.) Swingle, *Daucus carota*, *Ficus carica*, *Hypericum perforatum* (St. John's wort), *Petroselinum crispum*, and *Ranunculus acris* are reported to produce contact photosensitization [3].

3. Contamination of herbal medicines by tropane alkaloids

Tropane alkaloids that have been known as toxic and hallucinogenic are mainly seen in Solanaceae plants (*Atropa belladonna*, *Hyoscyamus niger*, *Datura stramonium*, etc.). All over the world, anticholinergic poisoning is observed due to the contamination of herbal teas and plants with tropane alkaloids. Tropane alkaloid poisoning can occur after consumption of any medicinal plant from Solanaceae family as contaminants. Globally, almost all reports from 1978 to 2014 include one of the herbs prescribed in herbal teas. Contamination is most likely to occur during harvesting or processing. For herbs, on-site inspection is required to exclude cross-contamination at the retail level and accidental mixing. The diagnosis is confirmed by screening for the presence of Solanaceae species and tropane alkaloids. Since, if these relatively heat-resistant alkaloids contaminate the herbal teas and other herbs in large quantities, significant health hazards may occur, the significance of good agricultural and collection practices (GACPs) for medicinal plants is accentuated by WHO repeatedly. The DNA barcode is also increasingly used to exclude the presence of pollutant (especially toxic species) and product substitution. All suspect cases should be reported to health authorities so that investigations throughout the supply chain and early intervention measures to protect the public can be taken [7].

4. Herb-drug interactions with the plants including furanocoumarins

Naturally occurring furanocoumarins are abundant in citrus fruits, vegetables, and medicinal herbs from the Apiaceae, Fabaceae, and Rutaceae families. Grapefruit-drug interactions were first discovered by chance in 1989 where 5-fold higher felodipine plasma concentrations were observed. Consumption of grapefruit juice has increased the oral bioavailability of various drugs, including calcium channel blockers (e.g., felodipine, nifedipine), HMG-CoA reductase inhibitors (simvastatin, lovastatin), benzodiazepines (midazolam, triazolam), antihistamines (terfenadines), and immunosuppressants (cyclosporine). In addition, phototoxicity developing with furanocoumarins occurs as a result of exposure to sunlight, following contact with the plant. Phototoxicity results in acute dermatitis, sometimes blisters, and vesicles. In many cases, prolonged hyperpigmentation is observed. Photochemotherapy for a long time with furanocoumarins can also cause cancer (skin and liver) [8].

5. Toxicity of pyrrolizidine alkaloids

Pyrrolizidine alkaloids (PAs) are common components of hundreds of plant species of unrelated botanical families scattered across many geographical regions of the world. In more than 6000 plants belonging to three large plant families, Asteraceae, Boraginaceae, and Fabaceae, above 660 PAs and PA *N-oxides* have been identified and about half of them are toxic. More than 10,000 cases of PAs poisoning have been documented worldwide, most of which resulted from exposure to food contaminated with PAs. Acute toxicity from PA is mainly seen in the liver, including hemorrhagic necrosis, hepatic megalocytosis, venous occlusion, liver cirrhosis, and hepatic carcinomas, and chronic exposure to PAs, from herbs/dietary products containing PAs, can lead to kidneys, pancreas, gastrointestinal tract, bone marrow, and brain. It is a worldwide public health problem due to the high risk of human exposure to genotoxic and tumorigenic PAs, and the International Program on Chemical Safety has concluded that PAs are a threat to human health and safety. Regulations have been constituted to restrict its use [8].

6. Adverse effects of anthraquinone derivatives

Anthraquinone derivatives with a laxative effect appear in a number of plants: *Sennae folium*, rhei rhizoma, frangulae cortex, and aloe. They have a laxative effect by directly stimulating the colonic smooth muscles. The adverse effects of laxative anthraquinone drugs are more likely to be caused by excessive loss of fluids and electrolytes, especially potassium loss, associated with the use of high doses. Higher doses also drain a larger portion of the colon, and the resulting natural absence of defecation over the next day leads to reuse of anthraquinone. Prolonged use of laxatives due to laxative addiction should be avoided, as it may have a detrimental effect on the intestinal mucosa, leading to a condition known as Melanosis coli. This is usually seen after at least 9–12 months of regular stimulant laxative use. Undesirable effects such as abdominal spasms and pain, urine color change by metabolites, and hemorrhoid congestion are common. A report from China reported that patients with senna leaf tea addiction as laxatives suffer from symptoms of fidgetiness, sleeplessness, dilated pupils, and loss of appetite while consuming 5–9 g of senna daily. Rare cases of hepatic inflammation induced by anthraquinone derivatives have been reported and may be dose dependent. Hypokalemia, which occurs as the effect of long-term use of laxative drugs, strengthens the effect of cardiac glycosides and interacts with antiarrhythmic drugs. Using other drugs (diuretics, adrenocorticosteroids, and licorice) that cause hypokalemia can speed up electrolyte imbalance. Contraindications for anthracene laxatives are intestinal obstruction and chronic intestinal inflammation such as stomach or duodenal ulcer or ulcerative colitis [9].

7. Adulterations

Many reports on the adulteration of herbal products with synthetic drugs have been systematically reviewed and published with case reports. The list of herbal products and adulterants produced in this way is quite impressive and caused serious side effects (**Table 3**). A case with the latest herbal product adulterated is related to a 56-year-old man from Indonesia. While visiting Australia, he was hospitalized in a mixed condition arising from hypoglycemia. He insisted that type II diabetes was controlled only by diet. However, despite dextrose infusions, glucose levels do not normalize. It was eventually discovered that he also received a TCM "Zhen Qi" from Malaysia. It was analyzed and shown to contain glibenclamide. Like that, in some cases, patients were severely damaged. Examples of serious side effects include agranulocytosis, Cushing's syndrome, coma, over-anticoagulation, gastrointestinal bleeding, arrhythmias, and various skin lesions. Due to the adulteration of herbal products with synthetic drugs, adequate and necessary procedures should be applied, and whole herbal products should be analyzed before marketing [10].

Acetaminophen	**Dexamethasone**	**Glibenclamide**
Aminopyrine	Dexamethasone acetate	Hydrochlorothiazide
Betamethasone	Diazepam	Hydrocortisone
Caffeine	Diclofenac	Indomethacin
Chlordiazepoxide	Ethoxybenzamide	Mefenamic acid
Chlorzoxazone	Fluocinolone acetonide	Methylsalicylate
Clobetasol propionate	Fluocortolone	Phenacetin
Corticosteroids	Fluocortolone	Phenylbutazone
Phenytoin	Prednisolone	Sibutramin
Sildenafil		

Table 3.
Adulterants found in herbal products.

8. Heavy metal contaminations

It is possible to come across heavy metals such as cadmium, cobalt, copper, iron, manganese, nickel, lead, zinc, and mercury in concentrations that are not produced within the framework of certain rules, especially the traditional Chinese herbal preparations. This contamination is probably caused by contamination during drying and preservation. With severe complications that may occur, these types of products are unlikely to cause adverse health effects, even if they are not consumed in large quantities for long periods of time [11].

9. Herb-drug interactions (HDI)

There are no molecules in nature that have no effect. Therefore, this diversity increases the variety of products while increasing the probability of interaction. If the effect of a drug is changed qualitatively or quantitatively by another substance (herbal medicine/product/ingredient), there is an interaction between these two drugs. It can be said as a rule that two drugs should be present at the same time in the body, especially in the place of interaction, for interaction to occur. But sometimes, if the drug causes a permanent effect on the body, interaction can occur even if such a drug is not found in the body. Interaction is sometimes deliberately created to increase the therapeutic effect of one drug with another drug or to reduce its side effects, which are useful interactions. In other cases, the interaction may occur undesirably as a result of unauthorized use of medicines or when the patient is starting treatment with a particular medication. Sometimes, unpredictable interactions due to new drugs may occur. Drug-related as well as disease-related factors (patient's age, gender, genetic characteristics, pathological condition), such as the posology and method of administration, pharmacokinetic, pharmacodynamic, and therapeutic properties of the drug may cause interactions between medicines and herbal medicines (**Figure 1**) [12].

It is observed that the use of herbal medicines/herbal products is more common in the geriatric group aged 65 and over, and the use in women in this adult population is higher than in men. Herbs/herbal products/drug interaction is higher in patients using drugs with narrow therapeutic index. Information on herbs-herbal products/drug/component interactions is based on *in vitro* tests, *in vivo* animal experiments,

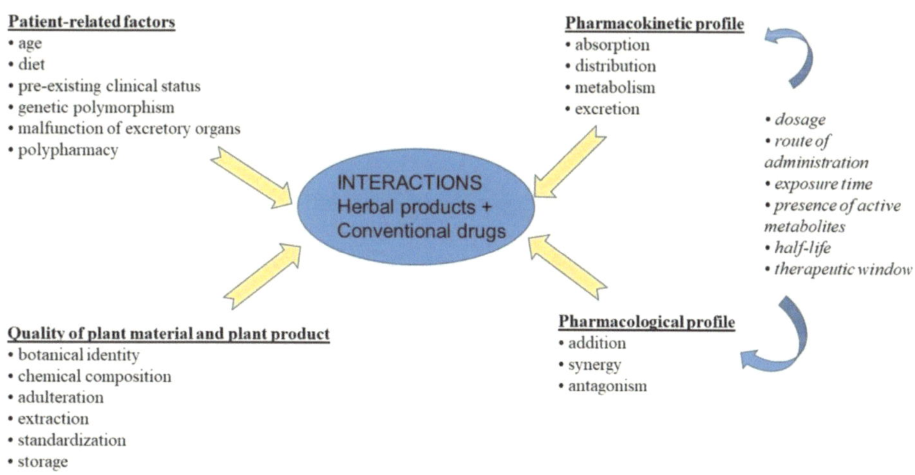

Figure 1.
The important risk factors that influence the occurrence of interactions between herbal products and conventional drugs [13].

and case reports. Many mechanisms play a role in these interactions, and interactions are seen in two main types as pharmacokinetic and pharmacodynamic interactions. Pharmacokinetic interactions result in changes in drug absorption, distribution, metabolism, and elimination. These interactions usually occur far away from the drug's effect and lead to a decrease or increase in effect as a result of the change in drug concentration in body fluids. In order to say that there is a pharmacokinetic interaction, the plasma level or half-life of the drug should be determined experimentally. Various interactions such as cytochrome P450, UDP-glucuronyl-transferase (UGTs), and carrier proteins such as P-glycoprotein (P-gp) are thought to play a role in these interactions. Pharmacokinetic interactions are the most common interactions as a cause of undesirable side effects. If the herb or natural products or its secondary metabolites inhibit an enzyme involved in drug metabolism, it may increase the potential for toxic effects, as it will reduce the metabolism of drugs that metabolize the enzyme and turn into an inactive metabolite as a result of metabolism. If the herbal drug induces an enzyme, a decrease in drug effect may be observed, since the metabolism of the drugs that are metabolized by this enzyme and converted into inactive metabolite as a result of metabolism will increase. Likewise, if the drug turns into an active metabolite as a result of metabolism, if the herbal drug induces the enzyme responsible for the metabolism of the drug, an increase in drug effect or toxic effect may be observed as a result of increased effective metabolite concentration [12].

Pharmacodynamic interactions occur when one drug changes the effect of another, that is, an effect opposite or in the same direction, chemically combined with it. That is, if the herbal medicine and drug affect the same receptor or the same site, interaction occurs and a synergic or antagonistic effect may occur. While the effect of the drug increases as a result of the additive effect, the effect of the drug decreases or disappears as a result of the antagonistic effect. The concentration of the drug in body fluids, plasma, is not changed by the second drug. Although most of the drug metabolism is carried out in the liver with cytochrome P450 enzymes, the metabolism of some drugs can be in the blood, kidney, skin, and intestine. Approximately 50 different cytochrome P450 enzymes have been identified. However, a small portion of these enzymes play a role in drug metabolism. Herbal drug-drug interactions are generally pharmacokinetic-type interactions that result from enzyme inhibition or induction [12].

The following are the evaluation parameters used to determine the probability of herb-drug interactions:

a. Adequate patient history.

b. Concurrent diseases, conditions, or other drugs associated with adverse events.

c. Concomitant medications are documented.

d. The description of the interactors is sufficient.

e. Clearly, alternative explanations are excluded.

f. Chronology is complete.

g. The time sequence of drug administration to adverse event is reasonable.

h. An adverse event has been sufficiently defined.

i. The event ends after stopping the medicine.

j. The activity repeats upon challenge again [3].

9.1. Herb-drug interactions in the treatment of cardiovascular disorders (CVDs)

In 2015, an estimated 422.7 million cases of cardiovascular disease (CVD) and 17.92 million CVD deaths were reported worldwide. And most people in the world still prefer complementary and alternative medicine (CAM) as their first treatment option. The consumption of over-the-counter CAM consumption increases the risk of HDI, which endangers the effective medical management of CVD. In cardiac therapy, the narrow therapeutic drug window and a wide range of cardiac drugs available for treatment are also a major cause of concern for HDI. People with chronic diseases often use CAM therapies inappropriately to manage their condition and thereby increase the potential or possibility of HDI formation [1].

This section of our review focuses on plants reported in the literature by preclinical or clinical studies (rats or humans) or cardiovascular drugs with appropriate case reports. These herbs are reported to affect the pharmacokinetics of some cardiovascular drugs through a variety of HDI mechanisms. Reported HDI studies of some plants commonly used for the treatment of CVDs are summarized in **Table 4** [1].

Herbs	Interacting drugs	CYP, P-gp induction/inhibition
Piper longum L.	Verapamil, digoxin, propranolol	CYP3A4, CYP2D6 and CYP1A2 (inhibition)
Curcuma longa L.	Losartan, rosuvastatin, warfarin, clopidogrel	CYP3A4, CYP1A2, CYP2B6, CYP2C19, CYP2C9 (inhibition)
	Talinolol	P-gp induction, intestinal P-gp in subjects with ABCB1 C3435T genotype inhibition
Fucus vesiculosus L.	Amiodarone, valsartan	CYP1A (induction), CYP2C9 (inhibition)
Zingiber officinale Roscoe	Nifedipine, phenprocoumon	CYP2C9 (potent inhibition) CYP2C19, CYP3A4 (moderate inhibition)
Terminalia bellirica (Gaertn.) Roxb.	Diltiazem	CYP3A4 CYP2D6
Salvia miltiorrhiza Bunge	Warfarin	CYP3A4 (induction) CYP1A2, CYP2C9, CYP1E1, CYP2C6, CYP2C11 (inhibition)
Allium sativum	Atorvastatin, cilostazol	CYP2C9, CYP3A4 and CYP2D6 (inhibition) P-gp induction
Ginkgo biloba	Diltiazem, cilostazol	CYP1A2, CYP3A, and CYP2C9 (P-gp inhibition inhibition) CYP2C19 (induction)
	Nifedipine	Unknown
	Talinolol	Intestinal P-gp inhibition
Glycrrhiza glabra	Atorvastatin, simvastatin, lovastatin	CYP2B6, CYP2C9, CYP2C19 (inhibition) CYP3A4 (induction)
Panax ginseng	Warfarin	CYP3A4 (induction), CYP2C11 (inhibition)
	Nifedipine	CYP3A4 (inhibition)
Pueraria montana (Lour.) Merr. var. *lobata* (Willd.) Sanjappa & Pradeep	Warfarin	CYP 1A2 (induction) CYP2D6, CYP3A4, and OATs (inhibition)
Citrus paradisi Macfad.	Felodipine	CYP3A4 (inhibition)
	Talinolol	OATP inhibition
	Aliskiren	OATP2B1 inhibition
	Atorvastatin	Intestinal CYP3A4 inhibition
	Lovastatin	Intestinal CYP3A4 inhibition
	Simvastatin	Intestinal CYP3A4 inhibition

Herbs	Interacting drugs	CYP, P-gp induction/inhibition
Mentha × piperita L.	Felodipine	CYP3A4 (inhibition)
Hypericum perforatum	Nifedipine	CYP3A4 (induction)
	Verapamil	
	Digoxin	P-gp induction
	Talinolol	P-gp induction
	Phenprocoumon	CYP2C9 induction, CYY3A4 induction
	Atorvastatin	CYP3A4 induction, P-gp induction
	Pravastatin	Intestinal CYP3A4 inhibition
	Simvastatin	CYP3A4 induction, P-gp induction
	Rosuvastatin	P-gp induction
Camellia sinensis (L.) Kuntze.	Digoxin	P-gp induction, digoxin uptake inhibition
	Nadolol	Intestinal OATP1A2 inhibition
	Rosuvastatin	Intestinal OATP1A2/OATB2P inhibition
Malus pumila Mill.	Atenolol	Unknown (possible mediated by OATP function and modulation of intestinal drug uptake)
	Aliskiren	OATP2B1 inhibition
Schisandra chinensis (Turcz.) Baill.	Talinolol	P-gp inhibition
Citrus × sinensis (L.) Osbeck	Aliskiren	OATP2B1 inhibition
Silybum marianum (L.) Gaertn.	Losartan	CYP2C9 inhibition

Table 4.
Reported HDI studies of some commonly used herbs for the treatment of CVDs [1, 13].

9.2 Herb-drug interactions with chemotherapeutic drugs

One of the most important risks associated with the combined use of herbal products and chemotherapeutic agents is herb-drug interactions. Patients with chronic illnesses who use more than one drug have a higher risk. Herb-drug interaction is undesirable in the treatment of cancer due to the perpendicular dose-effect relationship and toxicity of chemotherapeutic agents. The most common mechanism of herb-drug interaction is herbal mediated inhibition and/or stimulation of drug-metabolizing enzymes and/or transport proteins that lead to changes in the pharmacokinetic order of the victim drug. This focus on clinically significant herb-drug interaction should attract public attention, including practitioners, researchers, and cancer chemotherapy consumers (**Table 5**) [14].

9.3 Herb-drug interactions with attention-deficit/hyperactivity disorder (ADHD) medication

In some pediatric patients with attention deficit/hyperactivity disorder (ADHD), natural products such as herbal medicines are used. Although herbal remedies are thought to be safe when used appropriately, they may contain active ingredients that can interact with concurrently used medications and can lead to adverse events for natural products-drug interactions (**Table 6**) [15].

Herbs	Cancer drugs	Study type	Results
Echinacea	Etoposide	Case report	It was found that taking echinacea with etoposide rarely reduced platelet (16 × 103/L) compared to etoposide alone (44 × 103/L)
	Docetaxel	Prospective study in 10 cancer patients	Echinacea did not cause a significant change in the pharmacokinetics of docetaxel
Garlic	Docetaxel	Prospective, patient controlled, pharmacokinetic	Garlic was found to reduce docetaxel clearance. Although this reduction is not statistically significant, it can potentially increase side effects due to docetaxel accumulation
Ginseng	Imatinib	Case report	After receiving ginseng in patients receiving imatinib for 7 years, hepatotoxicity symptoms began to appear. Hepatotoxicity improved upon discontinuation of ginseng
Grapefruit juice	Docetaxel	Case report	Grapefruit juice has been found to reduce the clearance of docetaxel, while increasing the AUC and terminal half-life of docetaxel
	Nilotinib	Open label, randomized, 2 period crossover	It was found that grapefruit juice increased the AUC and the peak concentration of nilotinib, but did not affect the elimination half-life
Milk thistle	Irinotecan	Pharmacokinetic study	It has been found that milk thistle causes a statistically insignificant decrease in irinotecan clearance, which is unlikely to cause a clinical effect
St John's wort	Docetaxel	Pharmacokinetic study	St John's wort was found to cause a significant decrease in plasma docetaxel concentration
	Irinotecan	Unblinded, randomized crossover study	St John's wort caused a 42% reduction in plasma concentrations of the active metabolite (SN-38)
	Imatinib	Open-label, crossover pharmacokinetic study	St John's wort reduced the plasma concentration of imatinib by 32% and reduced the half-life of imatinib by 21%
		2-period, open-label, fixed sequence study	St John's wort increased the imatinib clearance by 43% and decreased the plasma concentration by 30%

Table 5.
Herbal interaction studies with chemotherapeutic agents conducted in human subjects [14].

9.4 Herb-drug interactions (HDI) with chronic kidney disease (CKD) medication

Chronic kidney disease (CKD) is defined as abnormalities in kidney structure or function that have been going on for more than 3 months, with adverse health consequences. The prevalence of CKD is estimated to be 8–16% worldwide.

Herbs	Drugs	Case
Ginkgo biloba	Strattera	An 8-year-old male patient with a history of ADHD, astigmatism, behavioral disorder, learning disorder, and asthma was using 25 mg Strattera for ADHD from October 2008 to September 2009. From May 2001 to November 2010, he was taking 85 mg of *G. biloba* daily. After starting Strattera, the patient experienced headaches and eye pain resulting in hospitalization. On ophthalmological examination, suspicion of glaucoma appeared. The reporting child psychiatrist stated that the incident was related to Strattera
Efalex evening primrose oil	Ritalin	A 7-year-old female was treated with Ritalin 10 mg/day orally for ADHD from October 2001. The patient has also been taking Efalex evening primrose oil since 2001. On March 7, 2002, she developed a tic including her both arms. It has become more complex. Ritalin was discontinued on March 7, 2002. There was an improvement in head, arm, neck, and leg movements after cessation, but movements were still present. There was no history of tic or movement disorders in the family. Before the tics, the patient had a nightmare for 1 week. She also had a skin rash and dry skin in her mouth. The case was considered medically significant
Evening primrose oil	Concerta	An 11-year-old male was using 36 mg of methylphenidate per day for ADHD for several years. The patient was also taking evening primrose oil for an unknown indication and duration. There was a history of moderate to severe developmental delay and slow learning. Methylphenidate was exhausted on December 30, 2002 and was brought to emergency with severe torticollis, rolling arm movements, lip chewing, and pharyngitis. On January 2, 2003, he presented to the pediatrician with the same symptoms and speech disorder, did not eat or drink, and was hospitalized. Torticollis improved with intravenous cetirizine hydrochloride. The patient was also diagnosed with pharyngeal abscess
St John's wort	Concerta	A 17-year-old female with a history of ADHD and depression was treated with methylphenidate for about a year. Concurrent medication included St. John's wort. The patient experienced psychotic symptoms on an unknown day. The patient saw and heard things that were not there and disturbed at night. The result was considered medically significant
	Ritalin	A 15-year-old male started 20 mg oral/day Ritalin for ADHD in 1998 and tolerated it well. He suffered a period of sadness from June 1, 2001, and he took St. John's wort (five drops) orally to treat his depression. A few hours later he presented agitation, unexplained crying, depression-changing aggression, and difficulty concentrating. On June 6, 2001, St. John's wort ceased and these symptoms subsided. Three weeks later, St. John's wort was restarted and the same symptoms appeared. St John's wort was quitted and symptoms were relieved again. The reaction was considered medically significant

Table 6.
Description of adverse status reports evaluated for the cause of natural product-drug interactions [15].

Most importantly, patients with CKD are advised to avoid over-the-counter products and herbal medicines according to the Kidney Disease Improving Global Outcome (KDIGO) guidelines. However, several studies have revealed that many patients with CKD have returned to complementary and alternative medicine (CAM) for a desperate treatment. The consumption of unregistered herbal products is more common today because these products can be easily purchased from on-line media, street markets, or stores. It is an alarming trend as it may be linked to an increase in the number of patients with liver and kidney failure in public hospitals. In addition, patients with CKD are at higher risk of developing cardiovascular disease. Most of them are prescribed with antiplatelet and anticoagulants. Anti-platelets and anticoagulants may interact with synergistic or additives with CAM products, which can cause blood-thinning effects that may later cause excessive bleeding (**Table 7**) [16].

Herbs	Dosage form/doses associated with safety concerns	Safety concerns
Panax ginseng	Crude and standardized *Ginseng* root extract, high doses, combined preparation	It may hypoglycemic effect and can cause hypertension, as well as may interact with anticoagulants
Ginkgo biloba	Standardized *Ginkgo* extract (EGb 761, 80 mg/day), crude *Ginkgo* plant parts (5 ppm of toxic ginkgolic acid)	It may interact with anticoagulants and can cause a severe allergic reaction
Cinnamomum cassia (L.) J.Presl	Cinnamon extract	It may have hypoglycemic effect and may cause worsen liver conditions
Zingiber officinale	Dried root, liquid extract, doses >10 g/day	It may interact with anticoagulants
Allium sativum	Fresh garlic, dried powder (>7 g/day), higher doses than usual dietary intake	It may interact with anticoagulants, antihypertensive, anti-hyperlipidemic, and hydrochlorothiazide
Andrographis paniculata (Burm.f.) Nees	*Andrographis paniculata* extract (50 and 100 mg/kg/day) for 14 days, standardized *Andrographis* extract	It may interact with hepatic metabolizing enzymes, anticoagulant, antiplatelet, anti-hyperglycemic, barbiturates
Momordica charantia L.	Bitter melon tea, bitter melon extract administered intravenously and intraperitoneally, high-dose bitter melon seed	It may hypoglycemic effect and may interact with hypoglycemic agents, death in children
Punica granatum L.	Pomegranate juice, pomegranate extract	It may possibly interact with anticoagulants
Angelica sinensis (Oliv.) Diels	Dong Quai extract (tablet), dose: 565 mg (1–2 tab/day) for 4 weeks	It may increase the risk of bleeding, increase cancer risk, as well as may interact with anticoagulants, antiplatelet, estrogen (augments the effect of estrogen)
Medicago sativa L.	Alfalfa seed products	It may cause autoimmune diseases (SLE, multiple sclerosis, rheumatoid arthritis), photosensitivity, estrogen-like and hypoglycemic effects, and may interact with immunosuppressants, warfarin, oral contraceptives, estrogen conjugates, oral hypoglycemic agents, iron, vitamin
Trigonella foenum-graecum L.	Fenugreek seeds, fenugreek seed powder (>5 g)	It may have a hypoglycemic and estrogen-like effects
Camellia sinensis	Tea (high dose >600 mg/day or 2.25–4.5 L/day)	It may cause liver problems, and may interact with nadolol (beta-blocker), diuretics
Morinda citrifolia L.	Noni juice, dose >400 mL	It may cause liver toxicity, and contains high potassium
Spirulina	A product containing blue-green algae	It may increase the risk of bleeding, may interact with immunosuppressant, antiplatelet, anticoagulants, NSAIDs, other herbs that reduce blood clotting (e.g., ginseng, garlic, ginkgo)

Table 7.
The herbs used by CKD patients and their safety concerns [16].

9.5 Herb-drug interactions with menopause medication

Herbal remedies are popular among women to relieve menopausal symptoms such as hot flashes, energy loss, depression, joint pain, and insomnia. As recently reviewed, a variety of herbs used to treat menopausal symptoms can cause herb-drug interactions (**Table 8**) [17].

Herbs	HID
Cimicifuga racemosa	Increase the activity of antihypertensive agents
Angelica sinensis	Inhibit platelet aggregation and increase risk of bleeding if co-medicated with anticoagulants
Oenothera biennis L.	Potentially interacts with anti-inflammatory drugs, corticosteroids, beta-blockers, antipsychotics and anticoagulants
Trifolium pratense L.	Increase the activity of CYP3A4 and alters the metabolism of drugs
Humulus lupulus L.	Interact with CNS depressants, antipsychotics, hormones and CYP-metabolized drugs

Table 8.
Herb-drug interactions with herbs for menopause.

10. Herb-micronutrient interactions

The ability of some foods to reduce or increase the absorption of various vitamins and minerals has been known for years. Almost half of the population regularly uses some herbal products as a dietary supplement, along with the vitamin and mineral supplements. The use of these products has increased significantly over the past two decades, and a number of clinically relevant herbal drug interactions have been identified during this time. Therefore, it is likely that the mechanisms underlying many herb-drug interactions may also affect micronutrient absorption, distribution, metabolism, and excretion. Not taking these eccentricities into account can negatively affect the outcome and interpretation of any advanced herb-micronutrient interaction studies [18] (**Table 9**).

Phytochemicals	Micronutrient affected	Effect and interaction mechanisms
Plant polyphenols (PPs) (tea catechins, phloretin, quercetin)	Iron	PPs reduce absorption through complexation
	Folate, ascorbate	PPs reduce absorption through uptake transporter inhibition
Silymarins	Iron	They reduce absorption through complexation
Phytic acid	Calcium, iron, zinc	It reduces absorption through complexation
Hyperforin (St. John's wort)	Vitamin D3	It enhances plasma clearance through induction of CYP3A4 metabolism

Table 9.
Herb-micronutrient interactions and their mechanisms.

11. Databases setup for plants/dietary supplements

The Integrative Medicine Service at Memorial Sloan Kettering Cancer Center has developed About Herbs (www.aboutherbs.com), which provides research information, including alleged uses, side effects, and herb-drug interactions for about 284 dietary supplements. Using Google Analytics, they have detected that more than 26,317,000 hits have been recorded since November 2002. According to these data, top 10 plant and/or dietary supplements in 2018 were chaga mushrooms, turmeric, ashwagandha, reishi mushroom, graviola, Active Hexose-Correlated Compound, boswellia, dandelion, green tea, and *Coriolus versicolor*. In **Table 10**, based on the literature researches in PubMed, their scientific and common names, plant-drug interactions and their appropriate use in the oncology environment are discussed. In the past 16 years, evidence of the use of these supplements is based on limited studies and mostly preclinical findings. It is important to inform healthcare professionals about popular dietary supplements so that patients can be informed to make decisions that maximize benefits and minimize risks [19] Hereby, important herb-drug interactions have been compiled in **Table 11**.

Common name	Scientific name of the plants/dietary supplements	Key interaction and concerns	Avoid in
Chaga	*Inonotus obliquus* (Ach. ex Pers.) Pilát	High in oxalates Anticoagulants Anti-platelets Antihyperglycemic agents	Renal disease Diabetic patients on treatment (acarbose)
Turmeric	*Curcuma longa*	High in oxalates CYP2C9 enzyme	Renal disease
Ashwagandha	*Withania somnifera* (L.) Dunal	Increase testosterone levels in men	Prostate cancer
Reishi mushroom	*Ganoderma lucidum* (Curtis) P.Karst.	Anticoagulants Anti-platelets	Radiation therapy
Graviola	*Annona muricate* L.	Antihyperglycemic agents	Diabetic patients on treatment
AHCC	*Active Hexose-Correlated Compound*	CYP2D6 enzyme inducer	Breast cancer patients on doxorubicin, zofran, and aromatase inhibitor (letrozole)
Boswellia	*Boswellia serrata* Roxb. ex Colebr.	Unknown	Contact dermatitis
Dandelion	*Taraxacum mongolicum* Hand.-Mazz., *T. officinale* (L.) Weber ex F.H.Wigg	CYP1A2 enzyme Diuretic Antihyperglycemic agents Estrogenic activity	Hormone-sensitive breast cancer
Green tea	*Camellia sinensis*	High doses or taken on an empty stomach can cause liver toxicity Bortezomib	Elevated liver function tests
Turkey tail mushroom	*Trametes versicolor* (L.) Lloyd	Unknown	Patients on immunosuppressants (in theory)

Table 10.
Top 10 monographs accessed from the "about herbs" database in 2018.

Plants	Effect and usage	Drugs	Interactions
Allium sativum	Antihypertensive, antithrombotic, fibrinolytic, antimicrobial, antidiabetic and lipid-lowering properties [20]	Anticoagulant	May lead to increased anticoagulation effect of warfarin and may increase the risk of bleeding [21–23]
		Antiretroviral (saquinavir)	May decrease the plasma level of protease inhibitor saquinavir [24, 25]
		Antidiabetic (metformin, chlorpropamide)	May occur greater reduction in blood glucose level [26, 27]
		Paracetamol (acetaminophen)	May change some pharmacokinetic variables of paracetamol [28]
Aloe vera L.	Laxative antidiabetic [20]	Corticosteroids and potassium-depleting diuretics	Laxative and potassium lowering effect may result in hypokalemia [29, 30]
		Cardiac glycosides and antiarrhythmic drugs	May enhance the hypokalemia-related arrhythmia [29, 30]
		Antidiabetics	Because of the glucose-lowering effects, diabetic patients should be careful when combining with an antidiabetic agent [31]
Cassia senna L.	Laxative [20]	Corticosteroids and potassium-depleting diuretics	May lead to hypokalemia, since senna can cause excessive water and potassium loss, theoretically [20]
		Digitalis glycosides	Risk of digitalis toxicity due to hypokalemic effect of senna, theoretically [20]
Echinacea purpurea (L.) Moench.	As immunostimulant and in treatment of upper respiratory tract infections [20]	Anabolic steroids, amiodarone (antiaritmic), methotrexate (chemotherapy agent-immunosuppressant), ketoconazole (antifungal), and acetaminophen	The risk of hepatoxicity by concomitant usage of potentially hepatoxic *Echinacea* [32, 33]
		Immunosuppressants	Might decrease the effects of immunosuppressants, theoretically [34]
		Midazolam (benzodiazepine)	May increase oral bioavailability of midazolam or [20]

DOI: http://dx.doi.org/10.5772/intechopen.92040

Plants	Effect and usage	Drugs	Interactions
Ginkgo biloba	To improve cognitive functions, cerebrovascular disorders and vertigo [20]	Phenobarbital	Reduces the therapeutic potency of phenobarbital [35]
		Ibuprofen (NSAID)	May cause fatal intracerebral bleeding [36]
		Anticoagulant (warfarin) and antiplatelet (aspirin) drugs	Possible additive inhibition on platelet aggregation [37, 38]
		Antidepressant (trazodone)	*Ginkgo* flavonoids increase the production of 1-(m-chlorophenyl) piperazine (mCPP), an active metabolite of trazodone. Flavonoids and mCPP may induce the enhancement of GABAergic activity [34]
		Thiazide diuretic (not specified in the original paper)	Further increase in blood pressure [39]
		Nicardipine (a calcium channel blocker)	Decreasing the hypotensive activity of drugs [40]
		Nifedipine, diltiazem (calcium channel blockers) and talinolol (β-blocker)	Possible increased antihypertensive activity resulting from high bioavailability [41–44]
		Cyclosporine	Decreased bioavailability of drug [45]
		Midazolam (benzodiazepine)	Decreased bioavailability of drug [46]
		Propranolol (β-blocker)	Decreased the plasma concentrations of propranolol [47]
		Theophylline	Less efficacy with *Ginkgo* [48]
		Omeprazole (proton pump inhibitor)	May induce the metabolism, and reduce the effect of omeprazole [49]
		Tolbutamide (an antidiabetic drug)	May increase or decrease the hypoglycemic effect of tolbutamide [50]
		Amikacin (aminoglycoside)	Amikacin ototoxicity may enhance [51]
Glycyrrhiza glabra	Expectorant, antispasmodic and anti-inflammatory properties and in treatment of peptic and duodenal ulcers [20]	Prednisolone (corticosteroid)	Glycyrrhizin increases the plasma concentrations and potentiates pharmacological effects of prednisolone [52, 53]
		Hydrocortisone (corticosteroid)	Glycyrrhetinic acid potentiates the activity the topical cutaneous vasoconstrictor effect [54]
		Dexamethasone (corticosteroid)	Dexamethasone induces the mineralocorticoid effects of glycyrrhizin [55]
		Antihypertensives	Mineralocorticoid effects (sodium and water retention and hypokalemia) of plant reduce the efficacy of the drugs that use to lower blood pressure. Hypokalemic effect of the plant may increase the effect of the loop and thiazide diuretics [20]

Plants	Effect and usage	Drugs	Interactions
Hypericum perforatum	To treat depression, seasonal affective disorder, anxiety and insomnia, especially related to menopause [20]	Gliclazide (an antidiabetic drug)	Increases the apparent clearance of gliclazide [56]
		Carbamazepine, phenytoin and phenobarbital (antiepileptics)	Clinically significant interaction is unlikely, but *Hypericum* should be used carefully with these antiepileptic drugs [20]
		Alprazolam, midazolam, triazolam and quazepam (benzodiazepines)	Since the main compound hyperforin induces the enzyme CYP3A4, bioavailability may decrease [20, 57]
		Indinavir (protease inhibitor) Nevirapine (nonnucleoside reverse transcriptase)	May decrease the antiretroviral drugs and may lead to development of drug resistance [58, 59]
		Cyclosporine, tacrolimus, (Immunosuppressants)	May decrease the blood levels and may lead the acute organ rejection in transplant patients [60–62]
		Warfarin and phenprocoumon (anticoagulants)	May cause a moderate reduction in the anticoagulant effects of the drugs [20]
		Simvastatin and atorvastatin (antihyperlipidemic agents)	May observe the increasing serum level of total cholesterol [63, 64]
		Nifedipine, verapamil (calcium channel blockers) and talinolol (a β-adrenoceptor blocker)	May decrease the bioavailability of drugs [65]
		Oral contraceptives	Associated with increased metabolism of ethinyl estradiol, norethindrone, and ketodesogestrel, and may cause bleeding and unwanted pregnancy [66–69]
		Carbamazepine (antiepileptic)	Should be considered a mild interaction between carbamazepine and *Hypericum*
		Sertraline, nefazodone (selective serotonin reuptake inhibitors)	May be occurred the symptoms of central serotonergic syndrome [70]
Linum usitatissimum L.	Demulcent for bronchitis and coughs, and topically used for burns [20]	Anticoagulant or antiplatelet drugs	In the view of the thought that omega-3 fatty acids such as linolenic acid have antiplatelet effects, should be concerned about the possibility of prolonged bleeding [20]

Plants	Effect and usage	Drugs	Interactions
Panax ginseng	Adaptogenic [20]	Phenelzine (MAO inhibitor)	Additive nervous system effect of drug such as headache, tremor, sleeplessness and mania [34]
		Warfarin (anticoagulant)	INR may decrease by concomitant usage [71]
		Warfarin, heparin, aspirin, and NSAIDs	There is no clear data, but due to the antiplatelet components in *P. ginseng*, it should be avoided concomitant using [32]
		Caffeine	Possible additive stimulant effects [20]
Piper methysticum	Anxiolytic, sedative, aphrodisiac	Barbiturates and benzodiazepines	Might potentiate the effects of central nervous system depressants [72]
		Alprazolam (benzodiazepine)	Risk of coma due to possible additive effect on GABA receptor [72]
		Levodopa	May reduce the efficacy due to possible dopaminergic antagonism [73]
		Acetaminophen	May enhance the risk of hepatotoxicity [33]
Valeriana officinalis	Used for stress and insomnia as sedative and anxiolytic [20]	Barbiturates	Excessive sedation. The active component valerenic acid seems to likely to have the additive effect to phenobarbital [74]
		Other central nervous system depressants such as benzodiazepines and opioids	Possible additive sedative effects [20]
		Caffeine	Possible reverse effect to the sedative effect of Valerian [20]
Zingiber officinale	To reduce nausea and emesis induced by pregnancy, chemotherapy, and postoperative ileus [75]	NSAIDs	May reduce the platelet aggregation and enhance the bleeding tendency [33]
		Nifedipine	May potentiate the antiplatelet effects [76]
		Metronidazole	May increase the bioavailability [77]
		Glibenclamide (antidiabetic)	May reduce the blood glucose level [26]

Table 11.
Some herb-drug interactions.

12. Criteria for risk assessment of herbal products

There have been an increasing number of herbal products as food ingredients or supplements, which are a commercially important part of the health food market. Herbal products can range from whole foods (e.g., cranberry against urinary infections) to pharmaceutical-like preparations in unit dose form, such as tablets, capsules, or drops, and are thought to provide additional benefits beyond basic nutrition. The regulatory position on food supplements is uncertain (food or medicine?), and there is concern about the safety assurance of these products. Several cases of poisoning have been reported with herbal products. In some cases, these were caused by contamination with other plant species, but this is not always the case. In addition, toxic components (e.g., pyrrolizidine alkaloids) are accumulated at different concentrations in different parts of the source plant, and climatic and agronomic differences lead to great variability in the composition [78].

Therefore, it is not possible to provide a simple checklist of suitable tests to ensure the safety of herbal products. International guidelines are available for the safety assessment of herbal product and should be designed to cover all life stages to ensure a lifelong intake that can be consumed without significant health risk [78].

Information relating to herbal product identification, characterization, and standardization:

A. Botanical source: identity to family (geographic origin), genus, and species of source plant (with authority), and, if relevant, variety and chemotype; common names as well as part(s) of plant used. Evidence from previous human exposure through food or other sources (ethnobotanical and folk medicine studies).

B. Growing conditions: wild or cultivated plant (Good Agricultural Practice—GAP), site and time of harvest; stage of growth at harvest, post-harvest treatment (drying, fermentation, etc.), storage conditions, phytosanitary measures pre- and postharvest (including use of and limits for pesticides) are very important.

C. Raw material (fresh or dried plant materials): specifications according to standard reference (e.g., herbal Pharmacopoeias), identity tests (macroscopic, microscopic, FT-IR, TLC, GC, HPLC, etc.), quantitative tests (especially constituents related for efficacy and/or toxicity).

D. Process applied to starting material: preparation steps (e.g., separation, extraction processes, solvents), methods used, handling specific precautions; e.g., light/temperature sensitivity, oxidation, etc.

E. Botanical preparation: standardization criteria (markers: active constituents, other related components; plant extract ratio), specifications: levels and range for markers, physico-chemical properties of relevant components; stability, purity criteria by chain control or analysis; microbiological, mycotoxins, pesticides, and environmental contaminants. Nature and level of excipients; formulation methodology, storage conditions should have been specified.

F. End product: formulated product.

G. Specification of the product.

H. Extent of use and estimated intake (posology and method of administration).

I. Bioavailability of active principles.

J. Toxicological assessment.

K. Preclinical and clinical studies. Clinical data including variability of response, adverse effects reports, and contraindications [78].

13. Possible ways to reduce the toxic effects of herbal products

Natural products/compounds are unique remedies, but as Paracelsus (1493–1541) stated that all substances are poison and this is just the correct dose that makes them medicine. There are some rules in the literature that can be summarized as follows:

a. If the herbal remedy is not prescribed by a registered physician, it should be considered unsafe.

b. The label and expiration date of the herbal products should be checked for the seal of the regulatory authority.

c. If the herbal medicine is consumed with allopathic medicines, the doctor should be informed.

d. Herbal products should not be used with drugs possessing narrow therapeutic index such as cyclosporin, digoxin, theophylline, and warfarin.

e. Herbal products containing heavy metals such as arsenic, lead, and mercury should not be used.

f. Pregnant or breastfeeding mothers should be careful when using herbal remedies such as black cohosh, chamomile, sage, Dong Quai root, feverfew, ginger, kava kava, St. John's wort, etc.

g. Excessive consumption of herbal/herbal medicine/natural products should be avoided and dosing instructions should be followed [3].

14. Conclusion

Herbal and traditional medicines are preferred as primary health care by three quarters of the world's population. Therefore, it is crucial in drug research to investigate the effectiveness and adverse effects of herbal medicine, to identify the active compounds in medicinal plants and to detect contamination from poisonous plants or herbal mixtures. In 2013, the World Health Organization (WHO) published the WHO traditional medicine strategy (2014–2023). It aims to support the use of Traditional Medicine (TM) and/or Complementary and Alternative Medicine (CAM) to improve public health, including phytotherapy using of medicinal product (MP) and/or herbal medicinal product (HMP) for medical practice. The plan aims to increase the safety, efficacy, and quality of TM and/or CAM by expanding its knowledge base and providing guidance on regulatory and quality assurance standards (WHO, 2013). In 2016, the National Complementary and Integrative Health Center (NCCIH) published a strategic plan to explore complementary and integrative health science. This plan has been published to inform the public, healthcare professionals, and health policy makers, with evidence-based information about the usefulness and safety of complementary and integrative health interventions and their role in health care development. The plan uses key research to facilitate understanding of the biological effects, mechanisms of action, effectiveness, and clinical effects of complementary health approaches. Both the WHO and NCCIH plans aim to improve TM and CAM knowledge, including phytotherapy. Therefore, understanding herb-drug interactions and the molecular mechanisms involved in these processes is a way to guarantee safe use of MP and/or HMP. In addition, this can help therapeutic planning and healthcare professionals to recommend the best treatment strategy to use.

In this review, some critical issues are also discussed. The botanical identification and labeling of the plant material are important for preventing undesirable health problems. The changes in the scientific definitions of the plants in traditional medicine in time can cause unwanted or toxicologic effects by the usage of the wrong plant. The contamination of the plants with the environmental contaminants (microorganisms, fungal toxins such as aflatoxins, pesticides, and heavy metals), inappropriate preparation process, and interaction of traditional herbs by concomitant or consecutive usage also endanger the safety of herbal medicine for human health. What makes herbal medicine research valuable is that it has the chance to research harmful and toxic plants for developing pharmacologically and therapeutically worth remedies, and to develop medicinal plant combinations as safe and efficient herbal medicines. Standardization and strict control mechanisms are essential to maintain the high quality of herbal products and to prevent from the contaminations for the safety of patients [17].

The following guidelines can be suggested to minimalize the risk of herbal uses:

1. Should not be used in case of pregnancy or a possibility of pregnancy and to babies.

2. Should not be used when breast-feeding.

3. Should not be used as daily and in large amounts.

4. Should be bought from the pharmacies and only in case the plant names are stated on the packages and sealed by the Ministry of Health.

Do not believe it is useless if it is natural or it is harmless if it is natural [79].

Conflict of interest

The authors declare that they have no known competing financial interests or personal relationships that could have appeared to influence the work reported in this chapter.

Author details

Cigdem Kahraman[1], Zekiye Ceren Arituluk[2] and Iffet Irem Tatli Cankaya[2*]

1 Faculty of Pharmacy, Department of Pharmacognosy, Hacettepe University, Ankara, Turkey

2 Faculty of Pharmacy, Department of Pharmaceutical Botany, Hacettepe University, Ankara, Turkey

*Address all correspondence to: itatli@hacettepe.edu.tr

References

[1] Shaikh AS, Thomas AB, Chitlange SS. Herb-drug interaction studies of herbs used in treatment of cardiovascular disorders—A narrative review of preclinical and clinical studies. Phytotherapy Research; 2020. DOI: 10.1002/ptr.6585

[2] Kleter GA, Groot MJ, Poelman M, Kok EJ, Marvin HJP. Timely awareness and prevention of emerging chemical and biochemical risks in foods: Proposal for a strategy based on experience with recent cases. Food and Chemical Toxicology. 2009;**47**(5):992-1008. DOI: 10.1016/j.fct.2008.08.021

[3] Nudrat F, Naira N. Toxic effects as a result of herbal medicine intake. In: Larramendy M, editor. Toxicology-New Aspects to This Scientific Conundrum. Rijeka: Intechopen; 2016. DOI: 10.5772/64468

[4] Brown AC. Kidney toxicity related to herbs and dietary supplements: Online table of case reports. Part 3 of 5 series. Food and Chemical Toxicology. 2017;**107**(Pt A):502-519. DOI: 10.1016/j.fct.2016.07.024

[5] Rasmussen CB, Glisson JK, Minor DS. Dietary supplements and hypertension: Potential benefits and precautions. The Journal of Clinical Hypertension. 2012;**14**(7):467-471. DOI: 10.1111/j.1751-7176.2012.00642.x

[6] Ernst E. Serious psychiatric and neurological adverse effects of herbal medicines—A systematic review. Acta Psychiatrica Scandinavica. 2003;**108**(2):83-91. DOI: 10.1034/j.1600-0447.2003.00158.x

[7] Chan TYK. Worldwide occurrence and investigations of contamination of herbal medicines by tropane alkaloids. Toxins. 2017;**9**(9). DOI: 10.3390/toxins9090284

[8] Wen B, Gorycki P. Bioactivation of herbal constituents: Mechanisms and toxicological relevance. Drug Metabolism Reviews. 2019;**51**(4):453-497. DOI: 10.1080/03602532.2019.1655570

[9] Bartnik M, Facey PC. Glycosides. In: Badal S, Delgoda R, editors. Pharmacognosy: Fundamentals, Applications and Strategy. London, UK: Elsevier Inc.; 2017. pp. 101-161. DOI: 10.1016/C2014-0-01794-7

[10] Ernst E. Risks of herbal medicinal products. Pharmacoepidemiology and Drug Safety. 2004;**13**(11):767-771. DOI: 10.1002/pds.1014

[11] Chan TYK, Critchley JAJH. Usage and adverse effects of Chinese herbal medicines. Human & Experimental Toxicology. 1996;**15**(1):5-12. DOI: 10.1177/096032719601500102

[12] Tatli II. Plant/Herbs-Drugs-Herbal Products-Components-Nutrient Interactions. Postgraduate Education Course, Nutrition and Dietetics Department, Hacettepe University; 2013

[13] Costache I-I, Miron A, Hăncianu M, Aursulesei V, Costache AD, Aprotosoaie AC. Pharmacokinetic interactions between cardiovascular medicines and plant products. Cardiovascular Therapeutics. 2019;**2019**:1-19. DOI: 10.1155/2019/9402781

[14] Fasinu PS, Rapp GK. Herbal interaction with chemotherapeutic drugs—A focus on linically significant findings. Frontiers in Oncology. 2019;**9**:1356. DOI: 10.3389/fonc.2019.01356

[15] Mazhar H, Foster BC, Necyk C, Gardiner PM, Harris CS, Robaey P. Natural health product-drug interaction causality assessment

in pediatric adverse event reports associated with attention-deficit/hyperactivity disorder medication. Journal of Child and Adolescent Psychopharmacology. 2020;**30**(1):38-47. DOI: 10.1089/cap.2019.0102

[16] Shamsuddin N, Karuppannan M, Hafiz Wan Md Adnan WA, Farooqui M, Gnanasan S. Pattern of complementary and alternative medicine (CAM) use among patients with chronic kidney disease. Complementary Therapies in Clinical Practice. 2019;**37**:86-92. DOI: 10.1016/j.ctcp.2019.09.003

[17] Efferth T, Kaina B. Toxicities by herbal medicines with emphasis to traditional Chinese medicine. Current Drug Metabolism. 2011;**12**(10):989-996. DOI: 10.2174/138920011798062328

[18] Gurley BJ, Tonsing-Carter A, Thomas SL, Fifer EK. Clinically relevant herb-micronutrient interactions: When botanicals, minerals, and vitamins collide. Advances in Nutrition. 2018;**9**(4):524S-532S. DOI: 10.1093/advances/nmy029

[19] Hou YN, Deng G, Mao JJ. Practical application of "about herbs" website: Herbs and dietary supplement use in oncology settings. The Cancer Journal. 2019;**25**(5):357-366. DOI: 10.1097/ppo.0000000000000403

[20] Williamson E, Driver S, Baxter K. Stockley's Herbal Medicines Interactions. 1st ed. London: Pharmaceutical Press; 2009

[21] Saw JT, Bahari MB, Ang HH, Lim YH. Potential drug-herb interaction with antiplatelet/anticoagulant drugs. Complementary Therapies in Clinical Practice. 2006;**12**(4):236-241. DOI: 10.1016/j.ctcp.2006.06.002

[22] Rose KD, Croissant PD, Parliament CF, Levin MB. Spontaneous spinal epidural hematoma with associated platelet dysfunction from excessive garlic ingestion: A case report. Neurosurgery. 1990;**26**(5):880-882. DOI: 10.1097/00006123-199005000-00026

[23] Burnham BE. Garlic as a possible risk for postoperative bleeding. Plastic and Reconstructive Surgery. 1995;**95**(1):213. DOI: 10.1097/00006534-199501000-00060

[24] Piscitelli SC, Burstein AH, Welden N, Gallicano KD, Falloon J. The effect of garlic supplements on the pharmacokinetics of saquinavir. Clinical Infectious Diseases. 2002;**34**(2):234-238. DOI: 10.1086/324351

[25] Hajda J, Rentsch KM, Gubler C, Steinert H, Stieger B, Fattinger K. Garlic extract induces intestinal P-glycoprotein, but exhibits no effect on intestinal and hepatic CYP3A4 in humans. European Journal of Pharmaceutical Sciences. 2010;**41**(5):729-735. DOI: 10.1016/j.ejps.2010.09.016

[26] Gupta RC, Chang D, Nammi S, Bensoussan A, Bilinski K, Roufogalis BD. Interactions between antidiabetic drugs and herbs: An overview of mechanisms of action and clinical implications. Diabetology & Metabolic Syndrome. 2017;**9**:59. DOI: 10.1186/s13098-017-0254-9

[27] Aslam M, Stockley IH. Interaction between curry ingredient (karela) and drug (chlorpropamide). Lancet. 1979;**1**(8116):607. DOI: 10.1016/s0140-6736(79)91028-6

[28] Gwilt PR, Lear CL, Tempero MA, Birt DD, Grandjean AC, Ruddon RW, et al. The effect of garlic extract on human metabolism of acetaminophen. Cancer Epidemiology, Biomarkers & Prevention. 1994;**3**(2):155

[29] Boudreau MD, Beland FA. An evaluation of the biological and toxicological properties of *Aloe barbadensis* (miller), *Aloe vera*. Journal

of Environmental Science and Health Part C, Environmental Carcinogenesis & Ecotoxicology Reviews. 2006;**24**(1):103-154. DOI: 10.1080/10590500600614303

[30] Foster M, Hunter D, Samman S. Evaluation of the nutritional and metabolic effects of *Aloe vera*. In: Benzie IFF, Wachtel-Galor S, editors. Herbal Medicine: Biomolecular and Clinical Aspects. 2nd ed. Boca Raton, FL: CRC Press/Taylor & Francis; 2011

[31] Yongchaiyudha S, Rungpitarangsi V, Bunyapraphatsara N, Chokechaijaroenporn O. Antidiabetic activity of *Aloe vera* L. juice. I. Clinical trial in new cases of diabetes mellitus. Phytomedicine. 1996;**3**(3):241-243. DOI: 10.1016/s0944-7113(96)80060-2

[32] Miller LG. Herbal medicinals: Selected clinical considerations focusing on known or potential drug-herb interactions. Archives of Internal Medicine. 1998;**158**(20):2200-2211. DOI: 10.1001/archinte.158.20.2200

[33] Abebe W. Herbal medication: Potential for adverse interactions with analgesic drugs. Journal of Clinical Pharmacy and Therapeutics. 2002;**27**(6):391-401. DOI: 10.1046/j.1365-2710.2002.00444.x

[34] Izzo AA, Ernst E. Interactions between herbal medicines and prescribed drugs: A systematic review. Drugs. 2001;**61**(15):2163-2175. DOI: 10.2165/00003495-200161150-00002

[35] Kubota Y, Kobayashi K, Tanaka N, Nakamura K, Kunitomo M, Umegaki K, et al. Pretreatment with *Ginkgo biloba* extract weakens the hypnosis action of phenobarbital and its plasma concentration in rats. The Journal of Pharmacy and Pharmacology. 2004;**56**(3):401-405. DOI: 10.1211/0022357022836

[36] Meisel C, Johne A, Roots I. Fatal intracerebral mass bleeding associated with *Ginkgo biloba* and ibuprofen. Atherosclerosis. 2003;**167**(2):367. DOI: 10.1016/S0021-9150(03)00015-7

[37] Rosenblatt M, Mindel J. Spontaneous hyphema associated with ingestion of *Ginkgo biloba* extract. The New England Journal of Medicine. 1997;**336**(15):1108. DOI: 10.1056/nejm199704103361518

[38] Matthews MK. Association of *Ginkgo biloba* with intracerebral hemorrhage. Neurology. 1998;**50**(6):1933-1934. DOI: 10.1212/wnl.50.6.1933

[39] Shaw D, Leon C, Kolev S, Murray V. Traditional remedies and food supplements. A 5-year toxicological study (1991-1995). Drug Safety. 1997;**17**(5):342-356. DOI: 10.2165/00002018-199717050-00006

[40] Shinozuka K, Umegaki K, Kubota Y, Tanaka N, Mizuno H, Yamauchi J, et al. Feeding of *Ginkgo biloba* extract (GBE) enhances gene expression of hepatic cytochrome P-450 and attenuates the hypotensive effect of nicardipine in rats. Life Sciences. 2002;**70**(23):2783-2792. DOI: 10.1016/S0024-3205(02)01530-8

[41] Yoshioka M, Ohnishi N, Sone N, Egami S, Takara K, Yokoyama T, et al. Studies on interactions between functional foods or dietary supplements and medicines. III. Effects of *Ginkgo biloba* leaf extract on the pharmacokinetics of nifedipine in rats. Biological & Pharmaceutical Bulletin. 2004;**27**(12):2042-2045. DOI: 10.1248/bpb.27.2042

[42] Fan L, Tao GY, Wang G, Chen Y, Zhang W, He YJ, et al. Effects of *Ginkgo biloba* extract ingestion on the pharmacokinetics of talinolol in healthy Chinese volunteers. The Annals of Pharmacotherapy. 2009;**43**(5):944-949. DOI: 10.1345/aph.1L656

[43] Fan L, Mao XQ, Tao GY, Wang G, Jiang F, Chen Y, et al. Effect of

Schisandra chinensis extract and *Ginkgo biloba* extract on the pharmacokinetics of talinolol in healthy volunteers. Xenobiotica. 2009;**39**(3):249-254. DOI: 10.1080/00498250802687657

[44] Ohnishi N, Kusuhara M, Yoshioka M, Kuroda K, Soga A, Nishikawa F, et al. Studies on interactions between functional foods or dietary supplements and medicines. I. Effects of *Ginkgo biloba* leaf extract on the pharmacokinetics of diltiazem in rats. Biological & Pharmaceutical Bulletin. 2003;**26**(9):1315-1320. DOI: 10.1248/bpb.26.1315

[45] Yang CY, Chao PD, Hou YC, Tsai SY, Wen KC, Hsiu SL. Marked decrease of cyclosporin bioavailability caused by coadministration of ginkgo and onion in rats. Food and Chemical Toxicology. 2006;**44**(9):1572-1578. DOI: 10.1016/j.fct.2006.04.008

[46] Robertson SM, Davey RT, Voell J, Formentini E, Alfaro RM, Penzak SR. Effect of *Ginkgo biloba* extract on lopinavir, midazolam and fexofenadine pharmacokinetics in healthy subjects. Current Medical Research and Opinion. 2008;**24**(2):591-599. DOI: 10.1185/030079908X260871

[47] Zhao LZ, Huang M, Chen J, Ee PL, Chan E, Duan W, et al. Induction of propranolol metabolism by Ginkgo biloba extract EGb 761 in rats. Current Drug Metabolism. 2006;7(6):577-587. DOI: 10.2174/138920006778017740

[48] Tang J, Sun J, Zhang Y, Li L, Cui F, He Z. Herb–drug interactions: Effect of *Ginkgo biloba* extract on the pharmacokinetics of theophylline in rats. Food and Chemical Toxicology. 2007;**45**(12):2441-2445. DOI: 10.1016/j.fct.2007.05.023

[49] Yin OQ, Tomlinson B, Waye MM, Chow AH, Chow MS. Pharmacogenetics and herb-drug interactions: Experience with *Ginkgo biloba* and omeprazole. Pharmacogenetics. 2004;**14**(12):841-850. DOI: 10.1097/00008571-200412000-00007

[50] Sugiyama T, Kubota Y, Shinozuka K, Yamada S, Wu J, Umegaki K. *Ginkgo biloba* extract modifies hypoglycemic action of tolbutamide via hepatic cytochrome P450 mediated mechanism in aged rats. Life Sciences. 2004;**75**(9):1113-1122. DOI: 10.1016/j.lfs.2004.02.020

[51] Miman MC, Ozturan O, Iraz M, Erdem T, Olmez E. Amikacin ototoxicity enhanced by *Ginkgo biloba* extract (EGb 761). Hearing Research. 2002;**169**(1-2):121-129. DOI: 10.1016/s0378-5955(02)00385-4

[52] Chen MF, Shimada F, Kato H, Yano S, Kanaoka M. Effect of glycyrrhizin on the pharmacokinetics of prednisolone following low dosage of prednisolone hemisuccinate. Endocrinologia Japonica. 1990;**37**(3):331-341. DOI: 10.1507/endocrj1954.37.331

[53] Chen MF, Shimada F, Kato H, Yano S, Kanaoka M. Effect of oral administration of glycyrrhizin on the pharmacokinetics of prednisolone. Endocrinologia Japonica. 1991;**38**(2):167-174. DOI: 10.1507/endocrj1954.38.167

[54] Teelucksingh S, Mackie ADR, Burt D. Potentiation of hydrocortisone activity in skin by glycyrrhetinic acid. Lancet. 1990;**335**(8697):1060-1063

[55] Kageyama Y, Suzuki H, Saruta T. Glycyrrhizin induces mineralocorticoid activity through alterations in cortisol metabolism in the human kidney. The Journal of Endocrinology. 1992;**135**(1):147-152. DOI: 10.1677/joe.0.1350147

[56] Xu H, Williams KM, Liauw WS, Murray M, Day RO, McLachlan AJ. Effects of St John's wort and CYP2C9

genotype on the pharmacokinetics and pharmacodynamics of gliclazide. British Journal of Pharmacology. 2008;**153**(7):1579-1586. DOI: 10.1038/sj.bjp.0707685

[57] Borrelli F, Izzo AA. Herb-drug interactions with St John's wort (*Hypericum perforatum*): An update on clinical observations. American Association of Pharmaceutical Scientists Journal. 2009;**11**(4):710-727. DOI: 10.1208/s12248-009-9146-8

[58] Piscitelli SC, Burstein AH, Chaitt D, Alfaro RM, Falloon J. Indinavir concentrations and St John's wort. Lancet. 2000;**355**(9203):547-548. DOI: 10.1016/S0140-6736(99)05712-8

[59] de Maat MMR, Hoetelmans RMW, Mathôt RAA, van Gorp ECM, Meenhorst PL, Mulder JW, et al. Drug interaction between St John's wort and nevirapine. AIDS. 2001;**15**(3):420-421

[60] Moschella C, Jaber BL. Interaction between cyclosporine and *Hypericum perforatum* (St. John's wort) after organ transplantation. American Journal of Kidney Diseases. 2001;**38**(5):1105-1107. DOI: 10.1053/ajkd.2001.28617

[61] Hebert MF, Park JM, Chen YL, Akhtar S, Larson AM. Effects of St. John's wort (*Hypericum perforatum*) on tacrolimus pharmacokinetics in healthy volunteers. Journal of Clinical Pharmacology. 2004;**44**(1):89-94. DOI: 10.1177/0091270003261078

[62] Mai I, Störmer E, Bauer S, Krüger H, Budde K, Roots I. Impact of St John's wort treatment on the pharmacokinetics of tacrolimus and mycophenolic acid in renal transplant patients. Nephrology Dialysis Transplantation. 2003;**18**(4):819-822. DOI: 10.1093/ndt/gfg002

[63] Andrén L, Andreasson A, Eggertsen R. Interaction between a commercially available St John's Wort product (Movina) and atorvastatin in patients with hypercholesterolemia. European Journal of Clinical Pharmacology. 2007;**63**:913-916. DOI: 10.1007/s00228-007-0345-x

[64] Sugimoto K, Ohmori M, Tsuruoka S, Nishiki K, Kawaguchi A, Harada K, et al. Different effects of St John's wort on the pharmacokinetics of simvastatin and pravastatin. Clinical Pharmacology and Therapeutics. 2001;**70**(6):518-524. DOI: 10.1067/mcp.2001.120025

[65] Di YM, Li CG, Xue CC, Zhou SF. Clinical drugs that interact with St. John's wort and implication in drug development. Current Pharmaceutical Design. 2008;**14**(17):1723-1742. DOI: 10.2174/138161208784746798

[66] Murphy PA, Kern SE, Stanczyk FZ, Westhoff CL. Interaction of St. John's Wort with oral contraceptives: Effects on the pharmacokinetics of norethindrone and ethinyl estradiol, ovarian activity and breakthrough bleeding. Contraception. 2005;**71**(6):402-408. DOI: 10.1016/j.contraception.2004.11.004

[67] Hall SD, Wang Z, Huang SM, Hamman MA, Vasavada N, Adigun AQ, et al. The interaction between St John's wort and an oral contraceptive. Clinical Pharmacology and Therapeutics. 2003;**74**(6):525-535. DOI: 10.1016/j.clpt.2003.08.009

[68] Pfrunder A, Schiesser M, Gerber S, Haschke M, Bitzer J, Drewe J. Interaction of St John's wort with low-dose oral contraceptive therapy: A randomized controlled trial. British Journal of Clinical Pharmacology. 2003;**56**(6):683-690. DOI: 10.1046/j.1365-2125.2003.02005.x

[69] Schwarz UI, Büschel B, Kirch W. Unwanted pregnancy on self-medication with St. John's wort

despite hormonal contraception. British Journal of Clinical Pharmacology. 2003;**55**(1):112-113. DOI: 10.1046/j.1365-2125.2003.01716.x

[70] Lantz MS, Buchalter E, Giambanco V. St. John's wort and antidepressant drug interactions in the elderly. Journal of Geriatric Psychiatry and Neurology. 1999;**12**(1):7-10. DOI: 10.1177/089198879901200103

[71] Vaes LPJ, Chyka PA. Interactions of warfarin with garlic, ginger, ginkgo, or ginseng: Nature of the evidence. The Annals of Pharmacotherapy. 2000;**34**(12):1478-1482. DOI: 10.1345/aph.10031

[72] Anke J, Ramzan I. Pharmacokinetic and pharmacodynamic drug interactions with kava (*Piper methysticum* Forst. f.). Journal of Ethnopharmacology. 2004;**93**(2):153-160. DOI: 10.1016/j.jep.2004.04.009

[73] Shi S, Klotz U. Drug interactions with herbal medicines. Clinical Pharmacokinetics. 2012;**51**(2):77-104. DOI: 10.2165/11597910-000000000-00000

[74] Hendriks H, Bos R, Woerdenbag HJ, Koster AS. Central nervous depressant activity of valerenic acid in the mouse. Planta Medica. 1985;**51**(1):28-31. DOI: 10.1055/s-2007-969384

[75] Lien H-C, Sun WM, Chen Y-H, Kim H, Hasler W, Owyang C. Effects of ginger on motion sickness and gastric slow-wave dysrhythmias induced by circular vection. American Journal of Physiology-Gastrointestinal and Liver Physiology. 2003;**284**(3):G481-G4G9. DOI: 10.1152/ajpgi.00164.2002

[76] Young HY, Liao JC, Chang YS, Luo YL, Lu MC, Peng WH. Synergistic effect of ginger and nifedipine on human platelet aggregation: A study in hypertensive patients and normal volunteers. The American Journal of Chinese Medicine. 2006;**34**(4):545-551. DOI: 10.1142/s0192415x06004089

[77] Okonta JM, Uboh M, Obonga WO. Herb-drug interaction: A case study of effect of ginger on the pharmacokinetic of metronidazole in rabbit. Indian Journal of Pharmaceutical Sciences. 2008;**70**(2):230-232. DOI: 10.4103/0250-474X.41462

[78] Walker R. Criteria for risk assessment of botanical food supplements. Toxicology Letters. 2004;**149**(1):187-195. DOI: 10.1016/j.toxlet.2004.03.001

[79] Huxtable RJ. The myth of beneficent nature: The risks of herbal preparations. Annals of Internal Medicine. 1992;**117**(2):165-166. DOI: 10.7326/0003-4819-117-2-165

Chapter 14

Analgesic Poisoning

Mahluga Jafarova Demirkapu

Abstract

According to the 2018 Annual Report of the American Association of Poison Control Centers (AAPCC), published in 2019, the most common cause of poisoning was medicines in all human exposures. According to the data in this report, the most common group of drugs that cause poisoning in humans are analgesics. The first three drugs that cause poisoning among analgesics are fentanyl, acetaminophen, and oxycodone, respectively. Fentanyl and oxycodone are analgesic drugs with an opioid nature. Opioid analgesics are the drugs of choice for acute and chronic pain management, but after repeated exposure, they cause addiction as a result of stimulation in the brain reward center, are used in higher doses to achieve the same effect, and lead to withdrawal syndrome when medication is not taken. Acetaminophen, which takes the second place in analgesic-related poisoning, is a non-opioid analgesic and antipyretic drug. Acetaminophen is often found in hundreds of over-the-counter (OTC) medications. In addition to being an OTC drug, acetaminophen often causes poisoning as it is cheap and easily accessible. This chapter reviews pharmacological properties of fentanyl, acetaminophen, and oxycodone, in addition to poisoning signs and treatments.

Keywords: fentanyl, acetaminophen, paracetamol, oxycodone, intoxication

1. Introduction

Poisoning is a medical emergency representing a major health problem worldwide, and the rate of poisoning of both prescription and over-the-counter (OTC) drugs is increasing day by day [1]. According to the American Association of Poison Control Centers (AAPCC) 2018 Annual Report, the most common cause of drug poisonings was analgesics in all human exposures [2]. Analgesics are used to manage mild, moderate, and severe, as well as acute and chronic, pain [3]. Generally, opioid and non-opioid drugs are used for analgesia [3]. According to the AAPCC 2018 Annual Report, most frequent causes of analgesic poisoning are fentanyl, acetaminophen, and oxycodone, respectively [2]. Fentanyl and oxycodone are opioid analgesics, whereas acetaminophen is a non-opioid analgesic [3].

Opioids are potent analgesics, but their use is limited as they cause addiction, withdrawal, and tolerance [4]. Opioids exert their effects by stimulating classical opioid receptors [μ (mu), δ (delta), and κ (kappa)] that are widely distributed in the body [5, 6]. These receptors show seven transmembrane domain structures specific to G-protein-coupled receptors, are induced by morphine and antagonized by naloxone (NLX), and had similar analgesic effect [4]. According to the studies, μ receptor was also related with addiction [7]. Opioid addiction develops in both psychic and physical dependence [4]. After physical dependence development, opioid consumption is maintained to prevent withdrawal symptoms [4]. Treatment of opioid addiction is long and difficult. For this purpose, opioid agonists, such as methadone and buprenorphine, an opioid antagonist naltrexone, or abstinence-based treatment may be preferred [8]. This disease, referred to as "opioid abuse and opioid dependence" in the Diagnostic and Statistical Manual of Mental Disorders, Fourth Edition, Text Revision (DSMIV-TR), has been changed to "opioid use disorder" in the Diagnostic and Statistical Manual of Mental Disorders, Fifth Edition (DSM-5) [9].

Classical opioid receptors are distributed in the peripheral tissue as well as central nervous system (CNS) [4]. Stimulation of these receptors in the central nervous system results in analgesia, drowsiness, euphoria, a sense of detachment, respiratory depression, nausea and vomiting, depressed cough reflex, and hypothermia [4]. When these receptors are stimulated in peripheral tissues, miosis, orthostatic hypotension, constipation, urinary retention, etc. emerge [4]. After stimulation of these Gi/0-coupled opioid receptors, the adenylate cyclase enzyme is suppressed, and the level of cyclic AMP decreases [4]. In addition, the voltage-gated calcium channels in the axon ends or neuron soma are closed, and intracellular calcium levels are reduced, and potassium channels are opened, leading to an increase in potassium conductance [4]. As a result, inhibition and hyperpolarization of neurons occur when opioid receptors are stimulated [10, 11]. Analgesic or antinociceptive effects, which are indicated for use of opioids, develop at the level of the brain and spinal cord [12]. At the brain level, attenuation of impulse spread is weakened and the perception of pain is inhibited, and at the spinal cord level, the transmission of pain impulses is suppressed [12].

Non-opioid or non-steroidal anti-inflammatory drugs (NSAIDs) are used to manage mild and moderate pain, as well as to reduce fever [13]. Although NSAIDs exact mechanism of action has not been fully established, according to the previous studies, it inhibits the cyclooxygenase pathways, which are involved in prostaglandin synthesis [14]. Prostaglandins are responsible for eliciting pain sensations [14]. NSAIDs do not cause addiction and withdrawal like opioid analgesics, and tolerance to analgesic effect does not develop [13].

Poisoning may lead to more dangerous consequences when taking more than one medication [2]. It is due to pharmacokinetic (PK) and pharmacodynamic (PD) drug-drug interactions (DDIs). According to Lexicomp, there are five DDI types (**Table 1**), which are clinically important (X, D, and C) and insignificant (B and A) [15].

DDI types	Approach	Explanation
X	Avoid combination	The risks associated with simultaneous use of this drug outweigh the benefits. Simultaneous use of this drug is contraindicated
D	Consider therapy modification	The rate of benefit and risk due to simultaneous use of this drug needs to be evaluated, and aggressive monitoring of the patient, empirical dosage changes, or selection of alternative agents should be considered
C	Monitor therapy	The benefits associated with simultaneous use of this drug outweigh the risks, and dosage adjustments of one or both drugs may be considered
B	No action needed	No intervention required
A	No known interaction	No intervention required

Table 1.
DDI types and treatment approach [15].

2. Analgesics that often lead to poisoning

2.1 Fentanyl

International Union of Pure and Applied Chemistry (IUPAC) name: N-phenyl-N-[1-(2-phenylethyl)piperidin-4-yl]propanamide.

Fentanyl is a synthetic and lipophilic phenylpiperidine opioid agonist with molecular formula $C_{22}H_{28}N_{20}$ and a molecular weight of 336.5 g/mol [16]. Fentanyl, 100 times more potent than morphine, was developed in the 1950s and approved by the FDA in 1968 [17]. Fentanyl is used for pain management, induction and maintenance of general anesthesia, recovery from general or regional anesthesia, and analgesia and sedation in intensive care unit patients [18–20]. It is applied by injection (i.v., i.m., epidural, intrathecal), transdermal (device and patch), transmucosal (buccal film and tablet, sublingual spray and tablet, lozenge), and intranasal means [16]. Pharmacodynamics and pharmacokinetics are summarized in **Table 2**.

Adverse effects (**Table 3**) occur when serum fentanyl concentration rises above 2 ng/mL [16]. CNS depression occurs above 3 ng/mL, whereas profound respiratory depression usually occurs at concentrations of 10 to 20 ng/mL [16].

Since it is an opioid drug, fentanyl has the potential for abuse [4]. As mentioned above, with repeated use of fentanyl, tolerance develops, which allows higher doses to achieve the same effect [4]. Therefore, fentanyl can be administered at toxic doses when abused. In addition, toxicity may develop with fentanyl used for therapeutic purposes [2]. These usually occur after accidental ingestion, following use in opioid non-tolerant patients and improper dosing [2]. Known and expected adverse reactions occur more severely, whether administered for abuse or therapeutic purposes [16]. The most important of these is respiratory depression, which can have fatal consequences. Concomitant use of fentanyl with drugs inhibiting CYP3A4 (e.g., erythromycin, ketoconazole, voriconazole, ritonavir) may cause potentially fatal respiratory depression (**Table 4**). Fentanyl may be associated with the development of serotonin syndrome. This risk increases when used concomitantly with

PDs and PKs	Routes of administration				
	Intranasal	i.m.	i.v.	Transdermal patch	Transmucosal
Onset of action	5–10 min	7–8 min	Immediately	6 h	5–15 min
Duration	—	1–2 h	0.5–1 h	72–96 h	—
Absorption	—	—	—	12–24 h	Rapidly
Distribution	—	—	4 L/kg	—	25.4 L/kg
Protein binding	Alpha-1-acid glycoprotein (mainly), albumin, and erythrocytes				
Metabolism	In the liver (primarily via CYP3A4) and intestinal mucosa • n-Dealkylation to *norfentanyl* (active metabolite) • Amide hydrolyzation to *despropionylfentanyl* • Alkyl hydroxylation to *hydroxyfentanyl*				
Bioavailability	64%				50–76%
Half-life elimination	15–25 h		Adults: 2–4 h Children: 2.4–36 h	20–27 h	3–14 h
Excretion	• Urine (primarily) • Feces				

Table 2.
PDs and PKs of fentanyl at therapeutic doses [16, 21–23].

Systems	Symptoms
CNS	Confusion, dizziness, drowsiness, fatigue, headache, sedation, abnormal dreams, abnormal gait, abnormality in thinking, agitation, altered sense of smell, amnesia, anxiety, ataxia, chills, depression, disorientation, euphoria, hallucination, hypertonia, hypoesthesia, hypothermia, insomnia, irritability, lack of concentration, lethargy, malaise, mental status changes, neuropathy, paranoia, paresthesia, restlessness, speech disturbance, stupor, vertigo, withdrawal syndrome
Respiratory	Dyspnea, atelectasis, cough, epistaxis, hemoptysis, flu-like symptoms, wheezing, hyperventilation/hypoventilation, pharyngolaryngeal pain, rhinitis, sinusitis, nasopharyngitis, pharyngitis, laryngitis, bronchitis, asthma, pneumonia, nasal discomfort, postnasal drip, rhinorrhea
Cardiovascular	Arrhythmia, pulmonary embolism (intranasal), chest pain, palpitations, deep vein thrombosis, hypertension/hypotension, myocardial infarction, edema
Gastrointestinal (GI)	Constipation, nausea, vomiting, abdominal distention, abdominal pain, anorexia, decreased appetite, diarrhea, dysgeusia, dyspepsia, flatulence, gingivitis, glossitis, stomatitis, tongue disease, xerostomia, gastroesophageal reflux, gastritis, gastroenteritis, hemorrhage, ulcer, hematemesis, intestinal obstruction, rectal pain
Hepatic	Ascites, increased serum alkaline phosphatase, increased serum AST, jaundice
Genitourinary (GU)	Renal failure, urinary retention, dysuria, erectile dysfunction, mastalgia, urinary incontinence, urinary tract infection, urinary urgency, vaginal hemorrhage, vaginitis
Ophthalmic	Blepharoptosis, blurred vision, diplopia, strabismus, swelling and drying of eye, visual disturbance
Hematologic and oncologic	Anemia, leukopenia, neutropenia, thrombocytopenia, lymphadenopathy
Dermatologic	Alopecia, cellulitis, decubitus ulcer, diaphoresis, erythema, hyperhidrosis, night sweats, pallor, pruritus, skin rash
Endocrine and metabolic	Dehydration, hot flash, hypercalcemia/hypocalcemia, hypokalemia, hypomagnesemia, hyponatremia, hypoalbuminemia, hyperglycemia, weight loss
Neuromuscular and skeletal	Asthenia, arthralgia, back pain, lower limb cramp, limb pain, myalgia, tremor
Miscellaneous	Hypersensitivity reaction, fever, abscess

Table 3.
Common adverse reactions of fentanyl [16, 21–26].

drugs at risk of serotonin syndrome (**Table 4**). Population that are particularly at risk and need attention are children; geriatric, cachectic, or debilitated patients; and patients with renal and hepatic impairment, underlying pulmonary conditions, known or suspected paralytic ileus and gastrointestinal obstruction, mucositis (sublingual spray), and cardiac bradyarrhythmias [16]. Clinically important DDIs are summarized in **Table 4**.

2.2 Acetaminophen

IUPAC name: N-(4-hydroxyphenyl)acetamide

Acetaminophen is an NSAID with molecular formula $C_8H_9NO_2$ and a molecular weight of 151.16 g/mol and approved by the FDA in 1951 [27]. Acetaminophen is used by oral, injection (i.v.), and rectal means for mild to moderate pain

Possible effects	Clinically important DDI types		
	X	**D**	**C**
Increase in the CNS depressant effects	Azelastine, bromperidol, orphenadrine, oxomemazine, paraldehyde, thalidomide, mifepristone	Blonanserin, chlormethiazole, CNS depressants, droperidol, flunitrazepam, lemborexant, meperidine, methotrimeprazine, opioid agonists, oxycodone, perampanel, phenobarbital, primidone, sodium oxybate, suvorexant, zolpidem, tramadol, tricyclic antidepressants (TCA), CYP3A4 inhibitors (strong, moderate)	Ethanol, alizapride, dimethindene, brimonidine, bromopride, tetrahydrocannabinol, cannabidiol, *Cannabis*, chlorphenesin carbamate, dronabinol, lisuride, lofexidine, magnesium sulfate, metoclopramide, minocycline (systemic), nabilone, piribedil, pramipexole, ropinirole, rotigotine, rufinamide
Enhancement in the serotonergic effects and serotonin syndrome	Dapoxetine, monoamine oxidase inhibitors (MAOI)	Linezolid, meperidine, methylene blue, nefazodone, ozanimod, tramadol, TCA	Almotriptan, alosetron, amphetamines, antiemetics (5HT3 antagonists), dexmethylphenidate-methylphenidate, dextromethorphan, eletriptan, ergot derivatives, buspirone, lorcaserin, ondansetron, oxitriptan, ramosetron, selective serotonin reuptake inhibitors (SSRI), serotonin 5-HT1D receptor agonists (triptans), serotonin/norepinephrine reuptake inhibitors (SNRI), St John's wort, Syrian rue
Constipation	Eluxadoline	—	Anticholinergic agents, ramosetron
Urinary retention	—	—	Anticholinergic agents
Enhancement in the bradycardia effects	Fexinidazole	Ceritinib, siponimod	Bradycardia-causing agents, ivabradine, lacosamide, midodrine, ruxolitinib, succinylcholine, terlipressin, tofacitinib
Enhancement in the psychomotor impairment	—	—	SSRI

Table 4.
Fentanyl and clinically important DDIs [15].

management and reduction of fever [27]. Acetaminophen is often found in hundreds of OTC and prescription medicines [28]. PDs and PKs are summarized in **Table 5**.

95% of acetaminophen undergoes biotransformation, while 5% is excreted unchanged into the urine [29]. Approximately 45–55% of acetaminophen transforms into glucuronide conjugates via UDP-glucuronosyltransferase, 30–35% into sulfate conjugates via sulfotransferase, and only 5% into toxic metabolite NAPQI

PDs and PKs	Routes of administration	
	Oral	**i.v.**
Onset of action	Above 1 h	5–10 min
Duration	4–6 h	4–6 h
Absorption	Small intestine (primarily) and stomach	
Distribution	Adults: 4–6 L/kg Children: 5–30 L/kg	
Protein binding	10–25%	
Metabolism	In the liver • Metabolism to glucuronide and sulfate conjugates (primarily) By CYP2E1 to toxic intermediate, N-acetyl-p-benzoquinone imine (NAPQI, **Figure 1**)	
Bioavailability	88%	
Half-life elimination	Adults: 2–3 h Children: 4–10 h	
Excretion	Urine (mainly)	

Table 5.
PDs and PKs of acetaminophen at therapeutic doses [29–31].

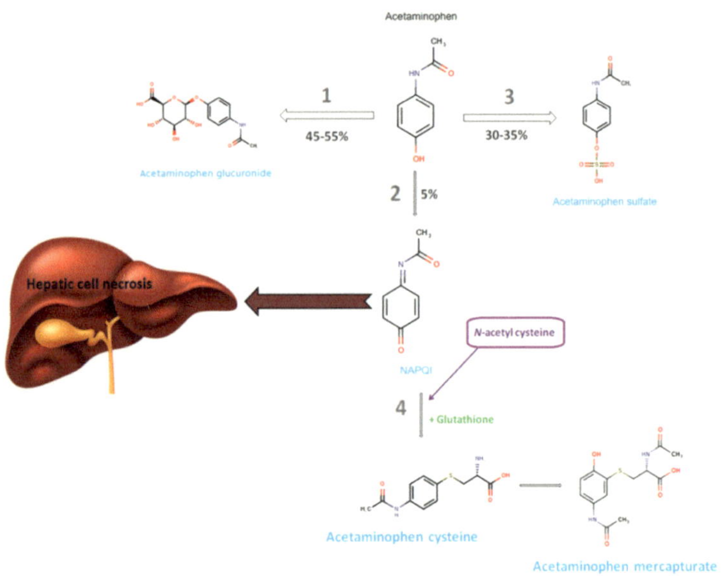

Figure 1.
Metabolism of acetaminophen. NAPQI, N-acetyl-p-benzoquinone imine; (1) UDP-glucuronosyltransferase (1-9, 1-6, 1-1, and 2B15 isoforms); (2) CYP2E1; (3) sulfotransferase (1A1 and 1A3/1A4 isoforms) and bile salt sulfotransferase; (4) glutathione S-transferase (P and theta-1 isoforms) [33–35].

through the CYP2E1 (**Figure 1**) [32–34]. NAPQI, produced in small amounts in therapeutic dose intakes, and hepatic glutathione are immediately transformed into nontoxic cysteine and mercapturate metabolites via glutathione S-transferase and excreted into the urine [34]. With intakes above the maximum daily dose (4 g in adults and 75 mg/kg in children), the increased formation of NAPQI depletes hepatic glutathione, covalently binds to critical cellular proteins and other vital molecules, and thereby causes acute liver toxicity (hepatic damage, liver failure) or even death [29, 35, 36]. Additional mechanisms such as mitochondrial injury, oxygen, and nitrogen stress deepen hepatic cell damage [37].

Mild to moderate elevations in serum aminotransferase (aspartate aminotransferase, alanine aminotransferase) levels are the first sign of liver damage; sometimes it can even occur in chronic treatment at the maximum daily dose [35, 36]. These elevations are generally asymptomatic and resolve rapidly with stopping therapy or reducing the dosage [35] and most commonly arise after taking more than 7.5 g as a single overdose [38]. If hepatotoxicity is not too severe, serum aminotransferase levels fall promptly, and recovery is rapid [39]. Instances of unintentional overdose in children are often due to errors in calculating the correct dosage or use of adult-sized tablets instead of child or infant formulations [39]. Concomitant use of acetaminophen (single) and acetaminophen-containing (combined) products may also cause toxicity [39]. Acetaminophen overdose may be manifested by renal tubular necrosis, hypoglycemic coma, and thrombocytopenia [39]. Acetaminophen has been associated with a risk of rare but serious skin reactions. These are Stevens-Johnson syndrome, toxic epidermal necrolysis, and acute generalized exanthematous pustulosis, and they can be fatal [39, 40]. Population that are particularly at risk and need attention are children, since they have less glucuronidation capacity of the drug than adults, and patients with alcoholism, hepatic impairment or active hepatic disease, chronic malnutrition, severe hypovolemia, and severe renal impairment [29, 38]. Adverse reactions and clinically important DDIs of acetaminophen are summarized in **Tables 6** and 7, respectively.

2.3 Oxycodone

IUPAC name: (4R,4aS,7aR,12bS)-4a-hydroxy-9-methoxy-3-methyl-2,4,5,6,7a,13-hexahydro-1H-4,12-methanobenzofuro[3,2-e]isoquinolin-7-one

Systems	Symptoms
CNS	Trismus, fatigue, headache, agitation, anxiety, insomnia
Respiratory	Atelectasis, hypoxia, pleural effusion, pulmonary edema, stridor, wheezing
Cardiovascular	Tachycardia, hypertension/hypotension, edema
GI	Constipation, nausea, vomiting, abdominal pain, diarrhea
Hepatic	Increased serum transaminases, hyperbilirubinemia
GU	Nephrotoxicity, hyperammonemia, oliguria
Ophthalmic	Periorbital edema
Hematologic and oncologic	Anemia
Dermatologic	Pruritus, skin rash
Endocrine and metabolic	Hypocalcemia, hyponatremia, hypokalemia, hypomagnesemia, hypophosphatemia, hyperchloremia, low bicarbonate levels, hypoalbuminemia, hyperuricemia, hyperglycemia, hypervolemia
Neuromuscular and skeletal	Muscle spasm, limb pain
Miscellaneous	Hypersensitivity reaction, fever

Table 6.
Common adverse reactions of acetaminophen [29, 38, 39].

Possible effects	Clinically important DDI types		
	X	D	C
Hepatotoxicity	—	Dasatinib, sorafenib, probenecid	Ethanol, barbiturates, carbamazepine, imatinib, mipomersen, fosphenytoin-phenytoin, isoniazid, metyrapone
Methemoglobinemia	—	—	Dapsone, local anesthetics, nitric oxide, prilocaine, sodium nitrite
High anion gap metabolic acidosis	—	—	Flucloxacillin
Enhancement in the anticoagulant effects	—	—	Vitamin K antagonists

Table 7.
Acetaminophen and clinically important DDIs [15].

Oxycodone is a semisynthetic opioid agonist, produced from thebaine and codeine found in the raw *Papaver somniferum L.* plant and approved by the FDA in 1968, with molecular formula $C_{18}H_{21}NO_4$ and a molecular weight of 315.4 g/mol [41–43]. It is used alone or in combination with acetaminophen in the management of moderate to severe pain [3]. It binds to classical opioid receptors such as fentanyl and mediates similar mechanisms of action [6]. Oxycodone also inhibits the release of vasopressin, somatostatin, insulin, and glucagon and nociceptive neurotransmitters, such as substance P, GABA, dopamine, acetylcholine, and noradrenaline [44]. The analgesic effects of oxycodone are mediated by both itself and its active metabolites, noroxycodone, oxymorphone, and noroxymorphone [21]. It can be applied both orally and rectally. PDs and PKs are summarized in **Table 8**.

Toxic effects occur when the serum oxycodone concentration is approximately 0.69 mg/L in single oxycodone administration and 0.72 mg/L in the oxycodone-combined drug administration [50]. When the serum oxycodone concentration is

PDs and PKs	Oral administration	
	Immediate release	**Extended release**
Onset of action	10–15 min	—
Duration	3–6 h	≤12 h
Distribution	Adults: 2.6 L/kg Children: 2.1 L/kg	
Protein binding	38–45% • Albumin (primarily) and alpha-1-acid glycoprotein	
Metabolism	In the liver • By CYP3A4 and CYP3A5 to noroxycodone and then by CYP2D6 to noroxymorphone. Noroxycodone (active) can also be reduced to alpha or beta noroxycodol • By CYP2D6 to oxymorphone and then by CYP3A4 to noroxymorphone (active). Oxymorphone (active) can also be reduced to alpha or beta oxymorphol 6-keto-reduced to alpha and beta oxycodol	
Bioavailability	60–87%	
Half-life elimination	3.2–4 h	4.5–5.6 h
Excretion	Urine (mainly)	

Table 8.
PDs and PKs of oxycodone at therapeutic doses [21, 45–49].

about 0.93 mg/L in a single-drug administration and 1.55 mg/L in the combined drug administration, it is fatal [51]. Common adverse reactions are summarized in **Table 9**.

Since oxycodone is an opioid drug, like fentanyl, it has the potential for abuse and develops tolerance. Repeated use of oxycodone causes the development of tolerance, which can lead to overdose and death [45–47]. Serious, life-threatening, or fatal respiratory depression may occur with use of oxycodone orally [45]. Accidental ingestion of even one dose of oxycodone preparations by children can result in death [47]. Long-term use during pregnancy can result in neonatal opioid withdrawal syndrome [45]. Concomitant use of oxycodone with CYP3A4 inducers (e.g., carbamazepine, phenytoin, and rifampin) may result in increasing clearance and decreasing plasma concentrations of oxycodone, with possible lack in therapeutic effectiveness [45]. Concomitant use of oxycodone with CYP3A4 inhibitors may result in reduced clearance and increased plasma concentrations of oxycodone, possibly resulting in increased or prolonged opiate effects, including an increased risk of fatal respiratory depression [52]. These effects could be more pronounced with concomitant use of oxycodone and inhibitors of both CYP2D6 and CYP3A4 [52]. Population that are particularly at risk and need attention are children; geriatric, cachectic, or debilitated patients; and patients with renal and hepatic impairment, underlying pulmonary conditions, and significant genetic variability in CYP2D6 activity [45, 53]. There is no evidence to prove hepatotoxicity when used alone, whereas oxycodone-acetaminophen and other opioid-acetaminophen combinations can lead to acute liver damage caused by unintentional overdose with acetaminophen [54]. Clinically important DDIs are summarized in **Table 10**.

Systems	Symptoms
CNS	Dizziness, drowsiness, headache, fatigue, abnormal dreams, twitching, abnormality in thinking, agitation, anxiety, chills, depression, hypertonia, hypoesthesia, insomnia, irritability, confusion, lethargy, nervousness, paresthesia, neuralgia, personality disorder, withdrawal syndrome
Respiratory	Dyspnea, cough, epistaxis, flu-like symptoms, oropharyngeal pain, rhinitis, sinusitis, pharyngitis, laryngismus, pulmonary disease
Cardiovascular	Flushing, tachycardia, palpitations, cardiac failure, deep vein thrombosis, hypertension/hypotension, edema
GI	Constipation, nausea, vomiting, hiccups, upper abdominal pain, abdominal pain, anorexia, diarrhea, dyspepsia, dysphagia, gingivitis, glossitis, xerostomia, gastroesophageal reflux, gastritis, gastroenteritis
Hepatic	Increased serum alanine aminotransferase
GU	Urinary retention, dysuria, urinary tract infection
Ophthalmic	Blurred vision, amblyopia
Hematologic and oncologic	Anemia, leukopenia, neutropenia, thrombocytopenia, hemorrhage
Dermatologic	Pruritus, diaphoresis, hyperhidrosis, skin rash, skin photosensitivity, excoriation, urticaria
Endocrine and metabolic	Hypochloremia, hyponatremia, hyperglycemia, weight loss, gout
Neuromuscular and skeletal	Asthenia, arthralgia, ostealgia, back pain, neck pain, limb pain, myalgia, tremor, arthritis, laryngospasm, pathological fracture
Miscellaneous	Hypersensitivity reaction, fever, infection, sepsis, seroma, accidental injury

Table 9.
Common adverse reactions of oxycodone [45–47].

Possible effects	Clinically important DDI types		
	X	D	C
Increase in the CNS depressant effects	Azelastine, bromperidol, orphenadrine, oxomemazine, paraldehyde, thalidomide	Blonanserin, chlormethiazole, CNS depressants, droperidol, flunitrazepam, lemborexant, methotrimeprazine, perampanel, phenobarbital, primidone, sodium oxybate, suvorexant, voriconazole, zolpidem, CYP3A4 inhibitors (strong)	Alizapride, brimonidine, bromopride, tetrahydrocannabinol, cannabidiol, *Cannabis*, dimethindene, dronabinol, lisuride, lofexidine, magnesium sulfate, metoclopramide, metyrosine, minocycline (systemic), nabilone, piribedil, pramipexole, ropinirole, rotigotine, rufinamide, CYP3A4 inhibitors (moderate)
Enhancement in the serotonergic effects and serotonin syndrome	MAOI	—	Serotonergic agents
Constipation	Eluxadoline	—	Anticholinergic agents, ramosetron
Urinary retention	—	—	Anticholinergic agents
Enhancement in the bradycardia effects	—	—	Succinylcholine
Enhancement in the psychomotor impairment	—	—	SSRI

Table 10.
Oxycodone and clinically important DDIs [15].

2.4 Fentanyl, acetaminophen, and oxycodone toxicity, clinical manifestations, and management

The toxicity, teratogenicity (FDA pregnancy category), and carcinogenicity (by the International Agency for Research on Cancer), clinical manifestations, and management of fentanyl, acetaminophen, and oxycodone poisoning are summarized in **Tables 11–13**, respectively.

Drugs	Fentanyl	Acetaminophen	Oxycodone
LD50 (mouse, i.p.) (mg/kg)	76	367	320
TDLo (human, oral) (mg/kg)	0.1	490	0.14
FDA pregnancy category	C	C	B
Classification by the IARC	NA	3	NA
LD50, median lethal dose; TDLo, lowest toxic dose; NA, not assigned [55–63]			

Table 11.
Toxicity, teratogenicity, and carcinogenicity of fentanyl, acetaminophen, and oxycodone.

Drugs	Clinical manifestations
Fentanyl	Respiratory depression, somnolence, sleepiness, stupor, coma, amnesia, skeletal muscle flaccidity, cold and clammy skin, constricted pupils, pulmonary edema, bradycardia, hypotension, partial or complete airway obstruction, atypical snoring, and death
Acetaminophen	Stage I (0.5 to 24 h): nausea, vomiting, diaphoresis, pallor, lethargy, malaise or asymptomatic
	Stage II (24 to 72 h): • Recovery in stage I symptoms • Increase in hepatic enzymes (aspartate aminotransferase, alanine aminotransferase) and total bilirubin, PT elongation, oliguria (occasionally)
	Stage III (72 to 96 h): • Jaundice, hepatic encephalopathy, a marked elevations of hepatic enzymes (exceed 10,000 IU/L) and total bilirubin (above 4.0 mg/dL), hyperammonemia, prolongation of the PT/INR, hypoglycemia, lactic acidosis, death (multiorgan system failure)
	Stage IV (4 days to 2 weeks): • Regression in symptoms and recovery phase
Oxycodone	Respiratory depression, sleepiness, stupor, coma, skeletal muscle flaccidity, cold sweat, constricted pupils, bradycardia, hypotension, QT interval prolongation, partial or complete airway obstruction, atypical snoring, and death

Table 12.
Clinical manifestations of fentanyl, acetaminophen, and oxycodone poisoning [16, 61, 64–71].

Management steps	Fentanyl	Oxycodone	Acetaminophen
ABC	Secure airway, breathing, and circulation as necessary		
Decontamination • GI • Patch	Activated charcoal: within 4 h of ingestion, unless contraindicated • Adult: 50 g orally Children: 1 g/kg orally or by nasogastric tube, max. 50 g • Must be removed		
Basic measures and treatment	1. Ensure adequate ventilation 2. Apply antidotal therapy with NLX. With a total of 5 to 10 mg, repeat administration until ventilation is adequate 3. Require supplemental oxygen, endotracheal intubation, and positive end-expiratory pressure, if response is inadequate to NLX or if pulmonary edema is present		1. Poisoning severity following an acute ingestion is quantified by plotting a timed serum acetaminophen concentration on the modified Rumack-Matthew nomogram 2. Antidotal therapy with N-acetyl cysteine (NAC)
Antidotal therapy dosing	Adults: • O_2 saturation is <90%: 0.05 mg i.v. or i.m. • For apneic patients: 0.2 to 1 mg i.v. or i.m. • Patients in cardiorespiratory arrest: min. 2 mg i.v. Children: • <20 kg: 0.1 mg/kg i.v. or intraosseous (i. o.), max. 2 mg per dose • ≥20 kg: 2 mg i.v. or i.o. Adolescents suspected of opioid addiction: • 0.04 to 0.4 mg per dose repeated every 3–5 min and titrated to patient response		**Oral dosing:** 140 mg/kg loading dose, followed by 17 doses of 70 mg/kg every 4 h **21 h i.v. protocol**: 150 mg/kg loading dose over 60 min, followed by 50 mg/kg infused over 4 h, with the final 100 mg/kg infused over the remaining 16 h • INR <2: 21 h i.v. protocol • INR >2: 21 h i.v. protocol, followed by a continuous i.v. NAC infusion at 6.25 mg/kg/h until INR is <2

Management steps	Fentanyl	Oxycodone	Acetaminophen
Supportive care	For possible coma, seizures, hypotension, and non-cardiogenic pulmonary edema		For vomiting

Table 13.
Management of acute fentanyl, acetaminophen, and oxycodone toxicity [72–82].

Antidotal therapy with NAC in acetaminophen poisoning should be applied orally (nonpregnant patients with a functional GI tract and no evidence of hepatotoxicity) or i.v. (patients with vomiting, contraindications to oral administration, and hepatic failure) if:

- Serum acetaminophen concentration is above the "treatment" line of the treatment nomogram
- Serum acetaminophen concentration is unavailable or will not return within 8 h of time of ingestion and acetaminophen ingestion is suspected
- Time of ingestion is unknown and serum acetaminophen level is >10 mcg/mL (66 μmol/L)
- There is evidence of any hepatotoxicity with a history of acetaminophen ingestion
- Patient has risk factors for hepatotoxicity, and the serum acetaminophen concentration is >10 mcg/mL (66 μmol/L) [80–82]

3. Conclusions

Drugs used in the treatment or prevention of diseases can lead to unintentional or intentional toxicity. Toxicity may be due to high-dose single-drug or multiple-drug intake. According to the AAPCC 2018 Annual Report, opioid and non-opioid analgesics often cause single-drug poisoning. The top three of analgesic poisoning are fentanyl, acetaminophen, and oxycodone, respectively.

Opioid analgesics, such as fentanyl and oxycodone, which are preferred in severe pain management, show central and peripheral effects by binding to classical opioid receptors that are widely distributed in the body. Repeated exposure causes an addiction; higher-dose usage to produce the same effect, i.e. tolerance; and withdrawal when stopping intake. Therefore, the dose and severity of toxicity differ between those who take opioid analgesics for the first time and those who are addicted. In poisoning with opioid analgesics, death due to respiratory depression is frequently observed. For this reason, in case of poisoning with opioid analgesics, first of all, adequate ventilation should be provided, subsequent antidote treatment with naloxone should be applied, the patient should be closely monitored for vital functions, and appropriate treatment should be performed when necessary. Since the effect of naloxone is short, application should be repeated when necessary. Supplementary oxygen, endotracheal intubation, and positive end-expiratory pressure should be considered if adequate response cannot be obtained despite a total of 5 to 10 mg of naloxone. Although high doses are not preferred, toxicity is more severe in patients using X and D interactive drugs together.

Acetaminophen, a non-opioid analgesic, found in hundreds of prescription and OTC medicines, with analgesia and antipyretic effects, often causes hepatotoxicity (hepatic damage, liver failure) or even death. Toxicity develops due to the overproduction of toxic NAPQI, which occurs during acetaminophen metabolism in the liver, which quickly consumes the glutathione necessary to convert it to the nontoxic metabolite and covalently binds to cell proteins and other vital molecules. Toxicity is more severe in patients with less glucuronidation capacity and/or concomitant use of X- and D-type interacting drugs. The use of activated charcoal within the first 4 h of acetaminophen poisoning and antidote treatment with NAC successfully heals liver damage.

After stabilizing the patient, it is necessary to investigate whether poisoning is performed unintentionally or intentionally. If there is substance abuse or suicidal tendency, the patient should be consulted to a psychiatrist, and psychosocial and/or medication for addiction treatment should be started. In unintentional poisonings, adults should be educated/warned by their health protectors about the drugs (effects, duration of action, daily maximum dose, conditions to be considered, side effects, and storage conditions) they use for themselves and/or their children, and additional arrangements should be made to increase the health literacy of the society. If poisoning has developed due to the X- and D-type interactions of the drugs used in therapeutic doses, it should be considered to be subject to periodical/continuous training of health protectors.

Author details

Mahluga Jafarova Demirkapu
Department of Medical Pharmacology, Faculty of Medicine, University of Tekirdag Namık Kemal, Tekirdag, Turkey

*Address all correspondence to: mjdemirkapu@nku.edu.tr

References

[1] Bakhaidar M, Jan S, Farahat F, Attar A, Alsaywid B, Abuznadah W. Pattern of drug overdose and chemical poisoning among patients attending an emergency department, western Saudi Arabia. Journal of Community Health. 2015;**40**(1):57-61. DOI: 10.1007/s10900-014-9895-x

[2] Gummin DD, Mowry JB, Spyker DA, Brooks DE, Beuhler MC, Rivers LJ, et al. 2018 Annual Report of the American Association of Poison Control Centers' National Poison Data System (NPDS): 36th Annual Report. Clinical Toxicology. 2019;**57**(12):1220-1413. DOI: 10.1080/15563650.2019.1677022

[3] Schug SA, Garrett WR, Gillespie G. Opioid and non-opioid analgesics. Best Practice & Research. Clinical Anaesthesiology. 2003;**17**(1):91-110

[4] Demirkapu MJ, Yananli HR. Opium Alkaloids [Online First]. IntechOpen; 2020. DOI: 10.5772/intechopen.91326. Available from: https://www.intechopen.com/online-first/opium-alkaloids [Published: 27 February 2020]

[5] Martin WR, Eades CG, Thompson JA, Huppler RE, Gilbert PE. The effects of morphine- and nalorphine-like drugs in the nondependent and morphine-dependent chronic spinal dog. The Journal of Pharmacology and Experimental Therapeutics. 1976;**197**:517-532

[6] Lord JA, Waterfield AA, Hughes J, Kosterlitz HW. Endogenous opioid peptides: Multiple agonists and receptors. Nature. 1977;**267**:495-499

[7] Hutcheson DM, Matthes HW, Valjent E, Sánchez-Blázquez P, Rodríguez-Díaz M, Garzón J, et al. Lack of dependence and rewarding effects of deltorphin II in mu-opioid receptor-deficient mice. The European Journal of Neuroscience. 2001;**13**:153-161. DOI: 10.1111/j.1460-9568.2001.01363.x

[8] Bart G. Maintenance medication for opiate addiction: The Foundation of recovery. Journal of Addictive Diseases. 2012;**31**(3):207-225. DOI: 10.1080/10550887.2012.694598

[9] American Psychiatric Association. Diagnostic and Statistical Manual of Mental Disorders. 5th ed. [DSM-5]. Arlington, VA: American Psychiatric Publishing; 2013. pp. 541-546

[10] Jordan B, Devi LA. Molecular mechanisms of opioid receptor signal transduction. British Journal of Anaesthesia. 1998;**81**:12-19. DOI: 10.1093/bja/81.1.12

[11] North RA, Williams JT, Surprenant A, Christie MJ. Mu and delta receptors belong to a family of receptors that are coupled to potassium channels. Proceedings of the National Academy of Sciences of the United States of America. 1987;**84**:5487-5491. DOI: 10.1073/pnas.84.15.5487

[12] Malaivijitnond S, Varavudhi P. Evidence for morphine-induced galactorrhea in male cynomolgus monkeys. Journal of Medical Primatology. 1998;**27**:1-9. DOI: 10.1111/j.1600-0684.1998.tb00061.x

[13] Hersh EV, Dionne RA. Nonopioid analgesics. In: Dowd FJ, Johnson B, Mariotti A, editors. Pharmacology and Therapeutics for Dentistry. 7th ed. St. Louis, Mosby: Elsevier; 2017. pp. 257-275

[14] Vane JR. Inhibition of prostaglandin synthesis as a mechanism of action for aspirin-like drugs. Nature: New Biology. 1971;**231**:232

[15] UpToDate, Inc. Lexi-Interact [Online]. Available from: www.uptodate.com/drug-interactions/?source=responsive_home#di-druglist

[16] Available from: https://www.uptodate.com/contents/fentanyl-drug-information?search=fentanyl&source=panel_search_result&selectedTitle=1~148&usage_type=panel&kp_tab=drug_general&display_rank=1#F52912015

[17] Raffa RB, Pergolizzi JV Jr, LeQuang JA, Taylor R Jr, Colucci S, Annabi MH. The fentanyl family: A distinguished medical history tainted by abuse. Journal of Clinical Pharmacy and Therapeutics. 2018;**43**(1):154-158. DOI: 10.1111/jcpt.12640

[18] Dowell D. Regarding CDC's Guideline for Prescribing Opioids for Chronic Pain [Written Communication]. Atlanta, GA: Centers for Disease Control and Prevention; 2019

[19] Casserly EC, Alexander JC. Perioperative uses of intravenous opioids in adults. In: Post TW, editor. UpToDate. Waltham, MA: UpToDate Inc. Available from: http://www.uptodate.com [Accessed: 21 August 2019]

[20] Devlin JW, Skrobik Y, Gélinas C, et al. Clinical practice guidelines for the prevention and management of pain, agitation/sedation, delirium, immobility, and sleep disruption in adult patients in the ICU. Critical Care Medicine. 2018;**46**(9):e825-e873. DOI: 10.1097/CCM.0000000000003299

[21] DePriest AZ, Puet BL, Holt AC, Roberts A, Cone EJ. Metabolism and disposition of prescription opioids: A review. Forensic Science Review. 2015; **27**(2):115-145

[22] Heikkinen EM, Voipio HM, Laaksonen S, Haapala L, Räsänen J, Acharya G, et al. Fentanyl pharmacokinetics in pregnant sheep after intravenous and transdermal administration to the ewe. Basic & Clinical Pharmacology & Toxicology. 2015;**117**(3):156-163. DOI: 10.1111/bcpt.12382

[23] Krinsky CS, Lathrop SL, Zumwalt R. An examination of the postmortem redistribution of fentanyl and interlaboratory variability. Journal of Forensic Sciences. 2014;**59**(5):1275-1279. DOI: 10.1111/1556-4029.12381

[24] Knoll J, Fürst S, Kelemen K. The pharmacology of azidomorphine and azidocodeine. The Journal of Pharmacy and Pharmacology. 1973;**25**(12):929-939

[25] Van Bever WF, Niemegeers CJ, Janssen PA. Synthetic analgesics. Synthesis and pharmacology of the diastereoisomers of N-(3-methyl-1-(2-phenylethyl)-4-piperidyl)-N-phenylpropanamide and N-(3-methyl-1-(1-methyl-2-phenylethyl)-4-piperidyl)-N-phenylpropanamide. Journal of Medicinal Chemistry. 1974;**17**(10):1047-1051

[26] US National Institutes of Health; DailyMed. Current Medication Information for Fentanyl Citrate (Fentanyl Citrate) Lozenge. 2012. Available from: http://dailymed.nlm.nih.gov/dailymed/drugInfo.cfm?setid=552ba162-76ed-4bc9-8c2c-fac7a1804da0 [Accessed: 01 June 2017]

[27] Available from: https://www.accessdata.fda.gov/drugsatfda_docs/label/2015/204767s000lbl.pdf

[28] Available from: https://www.fda.gov/drugs/information-drug-class/acetaminophen-information

[29] Available from: https://s3-us-west-2.amazonaws.com/drugbank/cite_this/attachments/files/000/004/124/original/Acetaminophen_monograph__suppository.pdf?1553636652

[30] Hardman JG, Limbird LE, Gilman AG. Goodman and Gilman's: The Pharmacological Basis of Therapeutics. 10th ed. New York, NY: McGraw-Hill; 2001. p. 704

[31] Ellenhorn MJ, Barceloux DG. Medical Toxicology—Diagnosis and

Treatment of Human Poisoning. New York, NY: Elsevier Science Publishing Co., Inc.; 1988. p. 157

[32] Mazaleuskaya LL, Sangkuhl K, Thorn CF, FitzGerald GA, Altman RB, Klein TE. PharmGKB summary: Pathways of acetaminophen metabolism at the therapeutic versus toxic doses. Pharmacogenetics and Genomics. 2015; **25**(8):416-426. DOI: 10.1097/FPC.0000000000000150

[33] McGill MR, Sharpe MR, Williams CD, Taha M, Curry SC, Jaeschke H. The mechanism underlying acetaminophen-induced hepatotoxicity in humans and mice involves mitochondrial damage and nuclear DNA fragmentation. The Journal of Clinical Investigation. 2012;**122**(4):1574-1583. DOI: 10.1172/JCI59755

[34] Whirl-Carrillo M, McDonagh EM, Hebert JM, Gong L, Sangkuhl K, Thorn CF, et al. Pharmacogenomics knowledge for personalized medicine. Clinical Pharmacology and Therapeutics. 2012;**92**(4):414-417. DOI: 10.1038/clpt.2012.96

[35] Watkins PB, Kaplowitz N, Slattery JT, Colonese CR, Colucci SV, Stewart PW, et al. Aminotransferase elevations in healthy adults receiving 4 grams of acetaminophen daily: A randomized controlled trial. Journal of the American Medical Association. 2006;**296**(1):87-93

[36] Mitchell JR, Jollow DJ, Potter WZ, Davis DC, Gillette JR, Brodie BB. Acetaminophen-induced hepatic necrosis. I. Role of drug metabolism. The Journal of Pharmacology and Experimental Therapeutics. 1973;**187**(1): 185-194

[37] Chiew AL, James LP, Isbister GK, McArdle K, et al. Early acetaminophen-protein adducts predict hepatotoxicity following overdose (ATOM-5). Journal of Hepatology. 2020;**72**(3):450-462

[38] US National Institutes of Health; DailyMed. Current Medication Information for OFIRMEV (Acetaminophen) Injection, Solution. 2013. Available from: http://dailymed.nlm.nih.gov/dailymed/lookup.cfm?setid=c5177abd-9465-40d8-861d-3904496d82b7 [Accessed: 06 March 2014]

[39] Available from: https://www.ncbi.nlm.nih.gov/books/n/livertox/Acetaminophen/

[40] Park HJ, Kim SR, Leem DW, Moon IJ, Koh BS, Park KH, et al. Clinical features of and genetic predisposition to drug-induced Stevens-Johnson syndrome and toxic epidermal necrolysis in a single Korean tertiary institution patients-investigating the relation between the HLA-B*4403 allele and lamotrigine. European Journal of Clinical Pharmacology. 2015; **71**:35-41

[41] Huang B-S, Lu Y, Ji B-Y, Christodoulou AP. Preparation of oxycodone from codeine. U.S. Patent US6008355. 1990

[42] Ruan X, Mancuso KF, Kaye AD. Revisiting oxycodone analgesia: A review and hypothesis. Anesthesiology Clinics. 2017;**35**(2):e163-e174. DOI: 10.1016/j.anclin.2017.01.022

[43] Bento AP, Gaulton A, Hersey A, et al. The ChEMBL bioactivity database: An update. Nucleic Acids Research. 2014;**42**(Database Issue):D1083-D1090

[44] Available from: https://ncit.nci.nih.gov/ncitbrowser/ConceptReport.jsp?dictionary=NCI_Thesaurus&ns=NCI_Thesaurus&code=C29309

[45] US National Institutes of Health; DailyMed. Current Medication Information Oxycodone Hydrochloride Capsule. 2017. Available from: https://dailymed.nlm.nih.gov/dailymed/drugInfo.cfm?setid=5df92fed-6194-4905-9ef

2-9eed0d2e8086 [Accessed: 09 November 2017]

[46] Romand S, Spaggiari D, Marsousi N, Samer C, Desmeules J, Daali Y, et al. Characterization of oxycodone in vitro metabolism by human cytochromes P450 and UDP-glucuronosyltransferases. Journal of Pharmaceutical and Biomedical Analysis. 2017;**144**:129-137. DOI: 10.1016/j.jpba.2016.09.024

[47] Ordóñez Gallego A, González Barón M, Espinosa AE. Oxycodone: A pharmacological and clinical review. Clinical & Translational Oncology. 2007;**9**(5):298-307

[48] Lalovic B, Phillips B, Risler LL, Howald W, Shen DD. Quantitative contribution of CYP2D6 and CYP3A to oxycodone metabolism in human liver and intestinal microsomes. Drug Metabolism and Disposition. 2004; **32**(4):447-454

[49] Riley J, Eisenberg E, Muller-Schwefe G, Drewes AM, Arendt-Nielsen L. Oxycodone: A review of its use in the management of pain. Current Medical Research and Opinion. 2008;**24**(1): 175-192

[50] Wolf BC, Lavezzi WA, Sullivan LM, Flannagan LM. One hundred seventy two deaths involving the use of oxycodone in Palm Beach County. Journal of Forensic Sciences. 2005; **50**(1):192-195

[51] Cone EJ, Fant RV, Rohay JM, Caplan YH, Ballina M, Reder RF, et al. Oxycodone involvement in drug abuse deaths. II. Evidence for toxic multiple drug-drug interactions. Journal of Analytical Toxicology. 2004;**28**(7): 616-624

[52] Available from: https://www.uptodate.com/contents/oxycodone-drug-information?search=oxycod&source=search_result&selectedTitle=1~2&usage_type=default&display_rank=1

[53] Foral PA, Ineck JR, Nystrom KK. Oxycodone accumulation in a hemodialysis patient. Southern Medical Journal. 2007;**100**(2):212-214

[54] Available from: https://www.ncbi.nlm.nih.gov/books/n/livertox/Oxycodone/

[55] Kurilenko VM, Khlienko ZN, Moiseeva LM, Sokolov DV, Praliev KD, Belikova NA. Synthesis and analgesic and psychotropic properties of piperidine and decahydroquinoline derivatives. III. 1-(3-phenylpropargyl)-4-phenyl-4-propionyloxypiperidine and its derivatives. Pharmaceutical Chemistry Journal. 1976;**10**:1193-1196

[56] Kadatz R, Ueberberg H. Pharmacological and toxicological studies of a new analgesic and antiphlogistic agent, 2-(2-methoxy-ethoxy)-5-acetaminoacetophenone. Arzneimittel-Forschung. 1965;**15**(5): 520-524

[57] Tullar PE. Comparative toxicities of 14-hydroxydihydromorphinone (oxymorphone) and other narcotic analgesic compounds. Toxicology and Applied Pharmacology. 1961;**3**:261-266

[58] Purucker M, Swann W. Potential for duragesic patch abuse. Annals of Emergency Medicine. 2000;**35**(3):314. DOI: 10.1016/s0196-0644(00)70091-6

[59] Carloss H, Forrester J, Austin F, Fuson T. Acute acetaminophen intoxication. Southern Medical Journal. 1978;**71**(8):906-908

[60] Available from: https://s3-us-west-2.amazonaws.com/drugbank/msds/DB00497.pdf?1557960957

[61] Available from: https://www.drugs.com/pregnancy/fentanyl.html

[62] Available from: https://s3-us-west-2.amazonaws.com/drugbank/fda_labels/DB00316.pdf?1553636682

[63] Available from: https://monographs.iarc.fr/agents-classified-by-the-iarc/

[64] Edinboro LE, Poklis A, Trautman D, Lowry S, Backer R, Harvey CM. Fatal fentanyl intoxication following excessive transdermal application. Journal of Forensic Sciences. 1997;**42**(4):741-743

[65] Available from: https://www.cdc.gov/drugoverdose/data/statedeaths.html

[66] Barash JA, Ganetsky M, Boyle KL, et al. Acute amnestic syndrome associated with fentanyl overdose. The New England Journal of Medicine. 2018; **378**:1157

[67] McBride PV, Rumack BH. Acetaminophen intoxication. Seminars in Dialysis. 1992;**5**:292

[68] Chun LJ, Tong MJ, Busuttil RW, Hiatt JR. Acetaminophen hepatotoxicity and acute liver failure. Journal of Clinical Gastroenterology. 2009;**43**:342

[69] Hendrickson RG, McKeown NJ. Acetaminophen. In: Nelson LS, Howland M, Lewin NA, Smith SW, Goldfrank LR, Hoffman RS, editors. Goldfrank's Toxicologic Emergencies. 11th ed. New York, NY: McGraw-Hill; 2019. p. 472

[70] Dart RC, editor. Medical Toxicology. 3rd ed. Philadelphia, PA: Lippincott Williams & Wilkins; 2004. p. 584

[71] Manini AF, Stimmel B, Vlahov D. Racial susceptibility for QT prolongation in acute drug overdoses. Journal of Electrocardiology. 2014;**47**:244

[72] Olson KR, editor. Poisoning and Drug Overdose. 6th ed. New York, NY: McGraw-Hill; 2012

[73] Osterwalder JJ. Naloxone—for intoxications with intravenous heroin and heroin mixtures—harmless or hazardous? A prospective clinical study. Journal of Toxicology: Clinical Toxicology. 1996;**34**:409

[74] Mills CA, Flacke JW, Flacke WE, et al. Narcotic reversal in hypercapnic dogs: Comparison of naloxone and nalbuphine. Canadian Journal of Anaesthesia. 1990;**37**:238

[75] Bertini G, Russo L, Cricelli F, et al. Role of a prehospital medical system in reducing heroin-related deaths. Critical Care Medicine. 1992;**20**:493

[76] Berlot G, Gullo A, Romano E, Rinaldi A. Naloxone in cardiorespiratory arrest. Anaesthesia. 1985;**40**:819

[77] Chamberlain JM, Klein BL. A comprehensive review of naloxone for the emergency physician. The American Journal of Emergency Medicine. 1994; **12**:650

[78] Available from: https://www.uptodate.com/contents/image?imageKey=EM%2F83590&topicKey=EM%2F318&search=acetaminophen%20overdose&source=see_link

[79] Buckley NA, Whyte IM, O'Connell DL, Dawson AH. Activated charcoal reduces the need for N-acetylcysteine treatment after acetaminophen (paracetamol) overdose. Journal of Toxicology. Clinical Toxicology. 1999;**37**:753

[80] Smilkstein MJ, Knapp GL, Kulig KW, Rumack BH. Efficacy of oral N-acetylcysteine in the treatment of acetaminophen overdose. Analysis of the national multicenter study (1976 to 1985). The New England Journal of Medicine. 1988;**319**:1557

[81] Prescott LF. Treatment of severe acetaminophen poisoning with intravenous acetylcysteine. Archives of Internal Medicine. 1981;**141**:386

[82] Prescott LF, Park J, Ballantyne A, et al. Treatment of paracetamol (acetaminophen) poisoning with N-acetylcysteine. Lancet. 1977;**2**:432

Section 5

Antidotes and Forensics

Chapter 15

Forensic Chemistry and Toxicology

Amarnath Mishra

Abstract

The current chapter deals with forensic chemistry & toxicology which is completely based on the introduction and classification of poisons and their impacts on the body and the factors affecting them and detection and examination of poisons. The purpose of this chapter is to discuss their mode of action and function once they reached in the human body. The impacts of poisons are severe and even cause death if not treated properly.

Keywords: poison, mode of action, alcohol, forensic analysis

1. Introduction

Four hundred years back, Paracelsus stated that, "All substances are poisons; there is none which is not a poison." If the right dose is taken, it could become a remedy, otherwise poisonous [1, 2]. The therapeutic index or ratio, i.e., LD50/ED50, tells whether the chemical is safe or not.

Poisons are generally found in cases of homicides, suicides, or accidents. They have a significant role to play as the silent weapon to destroy life mysteriously and secretively.

2. Action of poisons

Every poison has almost similar action on the victim's body. In many cases, they either stop the transfer of O_2 to the tissues or create an obstacle in the respiratory system by inhibition of enzymes which are associated with the process. In this, the myoneural junction and the ganglions and synapses are the sites of action. In some cases of insecticidal poisoning, hyperexcitement of voluntary and involuntary muscles can cause death. There are four categories of action of poisons—(i) local action, (ii) remote action, (iii) local and remote actions, and (iv) general action.

Local action: Local action means direct action on the affected site of the body. Examples include irritation and inflammation in strong mineral acids and alkalis, congestion and inflammation by irritants, the effect on motor and sensory nerves, etc.

Remote action: Remote action affects the person due to absorption of that poison into the system of that person. For example, alcohol is absorbed in the system and then it affects the person.

Local and remote actions: Some poisons can affect both local and remote organs. Thus, they not only affect the area with contact to the poison but also cause toxic effect after absorption into the system, for example, oxalic acid.

General action: General action means the absorbed poison affects more than one system of the body, for example, mercury, arsenic, etc.

3. Factors modifying the action of poisons

Toxicity of a poison depends upon its inherent properties such as physiochemical as well as pharmacological properties.

The action of poisons mainly depends upon the following factors discussed below:

1. **Forms of poison:** There are three forms of poison:

    - **Physical form:** Gaseous/volatile/vaporous forms of poisons act faster than liquid poisons as they are quickly absorbed. Similarly, liquid poisons act faster than solid poisons.

Gaseous or volatile > liquid > solid.

For solid poisons, powdered poisons act quickly than the lumps. For example, there are certain seeds that escape the gastrointestinal tract as they are solid, but when crushed, they can be fatal.

For solids: powdered > lumps

- **Chemical form:** Few substances like mercury or arsenic are not poisonous as they are insoluble and cannot be absorbed when they are in combination with other substances like mercuric chloride, arsenic oxide, etc.

  In other cases, the action is vice versa. For example, there are some substances that become inert in combination with silver nitrate and hydrochloric acid and are deadly and poisonous when present in pure forms.

- **Mechanical combination:** The effect of poisons is significantly altered when they are combined with inert substances.

2. **Quantity:** Large doses of toxin cause much lethal effect. But this statement is not always true. For example, sometimes when a toxin is taken in very large amount, the body produces a mechanism against it such as vomiting, and thus the intensity of the toxin is reduced.

3. **Concentration:** The absorption speed of poison is dependent on concentration; thus poison of higher concentration is fatal. However, there are still some exceptions. For example, a dilute oxalic acid is less corrosive, but the absorption rate is high and so it is more dangerous.

4. **Methods of administration:** It has a unique role in the process of absorption. It is fastest through inhalation and then through injection as compared to the oral mode.

5. **Condition of the body:** Different persons react differently when exposed to a poison. It is because the condition of our body is also responsible for the increase or decrease of the effect of a poison on the body:

    - **Age**: Children and older people are more affected than an adult by the same quantity of toxin.

- **Sleep**: The body functions are slower during sleep; thus toxin circulation in the body is also slower.

- **Health**: Healthy persons can tolerate a toxin better than a weak or ill person.

6. **Dosage:** The effect of the poison depends upon its dosage. It is said that the dose determines whether a substance is a poison or remedy. A substance is usually considered a poison after a certain fixed quantity. Although this quantity is not fixed for all people, it is considered according to the average effect on the population. There are two considerable effects of poison on the body of a person; these are the subtle long-term chronic toxicity and immediate fatality.

   Some poisons are lethal in microquantities, while others can affect in large doses. The significance of a dose can be understood by taking an example of a metal essential in the food, for example, iron, copper, manganese, zinc, etc.; if its dose is higher than the body requires, it can be lethal.

   - **Effective dose (ED)**: The effective dose is the quantity of a substance at which it shows its effect in the population. In most cases, ED50 is measured as a dose which induces a response in half of the targeted population.

   - **Lethal dose**: The lethal dose (LD) 50 is the amount of drug which is expected to cause death of 50% population.

7. **Hypersensitivity:** It is basically the type of reaction initiated by the body against any other substances. Sometimes, it could be related to allergy. There is an assumption that hypersensitivity does not depend on wrong doses. Every person who is hypersensitive to a particular substance has a dose related that defines the quantity required to cause hypersensitivity to that person. The allergic response is actually a toxic response and can be sometimes fatal.

8. **Idiosyncrasy:** It is defined as a reaction produced by the body to a chemical genetically. It is a type of person that affects only those people who are genetically sensitized to that particular chemical or substance but will show no effect on others. In such cases, the person experiences discomfort for several hours or if the dose is high can be fatal also. For example- peanut allergy in some people.

9. **Tolerance:** It is the capability of a person to not produce any effect against a chemical that usually causes reaction to normal persons. It is a state of reduced or no reaction to a chemical. There are basically two types of mechanism that induces tolerance. First is when the toxin reaches the effective site, its quantity is very less. This is called dispositional tolerance. The second is because the tissues show reduced response to the toxin.

   Tolerance can also be achieved if a drug is taken in a small quantity on a regular basis. This can be explained by taking the example of alcohol. When any human consume alcohol for the first time, he/she will show an effect even when the quantity is small, but eventually the effect will decrease and the person can tolerate a large amount also.

10. **Individual susceptibility:** It is defined as the different kinds of responses produced by different individuals to a particular harmful compound. It can be due to occupational or environmental factors and exposures. It is determined by complex genetic factors. Its effect depends upon the intensity of exposure. There is a gene uniqueness that varies from person to person; thus the same amount of exposure can show no effect in one individual, cause illness to other individual, and also could be fatal to someone as well.

4. Route of administration of poison

The route of administration is the path through which a drug, toxin, or poison is taken or administered into the body of a person which is distinguished by the location where any drug is applied. It is mostly classified on the basis of its target:

- Topical—which has a local effect
- Enteral—which has a wide effect, i.e., affect the whole system
- Parental—which follows a systemic action

Poisons are given or taken so that death can occur at once by shock due to stoppage of body's vital systems. Drug addicts take drugs through inhalation or injection.

Route of administration plays a very important role in determination of death by poison as time in which death occurs are fastest in inhaled poisons, relatively slow in injected and lastly when ingested orally.

Some important features that are considered during the administration of poisons and can make a poison fatal are:

- Rate of dissolution of the poison that depends upon the physical form of the poison, i.e., gaseous, vapors, liquid, solid, etc.
- The surface area affected at the site of administration of the poison
- The circulation rate of blood in that route
- The solubility of the poison, i.e., lipid soluble or water soluble
- The concentration of the poison
- The time required by the poison to be absorbed completely from the site of administration

Routes of administration can be classified into two categories:

1. Enteral routes/gastrointestinal routes.
2. Parenteral routes.

Enteral routes: When the drug is administered through the gastrointestinal tract, it is defined as an enteral route. It has both oral and rectal routes. It also includes sublingual and sublabial routes. It is comparatively a slower mode of action for absorption of drugs:

- **Oral route:** Generally absorption takes place in the tongue and the gums of the oral passage. The pH of the buccal cavity and mouth ranges from 4 to 5. Sublingual and supralingual routes have a significant role in absorption. The sublingual absorption is faster as the toxin is transformed directly to the heart, but it takes more time.

- **Rectal route:** Administration of drugs can be done through anus which directly absorbed in bloodstream through membrane of mucous. This administration can cause the burning of tissues or bleeding in rectum as the area is very sensitive.

- **Parental route:** It includes all the other routes that does not involve the gastrointestinal tract. It has a systemic effect on the body. It has the following categories of administration:

  - **Intradermal:** Here, the administration of drugs takes place from surface of skin. This type of poisoning is mostly found in chronic poisoning cases.

  - **Intravenous:** It is one of the fastest modes of drug administration as the injection is directly taken and the drug is transferred directly into the veins and thus is directly circulated into the blood quickly. Immediate death might be caused by this type of drug.

  - **Intraosseous:** It involves an administration of a drug directly into the bone marrow. This mode is actually used for administration of drugs for medical purposes.

  - **Intra-arterial:** It involves an administration of a drug into the artery directly through injection. It is a fast mode of administration.

  - **Intramuscular:** In this mode, the drug or poison is administered into the muscle of the thigh, upper arm, or buttock. The time required in this mode is greater than other parental modes.

  - **Subcutaneous:** In this mode, the drug is injected into the layer beneath the skin, i.e., the subcutaneous layer. The drug then goes to the small blood vessels and then to the bloodstream. This mode is used for mostly those protein drugs that would be destroyed if administered through the gastrointestinal tract.

  - **Inhalation:** In this mode, the nose is the primary path. Because of the presence of mucous membrane, the nasal aperture is very absorptive. The microparticles of poisons are easily absorbed and transported quickly to the lungs. From the lungs, they are circulated into the blood.

5. Classification of poisons

Poisons are classified into two ways:

i. Based on their action on the body.

ii. Based on their physical and chemical properties [1].

Classification based upon the effect of poison on the body:

1. Corrosive: The poisons burn the tissues or organs when they come in contact with them, e.g.:

    a. Strong acids such as H_2SO_4, HNO_3, HCL, etc.

    b. Strong alkalis such as hydroxides of Na, K, NH_4, etc.

2. Irritants: The poisons irritate the tissues or organs when they come in contact with them [3]:

    a. Inorganic:

    - Nonmetallic phosphorous, chlorine, bromine, iodine, etc.
    - Metallic salts of arsenic, antimony, mercury, copper, lead, zinc, etc.

    b. Organic:

    - Vegetable—castor oil, madar, croton oil, etc.
    - Animals—snake venom, cantharides, insect bites, etc.
    - Mechanical—glass powder, needles, diamond dust, hair, etc.

3. Neurotics: Poisons affect the nervous system and the brain [3]:

    a. Cerebral:

    - Narcotic—opium and its alkaloids
    - Inebriant (depressant)—alcohol, ether, chloroform, and chloral hydrate

    b. Spinal:

    - Excitant (stimulants)—nux vomica and strychnine
    - Depressant—gelsemium

    c. Cardiorespiratory:

    - Cardiac—aconite, digitalis, oleander, and hydrocyanic acid (HCN)
    - Asphyxiants—carbon monoxide, carbon dioxide, and hydrogen sulfide

4. Miscellaneous: A number of chemicals having diverse actions on their body are included in this group [4]:

    a. Animal poisons

    b. Curare (an arrow poison)

c. Poisonous food articles

d. Industrial poisons—methyl isocyanate (MIC)

e. Fuels—petroleum and kerosene

f. Insecticides—endrin, dichlorodiphenyltrichloroethane (DDT), and naphthalene

g. Radioactive substances

Classification of poisons based upon their properties:

A. Inorganic poisons

i. Metallic poisons:

a. Arsenic: It has been the most known and exclusively used throughout the ages to poison men and animals [1].

It is a white tasteless powder and a pinch of the poisons can kill two adult persons.

Arsenic for homicidal purposes is mixed with various food articles, e.g., cooked food, milk, tea, liquors, or medicines.

Arsenic in a metal form is not poisonous; its oxides are highly poisonous. It is extensively used in insecticides, etc. [5].

b. Mercury: Chloride and nitrites of mercury are highly poisonous. They are used in chemical industry and as fungicides.

c. Lead: Most of its compounds are poisonous. This is a slow poison, e.g., Sindoor adulterated with red lead oxide.

d. Copper: Its salts are used in electroplating; copper sulfate is a poison.

e. Thallium: Thallium salt is used as rat poison [6].

f. Antimony: Its effect is like that of arsenic.

ii. Nonmetallic poisons:

a. Cyanides: Cyanides of potassium and sodium are extremely poisonous, even in small quantities. They react with the acid of gastric juices in the stomach to form hydrocyanic acid, which paralyzes the respiratory center in the brain resulting in death due to respiratory failure [4].

b. Yellow phosphorus: In olden days it was used in match industry and several times proved highly poisonous.

c. Iodine: Only elemental iodine in high quantity is poisonous.

d. Strong acids and alkalis: These are highly poisonous with corrosive effects, e.g., sulfuric acid, nitric acid, sodium, potassium hydroxides, etc.

e. Gases: Phosphine gas kills rats when used on the rat holes and is poisonous for infants. MIC killed over 2000 persons and invalidated several others in a gas leak tragedy in Bhopal in 1984. Some other poisonous gases are HCN, carbon monoxide, hydrogen sulfide, arsine, etc. [3].

B. Organic poisons

i. Volatile poisons:

a. Ethyl alcohol: It is poisonous if taken in excess.

b. Other alcohols: Methyl alcohol and isopropyl alcohol are poisonous. Methanol, used in polish and chemical industries, is used in illicit liquor, and its intake causes paralysis, blindness, and death [3].

c. Phenol: Phenol or carbolic acid could be poisonous. It is mostly used as a disinfectant [6].

d. Miscellaneous substances: Various industrial chemicals like chlorinated hydrocarbons, benzene, chloral hydrate, etc. are poisonous. In several cases of poisoning, chloral hydrate could be used in illicit liquors.

ii. Nonvolatile substances:

a. Alkaloids: Several narcotics and vegetable poisons contain alkaloids, e.g., strychnine, morphine, cocaine, nicotine, etc.

b. Barbiturates: These drugs are synthetic and induce sleep [1].

c. Glycosides: These drugs can cause cardiac arrest and could be fatal such as aconite, oleander digitalis, etc.

d. Insecticides and pesticides

Poisoning: It is known as the injurious effect caused by the action of a poison or a detrimental chemical substance. It leads to the development of adverse reaction toward the harmful chemicals or drugs. It is basically differentiated in three categories: suicidal, homicidal, and accidental. Cattle poisoning is the poisoning related to animals. Accidental poisoning is caused by negligence and carelessness. Homicidal poisoning includes the killing of a person due to the poison. Suicidal poisoning refers to the use of toxic chemicals in order to kill oneself.

Corrosive poisoning: It is caused by poisons such as acids and alkalis. They produce a corrosive action on the human body by causing ulcers and acute inflammation.

Metallic poisoning: Metals such as arsenic, mercury, lead, etc., when ingested, cause a deleterious effect. This is known as metallic poisoning.

Plant poison: The study of plant poisons is known as phytotoxicology. Plant poisons, or phytotoxins, comprise a vast range of biologically active chemical substances, such as alkaloids, polypeptides, amines, glycosides, oxalates, resins, toxalbumins, etc.

6. Alcohol

An alcohol is a drink that contains ethanol. Ethanol is made by fermentation of grains, fruits, and some resources of sugar. Chemically, it is a group of compounds whose saturated carbon chain has a "-OH" group. Alcohol is also a depressant, and in low dose, it can reduce tension, cause euphoria, and improve sociability, but in high dose it can cause stupor, drunkenness, and even death. Regular alcohol intake can cause cancer, alcoholism, dependency, etc. 33% of the total people in the world consumes alcohol. Drinks containing alcohol are broadly classified into three classes, i.e., beer, spirit, and wine, whose alcohol content varies between 3% and 50%. When diluted, alcohol has nearly sweet taste, but when concentrated it gives a burning sensation. 90% of the absorbed alcohol is metabolized by the liver and broken down into less toxic metabolites. Alcohol acts on the central nervous system (CNS) as a depressant on the cells of the cerebral cortex. Its adverse effects like a decrease in cognitive and psychomotive skills are well documented. Alcohol percentage (ABV) differs from one brand to another, for example, beers contain 5%, wines contain typically 13.5%, fortified wines contain 15–22%, spirits contain 30–40%, fruit juice contains less than 0.1%, and cider/wine coolers contain 4–8% ABV [1].

7. Blood alcohol test

The goal of blood alcohol test is to check the concentration of alcohol in the body. This test result is known as blood alcohol concentration (BAC) which indicates alcohol % in the blood. It is directly proportional to the alcohol in the body, and alcohol hinders with people's decision, control on them and other characteristics [3]. This test can tell the presence of alcohol in blood for 12 hours [4]. Blood quickly absorbs alcohol and is measured within minutes of consuming alcoholic drink. The highest level of BAC result can be reached within an hour of consuming alcohol. Intake of food can vary the result. Liver breaks down almost 90% of alcohol and rest are given out from exhalation and urine [5].

8. Sample collection

In case of deaths due to alcoholic intoxication, the viscera is collected and preserved in saturated saline. Preservation of sample is very important as if wrongly preserved it can ruin the examination. Generally, urine and blood are taken as samples.

A sterile needle must be cleaned up by the swab of a nonalcoholic disinfectant like aqueous mercuric chloride and aqueous benzalkonium chloride (Zephiran) before the suspect's skin is punctured with it. The use of an alcoholic disinfectant either may give false-positive results or may contribute to falsely high alcohol contents of blood. About 5–10 ml of the sample (blood) is taken in a test tube; an anticoagulant such as potassium oxide and EDTA and a preservative such as NaF are added and stored in the refrigerator at 40°C. The anticoagulant will prevent blood from clotting, and the preservative will inhibit the presence of microorganisms. The urine sample is also collected in the usual manner and preserved with 30 mg of phenyl mercuric nitrate for every 10 ml of urine [6].

9. Extraction of ethyl alcohol from biological materials

Ethyl alcohol is isolated from biological materials by acid distillation. Viscera, vomit, stomach contents, and other materials should be analyzed separately. About 50–100 g of the viscera is taken and is finally minced by thin gruel and adding water (3–5 times) and sulfuric acid. It is passed to steam distillation which is generally heating it on the water bath. The condenser and the receiving flask should be well cooled with ice especially in the hot season, the outlet of the condenser being dipped in little water or NaOH solution. Some pieces of pumice stone are stored in the flask to avoid bumping. It is better to collect the distillate in 4–5 fractions, out of which the first one should not exceed 20 ml and the remaining fractions should be 50 ml each. The distillate contains alcohol and other volatile acids, etc. [6].

10. Chemical analysis of ethyl alcohol

There are some tests which show the presence of ethyl alcohol in the exhibits.

10.1 Iodoform test

Also known as triiodomethane reaction, it is used in the detection of CH_3CH (OH) which is present in alcohol. There are mainly two types of different mixtures used in this reaction which are mainly chemically equivalent. A pale yellow precipitate occurs if the result is positive [6].

In the above structure, "R" can be hydrogen or alkyl group or any other hydrocarbon group. In case when R denotes hydrogen, then the compound we have the possibility to find is primary alcohol ethanol. Ethanol is the only alcohol that gives an iodoform reaction. In case R is any hydrocarbon group, then it gives secondary alcohol groups. Tertiary alcohol is not able to contain R group because of the absence of hydrogen atom [7].

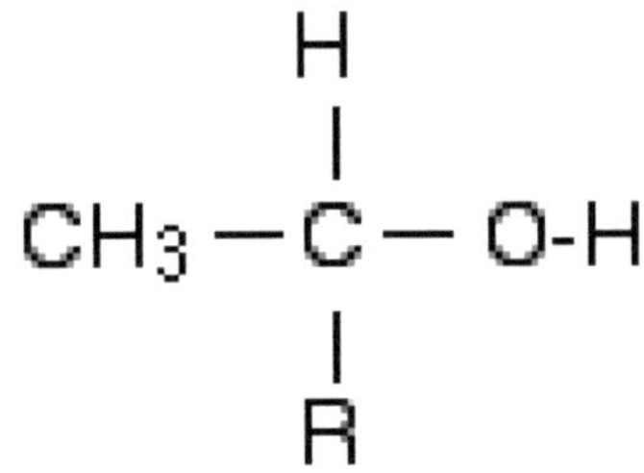

In 1 ml of distillate, a few drops of 10% NaOH are added dropwise till the solution becomes brown and warmed for a few minutes. A few drops of iodoform solution are added to change the color to yellow. The mixture has to be again heated on low flame/water bath; a yellow-colored precipitate is formed on standing. The precipitate has to be observed under a microscope. Characteristic hexagonal crystals of iodoform are seen which usually shows the presence of ethanol, acetaldehyde, isopropanol which on standing for long time breaks into flower like structure. This test initially involves oxidation followed by substitution and hydrolysis [6].

10.2 Sulphomolybdic acid test

Add 1 gm of molybdic acid in 25 ml of a concentrated sulfuric acid which has the reagent. Mix 2 ml of this reagent when hot and with 2 ml of distillate. At the junction of both liquids, a ring will be formed which is deep blue in color. On shaking, the whole mixture will become deep blue which is due to ethyl alcohol. This test is very sensitive and it gives a negative result with acetone, acetaldehyde, and dilute solution of methyl alcohol. Only the strong solution of methyl alcohol gives a light blue color after several minutes [6].

10.3 Ethyl benzoate test

Mix two drops of benzoyl chloride with 2 ml of the distillate. Add 10% of sodium hydroxide drop by drop till the solution becomes alkaline. By providing heat the irritating smell of benzoyl chloride will be replaced by sweet fruity odor of ethyl benzoate. Methyl alcohol gives this test also but not the iodoform test [6].

11. Determination of ethyl alcohol in blood/urine

In case of drunkenness, alcohol detection in the body is very important. Observing behavioral abnormalities of the suspect is the best method, but analyzing the breath, blood, and urine is the only way of confirming it. The analysis of breath alcohol can be performed on the spot with the help of breath-analyzer instruments like Alco-Sensor, Breathalyzer, etc. However, the alcohol content of the blood could be determined by using the modified version of the Kozelka and Hine/Cavett method [6].

In recent years, several methods in determining the alcohol in body fluids are described. Kent-Jones and Taylor reported the results of an investigation into the merits of two methods—the micro Cavett and that of Kozelka and Hine. The micro Cavett method is more accurate, but it suffered from serious inconsistencies in reproducibility, but the Kozelka and Hine method is less accurate and more time-consuming but gives good reproducibility.

Nickolls modified the micro Cavett method which appears to give a more accurate result in comparison with the unmodified method. The simplicity of this procedure increases its use for routine work in laboratory [8].

11.1 Cavett method/Kozelka and Hine method

The principle behind this method is the oxidation of alcohol, which is easy with acetic acid in the presence of oxidizing agents such as sulfuric acid and potassium dichromate. Reduction of each mL of N/20 potassium dichromate solution takes place that is equivalent to 0.575 mg of alcohol [6].

11.2 Widmark's formula

This formula is used to estimate the amount in which alcohol is present in the body.

a. For blood analysis

$$a = cpr.$$

Here, a = Total amount of alcohol absorbed in the body; p = Weight of the person; c = Concentration of alcohol in the blood; r = Constant which is 0.5 in women and 0.68 in men

b. In urine analysis.

$$a = 3/4qpr.$$

Here, a = Total alcohol content present in the body; p = Total weight of the person; q = Alcohol concentration in the urine; r = Constant, namely, 0.68 for men and 0.5 in women [6].

12. Instrumental technique of analysis of ethyl alcohol

12.1 Gas chromatography

There are several methods in determining ethanol in the blood, urine, and serum. One of the most important methods is gas chromatography (GC). The sample is injected in a heating chamber, and due to its high temperature, alcohol converts in vapors which are carried by inert carrier gas such as nitrogen through the column which is packed by an adsorbent material. Separation of different types of components depends on their different affinity, i.e., partition coefficient toward adsorbent phase which is stationary and later detected as shown in the figure below. A chromatogram so obtained helps in qualitative as well as quantitative analysis [6].

Various components of gas chromatography are [9]:

- Carrier gas
- Flow regulator
- Injector
- Column
- Stationary phase
- Oven
- Detectors
- Display device

The area covered by the peak represents the amount and position of a particular type of compound [6].

Operating conditions [10]:

Column: Porapak polymer bead 80–100 mesh or its equivalent, which can separate or resolve the ethanol.
Column temperature: 1600°C.
Carrier gas: Nitrogen.
Rate of gas flow: 50 ml/minute.
Detector: Flame ionization detector.

Alternative operating conditions:

Column: 0.3% Carbowax 20 M on 80–100 mesh Carbopak C, 2 m × 2 mm ID or its equivalent.
Column temperature: 350°C for 2 minutes and then programmed at 50°C per minute to 1750°C and hold for at least 8 minutes.
Carrier gas: Nitrogen at 30 ml/minute [6].

13. Conclusion

The purpose of this chapter is to discuss the mode of action and function of poisons once they reached in the human body. The impacts of poisons are severe and even cause death if not treated properly.

Author details

Amarnath Mishra
Amity Institute of Forensic Sciences, Amity University Uttar Pradesh, Noida, India

*Address all correspondence to: drmishraa1@gmail.com; amishra5@amity.edu

References

[1] Macht DI. A drug or poison? The Scientific Monthly. 1938;**47**(1):34-40

[2] Bajgar J. Organophosphates/nerve agent poisoning: Mechanism of action, diagnosis, prophylaxis, and treatment. Advances in Clinical Chemistry. 2004; **38**(1):151-216

[3] Prinzmetal M, Sommer H, Leake CD. The pharmacological action of "mussel poison". Journal of Pharmacology and Experimental Therapeutics. 1932;**46**(1): 63-73

[4] Wasserman D, Dawson CR. The toxic principle of poison ivy and other related plants. Journal of Chemical Education. 1943;**20**(9):448

[5] Yip L, Dart RC, Hurlbut KM. Intravenous administration of oral N-acetylcysteine. Critical Care Medicine. 1998;**26**(1):40-43

[6] Dedrick RL, Myers CE, Bungay PM, DeVita VT. Pharmacokinetic rationale for peritoneal drug administration. Cancer Treatment Reports. 1978;**62**:1-13

[7] De Boer AG, Moolenaar F, De Leede LGJ, Breimer DD. Rectal drug administration. Clinical Pharmacokinetics. 1982;**7**(4):285-311

[8] Peter JV, Sudarsan TI, Moran JL. Clinical features of organophosphate poisoning: A review of different classification systems and approaches. Indian Journal of Critical Care Medicine: Peer-reviewed, official publication of Indian Society of Critical Care Medicine. 2014;**18**(11):735

[9] Donaldson AE, Larsen GY, Fullerton-Gleason L, Olson LM. Classifying undetermined poisoning deaths. Injury Prevention. 2006;**12**(5):338-343

[10] Choi WY, Kim HJ, Na JY, Lee SJ, Lee YJ, Park JT, et al. Analysis of death due to poisoning in Gwangju and Jeollanam-do areas. Korean Journal of Legal Medicine. 2016;**40**(3):72-77

Chapter 16

Detoxification of Drug and Substance Abuse

Sreemoy Kanti Das

Abstract

Detoxification is a process of abolishing a substance of dependence from the body in a way which does not hinder the body's physiology. Detoxification often takes a couple of days and half a month to finish, which is contingent upon the substance being abused, the seriousness of reliance and the help accessible to the client. Metabolism plays an important role in an effective detoxification process; some of the eminent enzymes are discussed in this review, which helps in excretion of xenobiotics. Psychosocial treatments nearby pharmacological medicines are fundamental to improve result. The over reliance conditions considered in this review are detoxification from opioids with clonidine-naltrexone, buprenorphine and other procedures, detoxification of benzodiazepines through adjunctive therapies and medications. Detoxification of psychostimulants with propranolol and amantadine is also discussed in detail.

Keywords: opioids, cannabis, amphetamine, detoxification

1. Introduction

Detoxification is the process of disengaging a person from a specific psychoactive substance in a safe and effective manner. The choice of which strategy to use for detoxification can depend on many factors, involving clinical judgment, the user's personal preference and circumstances, lifestyle and expectations, degree of dependence and concomitant health problems. Detoxification does not imply that a patient has been given the diagnosis of substance use disorder such as addiction, abuse, or misuse of medications. Although addiction may necessitate detoxification in order to begin drug rehabilitation treatment, there are many reasons that patients must undergo detoxification. Detoxification refers to a decrease in biological activity of a drug after it has been metabolized in the body. Biotransformation is a critically essential pathway for drug detoxification and elimination in humans. Biotransformation of drugs leads to termination or alteration of their biologic activity, otherwise most drugs would have a prolonged duration of action. Despite the fact that probably every organ in the human body is capable of metabolizing drugs but the liver and small intestine serves as the dominant sites of expression of the major drug metabolizing enzymes. Broad spectrums of enzymes are present in a human that can catalyze biotransformation reactions, and they have been classified precisely into Phase I and Phase II processes. Whereas Phase I represents oxidation, reduction, and hydrolytic reactions, Phase II involves conjugation of the drug with an endogenous molecule that generally increases the hydrophilicity of the adducted

IntechOpen

metabolite. Ultimately, all drug metabolites are excreted primarily through the urine or bile. Many endogenous and Xenobiotics are lipophilic. They can easily cross lipid bilayers & transported by lipoproteins. Metabolism of endogenous compounds and xenobiotics allows organisms to convert lipophilic compounds to more water soluble forms which facilitate excretion. Many xenobiotic compounds contain aromatic rings and heterocyclic ring structures that we are unable to degrade or recycle because those are structures are hydrophobic in nature.

1.1 Detoxification as specific from substance abuse treatment

Detoxification is a lot of intercessions planned for overseeing intense inebriation and withdrawal. Directed detoxification may forestall conceivably hazardous complexities that may show up if the patient was left untreated. Simultaneously, detoxification is a type of palliative consideration (diminishing the force of a turmoil) for the individuals who need to get abstinent or who must watch obligatory forbearance because of hospitalization or legitimate contribution. At long last, for certain patients it speaks to a point of first contact with the treatment framework and the initial step to recuperation. Treatment/restoration, then again, includes a group of stars of continuous remedial administrations at last proposed to advance recuperation for substance misuse patients.

The accord board based on existing meanings of detoxification as an expansive procedure with three fundamental segments that may happen simultaneously or as a progression of steps:

Assessment involves testing for the nearness of substances of maltreatment in the circulation system, estimating their focus, and screening for co-happening mental and physical conditions. Assessment additionally incorporates an exhaustive evaluation of the patient's medicinal and mental conditions and social circumstance to help decide the proper degree of treatment following detoxification. Basically, the assessment fills in as the reason for the underlying substance misuse treatment plan once the patient has been pulled back effectively.

Adjustment incorporates the medicinal and psychosocial procedures of helping the patient through intense inebriation and withdrawal to the achievement of a therapeutically steady, completely upheld, sans substance state. This frequently is finished with the help of prescriptions, however in certain ways to deal with detoxification no drug is utilized. Adjustment incorporates acclimating patients with what's in store in the treatment milieu and their job in treatment and recuperation. During this time experts likewise look for the inclusion of the patient's family, bosses, and other huge individuals when fitting and with arrival of classification. Cultivating the patient's entrance into treatment includes setting up the patient for section into substance misuse treatment by focusing on the significance of finishing the total substance misuse treatment continuum of care. For patients who have exhibited an example of finishing detoxification administrations and afterward neglecting to participate in substance misuse treatment, a composed treatment agreement may energize entrance into a continuum of substance misuse treatment and care. This agreement, which is not legitimately official, is intentionally marked by patients when they are steady enough to do as such toward the start of treatment. In it, the patient consents to take an interest in a proceeding with care plan, with subtleties and contacts built up before the completion of detoxification.

The cytochrome P450 (CYP) catalysts are otherwise called microsomal blended capacity oxidases. The CYP compounds are layer bound proteins, present in the smooth endoplasmic reticulum of liver and different tissues. They are the most significant chemicals for Phase I biotransformation of medications. These catalysts contain a heme prosthetic gathering, where heme gathering is the iron-porphyrin

S. No.	CYP enzyme	Drug metabolized
1	1A2	Amitriptyline, clozapine
2	2A6	Acetaminophen, amodiaquine
3	2C8	Paclitaxel
4	2C9	Diclofenac, ibuprofen, phenytoin
5	3A4	Carbamazepine, erythromycin, zolpidem
6	2E1	Enflurane, halothane

Table 1.
List of drugs metabolized by various families of CYP enzymes.

unit. The oxidizing site in these chemicals is the heme focus, and is liable for the oxidation of hydrophobic mixes to hydrophilic or progressively polar metabolites for resulting discharge.

There are in excess of 300 distinctive CYP catalysts, which have been assembled into a few families and subfamilies dependent on the amino-corrosive arrangement. Out of these, 18 CYP families have been distinguished in warm blooded creatures, containing significantly of families CYP1, CYP2 and CYP3. Some of the CYP enzymes and their respective drugs are given in **Table 1**.

2. Detoxification of opioid poisoning

This section sets out the key aspects of the pharmacology of the opioids and other drugs used in detoxification, including the use of opioid agonists, partial agonists and opioid antagonists. The point of detoxification for a ward narcotic client is to kill the impacts of narcotic medications in a sheltered and viable way. Fitting organization of pharmacological operators assumes a significant job in improving the probability of a fruitful detoxification, while limiting the distress of withdrawal experienced by the administration client.

2.1 Opioid agonists

All narcotics, including heroin and methadone, are agonists that animate narcotic receptors. Numerous narcotic agonists are additionally endorsed for their pain relieving properties in torment the board, including morphine, codeine, dihydrocodeine, oxycodone, hydrocodone and fentanyl.

2.1.1 Partial agonists

Buprenorphine is a partial agonist at the narcotic receptor subtype, which implies that the framework is not completely animated in any event, when every one of the receptors are involved. This lesser impact is the primary contributory system hidden buprenorphine's better wellbeing profile when taken alone, since the edge for respiratory wretchedness is not come to in any event, when every one of the receptors are involved. As a fractional agonist, buprenorphine can likewise seem to go about as a rival (and all things considered may have been portrayed in more seasoned writing as a blended agonist-rival). In the event that buprenorphine is given to an individual who has taken a full agonist (for instance, heroin or methadone), it uproots the full agonist, because of buprenorphine's higher proclivity at the narcotic receptor, however just incompletely animates these receptors.

2.1.2 Antagonists

An antagonist, for example, naltrexone or naloxone, ties to the receptor yet does not invigorate it. Naltrexone and naloxone have a high fondness with narcotic receptors, to such an extent that they will dislodge existing agonists and keep further agonists from official to the receptors. Along these lines if an agonist is available animating the receptor, for instance heroin or methadone, taking naltrexone or naloxone will stop this incitement, coming about in accelerated (sudden) withdrawal. Thus, naloxone is usually utilized in crisis drug to switch narcotic overdose, while the more drawn out acting naltrexone is recommended as an upkeep treatment to anticipate detoxified administration clients from backsliding to narcotic use.

2.2 Clonidine-naltrexone detoxification

This technique joins a quick, hastened withdrawal by naltrexone delivering serious withdrawal manifestations, with high portions of clonidine and benzodiazepines when the naltrexone to improve the side effects. While shortening withdrawal to 2–3 days, proof is missing of longer restraint or naltrexone maintenance [1].

2.2.1 Rapid opioid withdrawal under general anesthesia

In the course of the most recent a very long while there has been a lot of progress understanding the atomic and cell premise of practices identified with nicotine addiction, and this comprehension has prompted focused on tranquilize disclosure prompting new therapeutics for smoking discontinuance, for example, varenicline [2]. These advances show that basic investigations of the neurobiological premise of medication misuse can build our insight into why people become dependent and what drives continuous smoking, however can likewise prompt novel techniques for mediation to assist individuals with stopping and remain abstinent. The information that has been increased about the systems fundamental nicotine support has been applied to understanding different practices that drive continuous smoking. Focusing on the multimodal reason for nicotine admission may in this way bring about progressively compelling medicines for smoking suspension going ahead.

2.2.2 Clonidine

The antihypertensive, α2-adrenergic agonist medicate clonidine has been utilized to encourage narcotic withdrawal in both inpatient and outpatient settings for more than 25 years. It works by official to α2 autoreceptors in the locus coeruleus and smothering its hyperactivity during withdrawal. Portions of 0.4–1.2 mg/day or higher decrease a considerable lot of the autonomic parts of the narcotic withdrawal disorder, however side effects, for example, a sleeping disorder, torpidity, muscle throbs, and fretfulness may not be sufficiently taken care of. Contrasted and methadone-helped withdrawal, clonidine has progressively symptoms, particularly hypotension, however is less inclined to prompt post-withdrawal rebound [3, 4]. Dropouts are bound to happen ahead of schedule with clonidine and later with methadone. In an investigation of heroin detoxification, buprenorphine improved on maintenance, heroin use, and withdrawal seriousness than the clonidine gathering. Since clonidine has gentle pain relieving impacts, included absence of pain may not be required during the withdrawal time frame for therapeutic narcotic addicts.

2.3 Toxicity mechanism of opioids

There are 3 primary narcotic receptors: delta, kappa, and mu. They happen all through the CNS yet especially in territories and tracts related with torment recognition. Receptors are likewise situated in some tactile nerves, on pole cells, and in certain cells of the GI tract.

Narcotic receptors are animated by endogenous endorphins, which for the most part produce absence of pain and a feeling of prosperity. Narcotics are utilized remedially, principally as analgesics. Narcotics fluctuate in their receptor movement, and a few (e.g., buprenorphine) have consolidated agonist and foe activities. Mixes with unadulterated rival action (e.g., naloxone, naltrexone) are accessible.

Exogenous narcotics can be taken by practically any course: orally, intravenously, subcutaneously, rectally, through the nasal layers, or breathed in as smoke. Pinnacle impacts are come to around 10 min after IV infusion, 10–15 min after nasal insufflation, and 90–120 min after oral ingestion, despite the fact that opportunity to top impacts and length of impact shift extensively relying upon the particular medication. Synapse discharge from neurons is regularly gone before by depolarisation of the nerve terminal and Ca++ section through voltage-touchy Ca++ channels. Medications may hinder synapse discharge by an immediate impact on Ca++ channels to diminish Ca ++ passage, or by implication by expanding the outward K + current, in this way shortening repolarisation time and the term of the activity potential. Narcotics produce both of these impacts in light of the fact that narcotic receptors are obviously coupled through G-proteins legitimately to K+ channels and voltage-touchy Ca++ channels. Narcotics additionally collaborate with other intracellular effector components, the most significant being the adenylate cyclase framework.

3. Detoxification of nicotine

Nicotine poisonous quality is frequently dismissed as far as helpful methodology regardless of most patients being smokers. The fundamental nicotine detoxification medications are considered beneath, yet likewise, clonidine can be considered as a second-line treatment. Tiagabine, baclofen, gabapentin, varenicline, mecamylamine (a non-particular NAch receptor foe) and topiramate have all been appeared in concentrates to effectively affect suspension.

Nicotine replacement treatment (NRT) ties to nicotine acetylcholinergic (NAch) receptors in the focal sensory system in a portion subordinate way. This diminishes the desire to smoke, withdrawal impacts and any reward from cigarettes if the client should backslide. It likewise gives a less destructive and less fortifying strategy for organization contrasted and smoking, and can improve end rates by 50–70%. The routine for detoxification treatment should begin 2 weeks before the end endeavor, as this has been demonstrated to be more successful than beginning treatment upon the arrival of suspension itself. NRT ought to be proceeded for at least 2 months, or for whatever length of time that vital. There is some proof that mental help is likewise valuable, as forbearance with NRT is higher on solution than when it is bought over the counter [5]. The slowest technique for conveying NRT is through transdermal patches. These come in differing portions, where higher dosages might be progressively advantageous for exceptionally subordinate smokers. Adequacy can be improved by utilizing patches related to a quicker conveyance technique. Biting gum, in portions of 2 and 4 mg, is a case of a quicker conveyance technique, as are inhalers, oral showers, sublingual tablets and capsules. The quickest conveyance technique is by nasal splash, which can supplant about a large portion of the blood nicotine levels of smoking inside 5–10 min [6]. All things being equal, NRT does not give nicotine as productively as smoking and does not copy the conduct ceremonies, which bargains its viability for cessation [7]. In the event that the client keeps on smoking during NRT, they may experience symptoms of nicotine poisonous quality, for example, queasiness, stomach torment, loose bowels, wooziness and palpitations, and mix-up these for nicotine withdrawal.

3.1 Nicotine receptor partial agonists

Nicotine receptor partial agonists check nicotine withdrawal side effects (by going about as an agonist) and lessen smoking fulfillment (by going about as an opponent), and might be valuable for improving long haul end. Varenicline is a particular fractional agonist for the a4-b2-NAch receptor with a moderate fondness for the 5-hydroxytryptamine-3 receptor. Cahill et al. [8] indicated varenicline improved long haul end by two to three times contrasted and fake treatment or bupropion, was as yet powerful at lower dosages which likewise decreased the symptoms of the medication, (for example, sickness). The suggested portion is 1 mg twice every day for 12 weeks, which is come to by continuously expanding the portion from 0.5 mg once day by day during the prior week smoking suspension starts. An additional 12 weeks of dosing can be utilized as backslide anticipation. It is hazy if these medicines are better than NRT and there have been unconfirmed connections between these medications and despondency with self-destructive speculation [9].

3.2 Toxicity mechanism of nicotine

Nicotine ties to nicotinic cholinergic receptors, coming about at first, by means of activities on autonomic ganglia, in overwhelmingly thoughtful anxious incitement. With higher portions, parasympathetic incitement and afterward ganglionic and neuromuscular bar may happen. Direct impacts on the mind may likewise bring about heaving and seizures. Extensive proof focuses to contribution of oxidative stress (OS), receptive oxygen species, lipid peroxidation, DNA harm, and advantageous impact of cancer prevention agents. Beforehand, a proposal was progressed for cooperation of iminium metabolites which may work, by means of electron transfer (ET) with redox cycling, to deliver radical elements. The conjugated iminium usefulness is one of the less notable ET types. The cationic metabolites emerge from a few courses, including oxidation of nicotine itself, and protonation of myosmine which starts from nornicotine through demethylation of nicotine. Decrease possibilities, which are in the range manageable to ET in vivo, loan assurance to the hypothetical structure. Another metabolic course involves hydrolysis of nicotine iminium to an open-chain ketoamine that, thusly, experiences nitrosation to shape a harmful nitrosamine. Thusly, the nitrosamine fills in as a DNA alkylator which can likewise produce conjugated iminiums by assault on specific nitrogen of DNA bases. During the previous 14 years, the speculation has delighted in generous help. Expanding proof focuses to a job for OS in danger by nicotine involving significant body organs, including the lung, cardiovascular framework, focal sensory system, liver, kidney, testicles, ovary, pancreas, and throat.

4. Detoxification of psychostimulants

Cocaine exerts its effects by interfering with the reabsorption of brain's natural neurotransmitters such as dopamine. Cocaine makes chemical changes in the brain that may take time to reverse. A safe and secure environment monitored around the clock by staff members may provide the smoothest possible detox. Physically, the body may need to stabilize. Cocaine suppresses appetite and may cause unhealthy weight loss, for example. A balanced diet plan can help restore a healthy body weight. Physical exercise is also beneficial during detox as it releases natural endorphins as well as increases physical strength and stamina, boosting self-esteem and confidence levels. Yoga and meditation have been proven to help reduce stress, and increase energy and focus naturally. Propranolol for cocaine detoxification is just more viable than fake treatment if the clients are follower to the medicine. Amantadine and other dopamine receptor agonists were seen as not any more powerful than placebo. [10, 11] GABA-ergic medications might be a superior course of examination, as glutamate exhaustion is related with rehashed cocaine administration [12]. For instance, progesterone, tiagabine, topiramate and gabapentin were found to diminish cocaine use in clients with low withdrawal seriousness.

Modafinil builds histamine discharge by means of the orexinergic framework and is a feeble monoamine re-take-up inhibitor. Modafinil may upgrade glutamate and hinder GABA, and has been seen as better than fake treatment regarding higher restraint levels [13]. It is thought to go about as an 'agonist substitution', hindering the dopamine transporter and, to a flimsier degree, the noradrenaline transporter, expanding extracellular dopamine and noradrenaline. Studies show modafinil may improve electrotonic coupling, whereby the associations over hole intersections turned out to be progressively viable. For amphetamine detoxification, mirtazapine and amineptine were seen as incapable. Anyway it very well may be inferred that bupropion and modafinil might be useful as an extra to conduct treatments.

5. Detoxification of cannabis

In detoxification for cannabis, anticonvulsants, for example, valproate semisodium and antidepressants, for example, bupropion, fluoxetine, mirtazapine and nefazodone have demonstrated little benefit [14, 15]. Yearnings are decreased, yet peevishness, uneasiness and tiredness are expanded. A significant issue in cannabis withdrawal is trouble dozing and has indicated this might be reduced with zolpidem. Examination into rimonabant, a cannabinoid receptor adversary, was ended because of unfortunate reactions. Some guarantee for cannabis detoxification has been appeared by oral tetrahydrocannabinol (THC or dronabinol) and lithium carbonate. A portion of 30–90 mg day by day of THC, especially when joined with lofexidine, has been appeared to lessen withdrawal manifestations, rest issues, uneasiness, longings and burdensome symptoms [16]. Dronabinol (δ-9-tetrahydrocannabinol) and lithium carbonate have been demonstrated to be helpful for reducing withdrawal [13]. Be that as it may, for unlawful medications including stimulants, cannabis and joy (MDMA), psychosocial treatments, for example, keyworking and possibility the executives remain the prescribed treatment. There is as yet a job for the clinician in the checking and treating of any emotional wellness issues, including psychosis, wretchedness or danger of suicide. Withdrawal manifestations from GHB and its forerunners (γ-butyrolactone, GBL and 1,4-butanediol, 1,4-CB) can incorporate serious neuropsychiatric issues and autonomic insecurity, which might be perilous and require escalated care. Less extreme yet continuing reactions incorporate a sleeping disorder, uneasiness and depression [17]. Ringer and Collins report pharmacological techniques to treat this incorporate the utilization of high portion benzodiazepines (for instance, 40–120 mg of diazepam), perhaps joined with baclofen or different narcotics like pentobarbital if there is no reaction to benzodiazepines. SSRIs ought to in a perfect world be maintained a strategic distance from in cocaine and amphetamine clients because of conceivable serotonin disorder, in spite of the fact that they are regularly utilized.

5.1 Toxicity mechanism for cannabis

Cannabis inebriation is a disorder perceived in DSM-IV and ICD-10, with both mental and conduct (rapture, unwinding, expanded craving, weakened memory and focus), and physical (engine incoordination, tachycardia, orthostatic hypotension), indications. Inebriation is generally mellow and self-restricting, not requiring pharmacological treatment. The most serious impacts (tension, alarm, psychosis) are best treated symptomatically with a benzodiazepine or second-age (atypical) antipsychotic prescription. No medicine is affirmed explicitly for treatment of cannabis inebriation.

Concentrates with the particular CB1 receptor opponent/opposite agonist rimonabant propose that CB1 receptors intercede a considerable lot of the intense impacts of cannabis in people. In a twofold visually impaired, fake treatment controlled investigation of 63 solid men with a background marked by cannabis use, single oral portions of rimonabant delivered noteworthy portion ward bar of the abstract inebriation and tachycardia brought about by smoking a functioning (2.64% THC) or fake treatment (twofold visually impaired) cannabis cigarette 2 hours after the fact. The 90-mg portion delivered about 40% decreases in appraisals of "high" "stoned" and "tranquilize impact" (on 100-mm visual-simple scales) and a 60% decrease in pulse. Rimonabant alone delivered no huge physiological or mental impacts and did not influence top THC plasma focus or its time course.

This example of discoveries proposes that the watched lessening of cannabis impacts was explicitly due to CB1 receptor bar, and not to decrease in cerebrum THC fixation or checking impacts of rimonabant. CB receptor adversaries, for example, rimonabant may be valuable in treating intense cannabis inebriation, in the way that the mu-narcotic receptor (mOR) foes naloxone and naltrexone are utilized to treat sedative inebriation. Be that as it may, such meds are never again accessible for clinical use. Rimonant and comparable CB1 receptor rivals were pulled back from clinical advancement and use in view of mental reactions related with their long haul use.

6. Detoxification of benzodiazepine

Long haul endorsing of high portions of benzodiazepines (more than 30 mg of diazepam) can be destructive. Benzodiazepine reliance is normally treated in optional consideration, however may display close by other medication reliance. It is suggested that clients of methadone and benzodiazepines ought to experience detoxification from benzodiazepines first. Anyway there is proof that narcotic/benzodiazepine clients may have less withdrawal impacts if buprenorphine is utilized for detoxification. Benzodiazepine reliance is not just by means of rehash solution. They are additionally obtained and abused unlawfully and there might be some an incentive in "support" endorsing for high portion illegal clients before withdrawal. Solutions for benzodiazepines ought to be diminished gradually to the most minimal portion to control the reliance. There is no proof that week-on week-off (beat) dosing is successful. Reliance on high dosages may require authority treatment however can have a quicker pace of decrease, for example, lessening portions significantly more than about a month and a half, without a danger of seizures. Decrease of high portion use to a remedial portion level might be a helpful restorative goal in some needy clients. Medications, for example, zolpidem, or melatonin might be useful for any subsequent a sleeping disorder. The DH Drug Misuse and

Dependence rules prescribe changing over all benzodiazepines to a proper portion of diazepam, which has a long half-life, and afterward decreasing the portion by an eighth at regular intervals. Phenobarbital can likewise be utilized along these lines. Different methodologies incorporate changing to a nonbenzodiazepine anxiolytic, or the solution of aide drugs, for example, antidepressants or anticonvulsants. For instance, pregabalin at higher dosages of 225–900 mg have been seen as powerful, and an ongoing Cochrane survey recognized carbamazepine as a potential extra to lessen withdrawal impacts. Flumazenil, the benzodiazepine enemy, additionally shows guarantee when given by moderate imbuement, and has the bit of leeway that both high and low portions can be detoxified similarly well, and patients feel well after the detoxification.

Detoxification of benzodiazepines has different therapeutic regimes depending on the patient's condition. Some of the protocols are discussed below.

- Need to institute a excellent therapeutic relationship between the general practitioner and the patient—the process of benzodiazepine weaning is often interminable and benzodiazepine doses may need to be continually negotiated.

- Need to treat earnestly any clinically significant anxiety and depression with appropriate pharmacological or non-pharmacological methods. This is so as to diminish the degrees of nervousness and discouragement while the patient keeps on getting his/her standard benzodiazepine portion. There will be cutoff points to what can be accomplished at times in light of the fact that the nervousness and gloom indications might be a sign of benzodiazepine reliance.

- Need to prescribe a dose of diazepam equivalent to their usual regime and maintain this dose for 1 week. The dose of diazepam can then be reduced by approximately 10–15% at weekly intervals until withdrawal symptoms develop. If withdrawal symptoms develop smaller decrements and longer intervals between dose reductions may be necessary. It may be very difficult for patients to discontinue the final few milligrams. Although complete cessation is preferable, a single daily dose of 2 mg diazepam is sometimes acceptable.

A few patients may turn out to be progressively upset with regards to step-wise decrease and it might become clear that they have under evaluated their portion. It is basic that the believing relationship is kept up and portions renegotiated by seriousness of withdrawal.

6.1 Adjunctive therapies and medications

During the withdrawal organize, adjunctive medications, for instance, scholarly social treatment (CBT), loosening up treatment and planning in pressure the board have exhibited to be simply humbly effective. If downturn ascends during the withdrawal organize, the patient should be eagerly watched for reckless ideation. Stimulant treatment may ought to be considered. Mental interventions, for instance, CBT may be completed to address the scholarly signs of melancholy. Carbamazepine at a portion of 200–800 mg every day during withdrawal might be fruitful in averting benzodiazepine reuse despite the fact that it has no announced impact on the seriousness of withdrawal indications. Propranolol may help when substantial indications, for example, tremor and uneasiness are lessened. Cyproheptadine 4 mg daily is useful for rest unsettling influence or a sleeping disorder which is a typical element during detoxification.

6.1.1 Symptomatic relief

Symptomatic help is fundamental for some patients in benzodiazepine withdrawal notwithstanding sedation, especially when muscle issues or gut manifestations are noticeable. Side effects ought to be treated on an as required premise, as per the specific side effect complex. Metoclopramide is recommended orally or IM at a portion of 10 mg at regular intervals as required for sickness as well as spewing. An acid neutralizer 15-20 ml orally is allowed at regular intervals as required for indigestion or heartburn. Propantheline 15 mg orally is allowed like clockwork as required for stomach issues. Kaolin blend 15–20 ml orally is allowed at regular intervals as required for the runs. Quinine sulfate 300 mg orally is given twice day by day as required for muscle spasms. In any case, overabundance quinine sulfate is dangerous to the heart. Paracetamol 1 g orally is given each 4–6 hours as required for cerebral pains and other minor torments. Increasingly extreme a throbbing painfulness can be treated with nonsteroidal calming drugs (NSAIDS, for example, Ibuprofen 400 mg orally at regular intervals as required gave there is no history of ulcers, gastritis or asthma. A cox-2 inhibitor, for example, Celecoxib is a suitable elective where there is a contra-sign for vague NSAIDS.

6.2 Mechanism of cellular toxicity of benzodiazepines

Benzodiazepines (BZD) are natural bases with a benzene ring and a seven part diazepine moiety; different side chains decide the strength, length of activity, metabolite movement, and pace of disposal for explicit operators. BZDs apply their impact by means of tweak of the gamma-aminobutyric corrosive A (GABA-A) receptor. Gamma-aminobutyric corrosive (GABA) is the boss inhibitory synapse of the focal sensory system.

The GABA-A receptor is made out of five subunits (alpha, beta, and gamma) orchestrated in different mixes. The organization of subunits decides the liking of the different xenobiotics that quandary to the receptor. Benzodiazepines tie at the interface of the alpha and gamma subunits and, when bound, lock the GABA-A receptor into an adaptation that builds its partiality for GABA. BZDs do not modify the amalgamation, discharge, or digestion of GABA yet rather potentiate its inhibitory activities by increasing receptor authoritative. This coupling builds the progression of chloride particles through the GABA particle channel, causing postsynaptic hyperpolarization and a diminished capacity to start an activity potential. The low occurrence of respiratory sadness with orally ingested BZDs has all the earmarks of being identified with the low thickness of restricting locales in the brainstem respiratory focus.

7. Detoxification from alcohol

Withdrawal from liquor may not require pharmacological mediation, if the seriousness of reliance and withdrawal manifestations do not require it. In any case, thiamine enhancements might be important to keep away from the Wernicke-Korsakoff disorder. Those with liquor reliance will in general have a diminished dimension of thiamine in their eating regimen and ethanol can upset thiamine stockpiling and use. Notwithstanding the medicines sketched out beneath, it tends to be contended that different medications have a job in detoxification, for example, naltrexone, nalmefene, acamprosate, baclofen and disulfiram, despite the fact that these are progressively fit to backslide aversion [9]. Another treatment with a potential job in liquor detoxification is the psychotropic pain relieving nitrous oxide (PAN), which

S. No.	Substance of abuse	Detoxification process
1	Opioids (morphine)	Clonidine-naltrexone detoxification, rapid opioid withdrawal under general anesthesia
2	Nicotine	Nicotine replacement therapy (NRT); e.g., tiagabine, baclofen, gabapentin, varenicline, mecamylamine.
3	Benzodiazepine	Flumazenil as an antidote.
4	Cannabis	Antagonist approach, e.g., rimonabant
5	Alcohol	Disulfiram
6	Cocaine	Bupropion
7	Amphetamine	Modafinil

Table 2.
Summary of detoxification process of different substance of abuse.

has been distinguished by a Cochrane survey for mellow to direct liquor withdrawal. This may have a quick remedial impact with negligible sedation (**Table 2**).

7.1 Alcohol toxicity

Alcohol is a lethal substance and its danger is identified with the amount and term of alcohol utilization. It can affect each organ in the body. In the mind, in a solitary drinking scene, expanding levels of liquor lead at first to incitement (experienced as joy), fervor and garrulity. At expanding fixations liquor creates sedation prompting uproars of unwinding, afterwards to slurred discourse, instability, loss of coordination, incontinence, trance state and eventually Alcohol reliance and unsafe liquor use demise through liquor harming, because of the sedation of the essential mind works on breathing and flow. The reliance delivering properties of liquor have been examined widely over the most recent 20 years. Liquor influences a wide scope of synapse frameworks in the mind, prompting the highlights of liquor reliance. The principle synapse frameworks influenced by liquor are gamma-amino-butyric corrosive (GABA), glutamate, dopamine and narcotic. The activity of liquor on GABA is like the impacts of different narcotics, for example, benzodiazepines and is answerable for liquor's calming and anxiolytic properties. Glutamate is a major neurotransmitter responsible for brain stimulation, and alcohol affects glutamate through its inhibitory action on N-methyl D-aspartate (NMDA)-type glutamate receptors, producing amnesia (for example, blackouts) and sedation. Chronic alcohol consumption leads to the development of tolerance through a process of

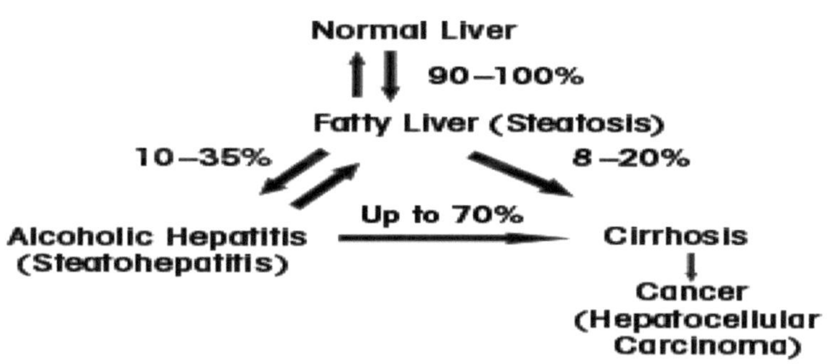

Figure 1.
Progression of liver disease in chronic alcoholism.

neuroadaptation: receptors in the brain gradually adapt to the effects of alcohol, to compensate for stimulation or sedation (**Figure 1**). This is experienced by the individual as the same amount of alcohol having less effect over time. This can lead to individual increasing alcohol consumption to achieve the desired psychoactive effects. The key neurotransmitters involved in tolerance are GABA and glutamate, with chronic alcohol intake associated with reduced GABA inhibitory function an increased NMDA-glutamatergic activity.

This GABA—glutamate unevenness is adequate within the sight of liquor, which expands GABA and lessens NMDA-glutamate movement. Be that as it may, when the liquor subordinate individual quits drinking, the irregularity between these synapse frameworks brings about the cerebrum getting overactive following a couple of hours prompting horrendous withdrawal manifestations, for example, uneasiness, perspiring, longing for, seizures and mental trips. This can be hazardous in extreme cases and requires critical medicinal treatment. Rehashed withdrawal is additionally thought to

S No	Structure of Substance abuse	Structure of drugs used in detoxification process
1	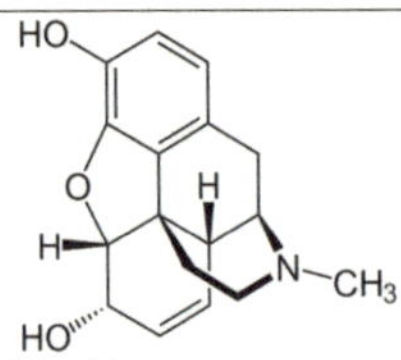 Morphine	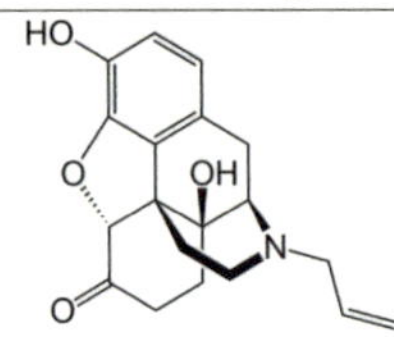 Naloxone
2	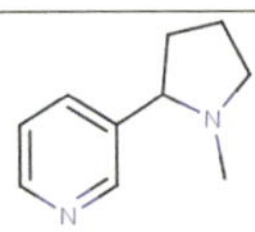 Nicotine	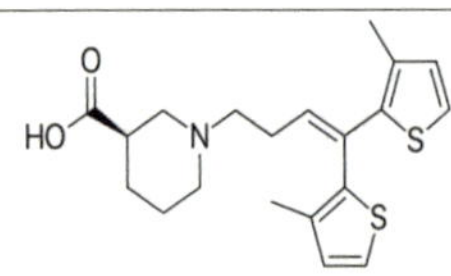 Tiagabine
3	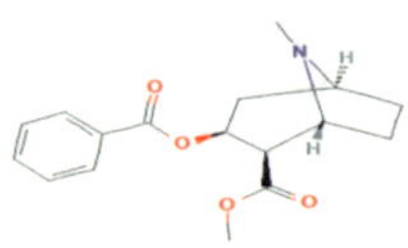 Cocaine	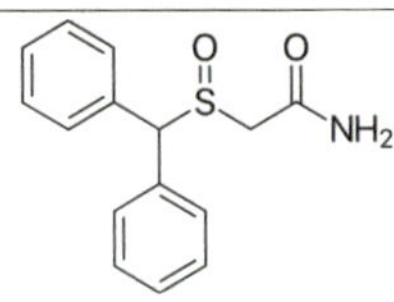 Modafinil
4	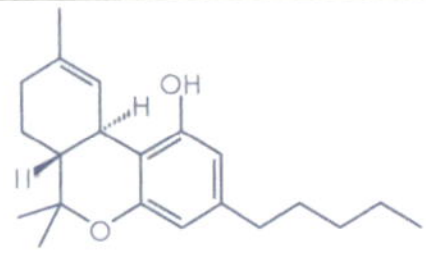 Cannabis	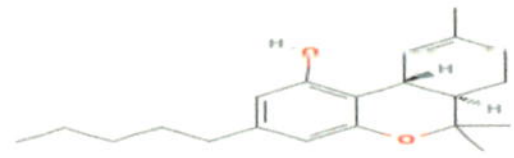 Dronabinol
5	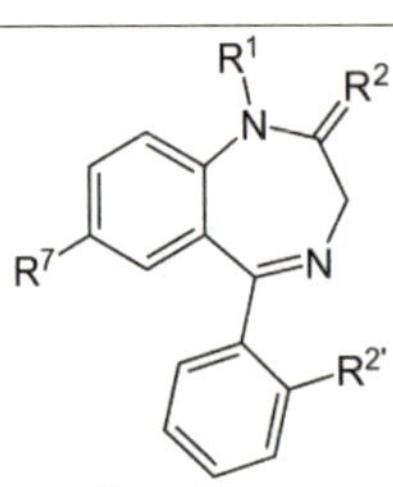 Benzodiazepine	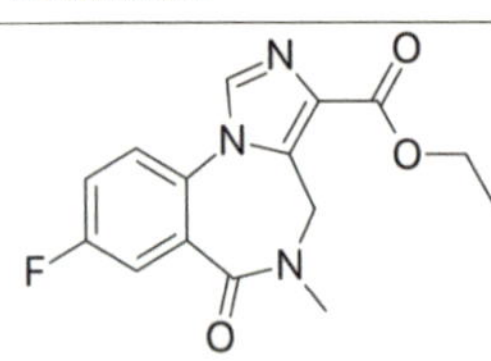 Flumazenil

Table 3.
Molecular structure of substance abuse and drugs used in detoxification.

underlie the lethal impact of liquor on neurons, prompting subjective disability and cerebrum harm. The impacts of liquor withdrawal can take up to between 3 months and 1 year to completely recuperate from (alluded to as the extended withdrawal disorder). That being said, the mind remains strangely delicate to liquor and, when drinking is continued, resistance and withdrawal can return inside a couple of days (known as restoration). This makes it amazingly hard for an individual who has created liquor reliance to come back to supported moderate drinking (**Table 3**).

8. Conclusion

Detoxification is not an end in itself, however a transitional state among reliance and restraint or decreased use. It can give a chance to restraint as a major aspect of the recuperation venture, yet for certain medications may build the danger of overdose and supported backslide. It is a harmony between the substance client's needs and inclination, decision of medicine, strategies for organization, and the force of key working and psychosocial programs. Proof has appeared pharmacological treatment for substance abuse works; however that it should be joined with psychosocial treatment. We should now ask how we can best tailor built up medicines to suit the requirements of people in distinction conditions. Questions remain with respect to examinations between medicines, mixes of medications and ideal treatment regimens. Much consideration has been given to affirmed medicines, for example, methadone decreasing for narcotic reliance and benzodiazepines for liquor reliance, and more research is required into rising treatment potential outcomes, for example, oxytocin and flumazenil. Different medications for abuse are less all around inquired about, to some degree because of the administrative obstacles associated with setting up investigations of substances of abuse and controlled medications. Ebb and flow investigation into extra or elective medicines is not vigorous enough for significant survey bodies, which mean suggestion, are difficult to accomplish. The decision of which technique to use for detoxification can rely upon numerous elements, including clinical judgment, the client's close to home inclination and conditions, way of life and desires, level of reliance and associative medical issues. Clinicians may need to tailor pharmacological medicines, for instance, in connection to danger of overdose if detoxification treatment can be occupied for infusion, or if there are any dangers to kids living with the client if the treatment can be brought home. For viable treatment plans, clients ought to be associated with their treatment decisions. The choice of medication for detoxification in case of opioid poisoning is very important. Methadone or buprenorphine should be offered as the first-line treatment in opioid detoxification.

It should take into account whether the service user is receiving maintenance treatment with methadone or buprenorphine if so, opioid detoxification should normally be started with the same medication. Lofexidine may be considered for people who have made an informed and clinically appropriate decision not to use methadone or buprenorphine for detoxification or who have made an informed and clinically appropriate decision to detoxify within a short time period with mild or uncertain dependence (including young people). Clonidine should not be used routinely in opioid detoxification.

Dihydrocodeine should not be used routinely in opioid detoxification.

Dosage and duration of detoxification has a crucial role. When determining the starting dose, duration and regimen (for example, linear or stepped) of opioid detoxification, healthcare professionals, in severity of dependence (particular caution should be exercised where there is uncertainty about dependence) stability of the service user (including polydrug and alcohol use, and comorbid mental health problems), pharmacology of the chosen detoxification medication and any adjunctive medication. The duration of opioid detoxification should normally be up to 4 weeks in an inpatient/residential setting and up to 12 weeks in a community setting. In the course of the most recent a very long while there has been a lot of progress understanding the atomic and cell premise of practices identified with nicotine addiction, and this comprehension has prompted focused on tranquilize disclosure prompting new therapeutics for smoking discontinuance, for example, varenicline. These advances show that basic investigations of the neurobiological premise of medication misuse can build our insight into why people become dependent and what drives continuous smoking, however can likewise prompt novel techniques for mediation to assist individuals with stopping and remain abstinent. The information that has been increased about the systems fundamental nicotine support has been applied to understanding different practices that drive continuous smoking. Focusing on the multimodal reason for nicotine admission may in this way bring about progressively compelling medicines for smoking suspension going ahead. Restraint of synapse discharge is viewed as the significant system of activity liable for the clinical impacts of narcotics. By the by, notwithstanding broad examination, comprehension of the cell activities of morphine and different narcotics is inadequate. This is astounding for a gathering of medications with such amazing impacts, and is an impression of the unpredictability of the instruments associated with synapse discharge. Affirmation of current speculations with respect to components of narcotic hindrance of synapse discharge must anticipate the use of progressively refined methods. Ongoing progresses in the atomic science of narcotic receptors guarantee critical propels in narcotic pharmacology and should help disclosure of narcotics with increasingly specific activities.

Conflict of interest

The authors declare no conflict of interest.

Author details

Sreemoy Kanti Das
Faculty of Pharmacy, Lincoln University College, Malaysia

*Address all correspondence to: sreemoy_das@yahoo.com

References

[1] Kleber HD. Pharmacologic treatments for opioid dependence: Detoxification and maintenance options. Dialogues in Clinical Neuroscience. 2007;**9**(4):455

[2] Cucchia AT, Monnat M, Spagnoli J, Ferrero F, Bertschy G. Ultra-rapid opiate detoxification using deep sedation with oral midazolam: Short and long-term results. Drug and Alcohol Dependence. 1998;**52**(3):243-250

[3] Kleber HD, Riordan CE, Rounsaville B, Kosten T, Charney D, Gaspari J, et al. Clonidine in outpatient detoxification from methadone maintenance. Archives of General Psychiatry. 1985;**42**(4):391-394

[4] Jasinski DR, Johnson RE, Kocher TR. Clonidine in morphine withdrawal: Differential effects on signs and symptoms. Archives of General Psychiatry. 1985;**42**(11):1063-1066

[5] Lingford-Hughes AR, Welch S, Peters L. Nutt D. BAP updated guidelines: Evidence-based guidelines for the pharmacological management of substance abuse, harmful use, addiction and comorbidity: Recommendations from BAP. Journal of Psychopharmacology. 2012;**26**(7):899-952

[6] Frishman WH. Smoking cessation pharmacotherapy—Nicotine and non-nicotine preparations. Preventive Cardiology. 2007;**10**:10-22

[7] Roll JM, Higgins ST. A within-subject comparison of three different schedules of reinforcement of drug abstinence using cigarette smoking as an exemplar. Drug and Alcohol Dependence. 2000;**58**(1-2):103-109

[8] McGregor IS, Bowen MT. Breaking the loop: Oxytocin as a potential treatment for drug addiction. Hormones and Behavior. 2012;**61**(3):331-339

[9] Lingford-Hughes A, Welch S, Nutt D. Evidence-based guidelines for the pharmacological management of substance misuse, addiction and comorbidity: Recommendations from the British Association for Psychopharmacology. Journal of Psychopharmacology. 2004;**18**(3):293-335

[10] Kampman KM, Dackis C, Lynch KG, Pettinati H, Tirado C, Gariti P, et al. A double-blind, placebo-controlled trial of amantadine, propranolol, and their combination for the treatment of cocaine dependence in patients with severe cocaine withdrawal symptoms. Drug and Alcohol Dependence. 2006;**85**(2):129-137

[11] Minozzi S, Amato L, Pani PP, Solimini R, Vecchi S, De Crescenzo F, et al. Dopamine agonists for the treatment of cocaine dependence. Cochrane Database of Systematic Reviews. 2015;(5). Available from: https://doi.org/10.1002/14651858.CD003352.pub4

[12] Keys AS, Mark GP, Emre N, Meshul CK. Reduced glutamate immunolabeling in the nucleus accumbens following extended withdrawal from self-administered cocaine. Synapse. 1998;**30**(4):393-401

[13] Bowen R, McIlwrick J, Baetz M, Zhang X. Lithium and marijuana withdrawal. The Canadian Journal of Psychiatry. 2005;**50**(4):240-241

[14] Haney M, Hart CL, Vosburg SK, Comer SD, Reed SC, Cooper ZD, et al. Effects of baclofen and mirtazapine on a laboratory model of marijuana withdrawal and relapse. Psychopharmacology. 2010;**211**(2): 233-244

[15] Zuardi AW, Crippa JAS, Hallak JE. Cannabis sativa: The plant

that can induce unwanted effects and also treat them. Revista Brasileira de Psiquiatria. 2010;**32**:51-52

[16] Moreira FA, Crippa JAS. The psychiatric side-effects of rimonabant. Revista brasileira de psiquiatria. 2009;**31**(2):145-153

[17] Lin S-K, Chen C-H, Pan C-H. Venlafaxine for acute heroin detoxification: A double-blind, randomized, control trial. Journal of Clinical Psychopharmacology. 2008;**28**(2):189-194

Chapter 17

Antidotes Network

Alberto Frutos Pérez-Surio

Abstract

Antidotes are essential medicines for the management of some of the emergencies attended in the hospital environment, and the speed of administration can be a key element for the survival of the patient. The Hospital Pharmacy Services are responsible for guaranteeing its availability. However, this availability can be affected by some aspects like the frequency of presentation of an intoxication in a geographical area, urgency in administration, difficulties of acquisition, cost, and period of validity, among others. In Spain, a web-based application was developed (www.redantidotos.org). It includes a public site with general information, an updated antidote guide and a section where non-urgent toxicological consultations could be submitted. Design a virtual antidote network between hospitals could be really useful to help the location online of the hospitals that stocked those antidotes with the highest difficulty in terms of availability, and ensured that the medication will be loaned in case of necessity. Therefore, it is necessary to create a tool that facilitates the exchange of antidotes between hospitals and ensures their availability. The aim is to continue improving communication between professionals involved in intoxication management at national, European and international level, sharing knowledge and improving the care we offer to our patients.

Keywords: antidotes, poisonings, virtual network, emergency, hospital pharmacy services

1. Introduction

1.1 Antidotes

Poisoning is the second leading cause of injury-related morbidity and mortality in the United States, with more than 2.4 million toxic exposures reported each year [1].

Antidotes, remedies or agents counteracting or neutralizing the action of poisons (MeSH and Emtree definitions, from Dorland's Medical Dictionary, 32nd edition), apply their useful impacts through an assortment of components, including the development of an inactive complex with the venom, the speeding up of venom detoxification, the decrease of venom transformation rate to a progressively dangerous compound, rivalry with venom for fundamental receptor locales, blockage of basic receptors through which lethal impacts are intervened, and avoidance of venom impact. There are explicit antidotes for few toxins, and a couple of counteractants are routinely utilized in clinical practice. These are acetylcysteine, naloxone and flumazenil.

Antidotal therapy is a critical aspect of the poisoning management in emergency setting: prompt availability and sufficient amount are essential, particularly when these molecules represent life-saving therapy for the acute poisoned patient.

Pharmacists can help reduce morbidity and mortality due to poisonings and overdoses by recognizing the signs exposure, guiding emergency room staff on the appropriate use of antidotes and supportive therapies, helping to ensure appropriate monitoring of patients for antidote response and adverse effects and managing the procurement and stocking of antidotes to ensure their timely availability [2].

1.2 Justification and background

Antidotes are essential medicines for the management of some of the emergencies attended in the hospital environment, and the speed of administration can be a key element for the survival of the patient. The Hospital Pharmacy Services are responsible for guaranteeing its availability [3–6].

However, it can be affected by several causes:

- Frequency of presentation of an intoxication in a geographical area
- Urgency in administration
- Difficulties of acquisition
- Cost
- Period of validity

Therefore, it is necessary to create a tool that facilitates the exchange of antidotes between hospitals and ensures their availability.

For example, in other countries like in the USA, to appropriately prepare for bioterrorism response, the governmental Agency that optimally provides the surveillance and planning guidance is the Centers for Disease Control and Prevention (CDC). Pharmacists can play a key role in reducing poisoning and overdose injuries and deaths by assisting in the early recognition of toxic exposures and guiding emergency personnel on the proper storage, selection, and use of antidotal therapies. The clinical pharmacist for a hospital is creating a protocol for the pharmacy department in the event of a biological disaster. Five elements that are critical to the protocol follow the National Preparedness Goal (NPG) created to prepare the United States for threats that pose risks to the nation, including acts of terrorism. The five mission areas that were identified in order to achieve the NPG are: Prevention, protection, mitigation, response, and recovery. The pharmacy department of a given hospital stores a Strategic National Stockpile (SNS) cache for use in a disaster. The person that authorizes deployment of the stockpile is the State governor's office, and thereafter, Pharmacy director and Hospital Incident Command System (HICS).

Inadequate stock or insufficient number of antidotes is a common and diffused problem in the Emergency Departments in many countries. In Italy, based on this consideration, from 2003 to 2012 two National surveys has been conducted from Pavia Poison Control Centre (Pavia-PCC) with the grant of the Italian Ministry of Health. The aim of these surveys was to evaluate antidotes availability in the Emergency Services (PCCs, EDs, intensive care units) and Hospital Pharmacies of the National Health System (NHS) throughout the Italian country. As a result of this initiative, since 2006, the collected data were organized in a specific "National database of antidotes" (BAnDA), available online (www.cavpavia.it) for the registered services that provided their data and with optimal and effective results.

Regarding Spain, in July 2015, the Xarxa d'Antídots de Catalunya was created to interconnect public and private hospitals throughout the community. It includes the provision, in these centers, of 18 antidotes for which there may be problems of availability due to the aforementioned factors.

The experience of the first few years has been very positive, both in terms of the number of hospitals adhered to and the toxicological consultations received, and loans made. For this reason, and with the intention of extending this project throughout the country, the Antidote Network was created. The Balearic Islands has been the first community to join and it is planned to expand with more regions in the near future.

1.3 Objectives

- To describe and to make a revision of Antidotes and their importance as an essential drug for management of acute intoxications.

- To give several evidences that the availability problems about stocking of antidotes in hospitals are an important concern, due to the lack of a National Regulation.

- To show the importance and responsibility that Pharmacy Departments are for warranting an optimal qualitative and quantitative stock of these drugs.

- In this context, the main objective is to propose a detailed review of the Antidotes Network that has been created in the Spanish territory.

2. Methodology

Within the framework of the Catalan Society of Clinical Pharmacy, a working group formed by pharmacists and doctors with experience in the field of Clinical Toxicology was created to develop the network. First, the group prepared a document with recommendations on the storage of antidotes according to the complexity and location of the hospital. An online application was then intended to be utilized as a specialized instrument between centers.

The application collects information on 15 antidotes, selected according to criteria of availability, urgency, frequency of use or cost (fragments of digoxin antibodies, methylene blue, deferoxamine, dimercaprol, calcium sodium edate, ethanol, physostigmine, fomepizole, glucagon, hydroxocobalamin, pyridoxine, pralidoxime, silibinin, botulinum antitoxin and snake venom antiserum). This tool provides information on the stock of each center (including the expiration date) and facilitates the loan of antidotes between hospitals.

3. Results

3.1 Antidotes network

The online application "Red de Antidotos" was propelled in July 2015. It has an open region with data about the task and offers the probability of non-dire toxicological discussions to the specialists of the gathering, and a private zone available with username and secret key for the focuses that have joined the network. So far 34 Catalan clinics offering crisis care have been fused. In each inside there is a drug specialist and a specialist from the Emergency Department in charge of the network. These figures are designated "farmatox" and "urgetox". The "farmatox" is responsible for the support of the stocks, refreshes the developments of medications and arranges and loan antidotes between emergency clinics. The "urgetox" builds up the elements of toxicology referent of the Emergency Department.

The network of antidotes is a really intuitive and helpful device. The private region is separated into four segments. The Antidote segment contains data on antidotes, which can be counseled on the web. It is a powerful list, kept up by the individuals from the gathering, which gathers information on toxicological signs, measurements with the best agreement for the two grown-ups and kids, accessible definitions, perceptions on organization, strength, unfriendly responses and different contemplations to be considered, just as the prescribed amounts to be put away relying upon the multifaceted nature of every medical clinic.

The Antidote Stock Management segment gathers the accessible measure of antitoxins in the network put away in every emergency clinic. The application permits the "farmatox" to enter any section and leave development. Every passage must include: medicine, number of units, bunch, lapse date and sort of development. For the last mentioned, two sorts of passage developments have been characterized (buy of drugs and return of the advance to another medical clinic), and three kinds of leave developments (claim use, termination and credit).

All developments for stock refreshing (credit developments just as for possess use) must be done physically by the drug specialist mindful in every emergency clinic. To encourage this stock upkeep, the application enables you to print a record with the units entered for each clump and the lapse date for each group. Lapsed units are featured in red.

The application enables you to scan for antidotes by drug or by medical clinic, in the area of the guide that demonstrates the data of the considerable number of emergency clinics incorporated into the network. At the point when the inquiry is done by clinic, the accompanying information can be counseled on the guide: name of the "farmatox" and the "urgetox", address, phone, email, fax and opening times of the Pharmacy, Department and phone of the Emergency Unit. It likewise demonstrates every one of the antidotes accessible in the inside, with their number of units and the following expiry date. At the point when the antitoxin search is played out, all clinics in which the cure is accessible will be shown, just as the quantity of accessible units and the following termination date.

3.2 Centers

The network was first implemented in Catalonia and now the project is being extended to other Spanish regions (currently it has been implemented in three out of 17 regions, **Figure 1**), with the aim to continue improving communication between professionals involved in intoxication management, sharing knowledge and improving the care we offer to our patients.

There are presently 63 Spanish emergency clinics incorporated into the Antidotes Network. It has been utilized multiple times to find a remedy that was vital and to apply for an advance between focuses. Up until this point, 13 counteractants have been engaged with these developments. The most requested drugs are represented in the image below (**Figure 2**). Likewise, proposals on stock accessibility and utilization of antidotes as indicated by the multifaceted nature of the medical clinic were distributed and are accessible in the Emergencias Journal.

3.3 Antidotes stocks

As a result of this project, "the Antidotes Guide" was published, that includes recommendations for the availability of 38 antidotes depending on the level of

DOI: http://dx.doi.org/10.5772/intechopen.89816

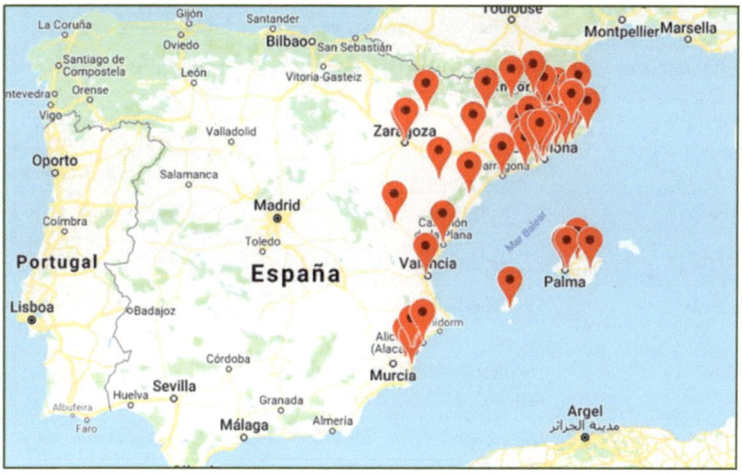

Figure 1.
Centers of the Antidotes Network in Spain.

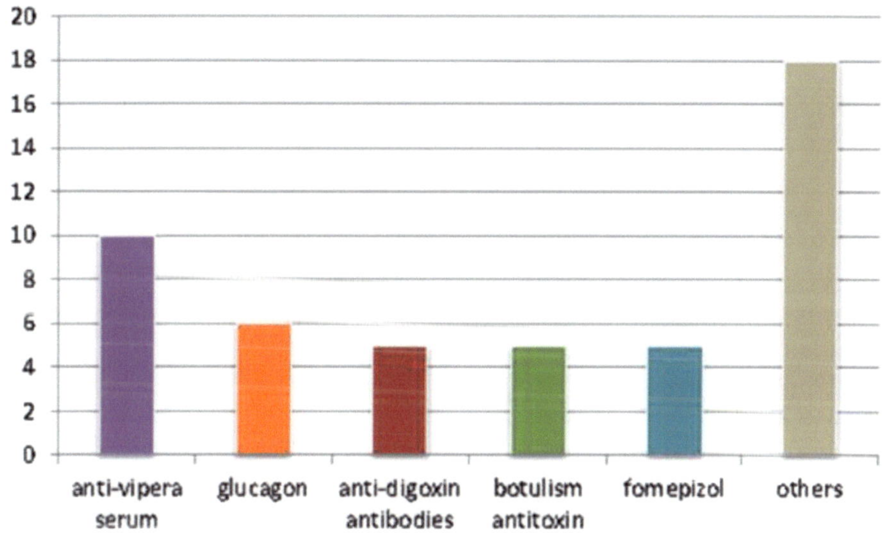

Figure 2.
Most request drugs. Source: Aguilar-Salmerón et al [7].

complexity of the hospitals and information on toxicological indications, posology and other observations of interest.

In the private part of the Antidotes Network, the stocks of the adhered hospitals are available for those antidotes in which availability problems may occur. Currently there are 18 antidotes included in the private part of the Network (**Table 1**).

Note also that the list of antidotes included in the network will change according to the needs of its hospitals, any epidemiological changes in poisoning, the launch of new antidotes, and problems for supply of others.

3.4 Consultations section

The consultations section is a tool very useful that the Antidote Network offers to any Health Professional the possibility of carrying out various types of toxicological consultations, as: (i) intoxications in which an antidote could be used, (ii) antidotes

Antidotes	Commercial presentations	Initial dosing
Antidigoxin antibodies	Digifab® 40 mg vial Refrigerator. Foreigner	IV 40 mg per 0.5 mg digoxin. If unknown digoxin quantity 400 mg (10 vials). To reconstitute with 4 mL of water + 250 mL PS 30 minutes inf. It may be necessary to repeat doses
Dantrolene	Dantrolen® 20 mg vial	IV 2.5 mg/kg (each vial in 3 min) preferably via central. Maximum doses reached 10 mg/kg
Deferoxamine	Desferin® vial 500 mg	IM 2 g in 10 mL Water or IV 15 mg/Kg/h (max. 80 mg/Kg/24 h)
Defibrotide	Defibrotide® 200 mg/2.5 mL vial	IV 6.25 mg/kg/h in 2 h
Dimercaprol (bal, British anti-lewisite)	Dimercaprol® amp. 200 mg c/12 amp 2 mL. Foreigner	IM 3 mg/Kg/4 h for 2 days
Calcium edetate sodium (EDTA)	Calcium Edetate sodium® amp.500 mg/10 mL c/10 amp. Foreigner	IV 1000 mg in 250 mL SF 6 hours infusion. Repeat every 12 h for 5 days
Ethanol (absolute ethanol)	Absolute ethanol® amp 10 mL Pharmaceutical Compounding	IV. 1 mL/Kg in D 5% 50 mL in 1 h. Continue with 0.1 mL/Kg/h. If alcoholic, double dose. Requires analytical control e/6h
Physostigmine	Anticholium® 2 mg/5 mL amp	IV 1–2 mg in 2 min. Repeat each bolus every 10–30 min. Alternatively: 2 mg/h up to a maximum of 8 mg/h
Fomepizole	Fomepizol® vial 100 mg	IV Loading dose of 15 mg/kg in 100–250 mg of NaCl 0.9% or D 5% and administered in 30–45 min
Glucagon	Glucagon Gen Hypokit® 1 mg syringe	IV 5 mg in 1 min. Repeat, if needed, in 10 min
Glucarpidase	Voraxazane® 1000 U vial	IV 50 U/kg in 5 min injection
Hydroxocobalamin	Cyanokit® 5 g vial	IV 5 g in 10 min (2.5 g if <35 Kg). If cardiac arrest 10 g in 10 min. If after 1 h there is no change, 5 more grams in 15 min
Idarucizumab	Praxbind® 2.5 g injectable solution	IV 5 g (2 vials) in two consecutive infusions or in one infusion
Pralidoxime (pam)	Contrathion® vial 200 mg/10 mL c/10 vials-amp. Foreigner	IV 1 g in 100 mL G 5 % 1 h infusion. If necessary, continue with the same dose every 6 h for 2–3 days.
Silibinin	Legalon® vial 350 mg	IV 5 mg/kg in 500 mL NaCl 0.9% or D 5% in 2 h. Repeat each 6 h (3–4 days)
Antibotulinum serum	Botulism Antitoxin Heptavalent A, B, C, D, E, F, G (BAT) 50 mL injectable solution	IV dilute 1 vial 1:10 and administer at 0.5 mL/min during 30 min. Maximum rate of 2 mL/min
Antiophidic serum	Snake venom antiserum (Bulbio®) vial 100 UI (5 mL). Foreigner	One dose corresponds to 100 IU (1 vial). First dose given via SC at the site of the sting, second dose via IM in the buttock. Further doses may be necessary at a later time as clinically determined.
Uridine triacetate	Vistonuridine® 10 g sachet	PO 10 g each 6 h, 20 doses

Table 1.
Antidotes included in the private part of the Network.

that could be used in some types of poisonings, (iii) agents used for digestive, cutaneous or ocular decontamination (iv) recommendations on qualitative and quantitative availability of antidotes.

Also, this section offers the possibility that the answer to some of these questions can be found by the reader in the Antidote Guide that can be found in this website.

For urgent medical consultations due to poisonings and toxicological emergencies, it is possible to contact by telephone the Toxicological Information Service of the National Institute of Toxicology and Forensic Sciences as this Service offers toxicological advice 24 h a day, 365 days a year. Otherwise, for non-urgent consultations on Clinical Toxicology, pharmacological aspects of antidotes or on drugs that can cause intoxications, it is possible to contact the experts of the Group of antidotes, specialized in assistance to acute intoxications in both adults and pediatrics, via an official email published on the official website.

4. Discussion

It is necessary to guarantee an adequate stock of antidotes in those hospitals managing poisoned patients; however, this is not always simple to realize.

Making a database of refreshed supplies of antitoxins open to all medical clinics overseeing clinic crises is definitely not another thought. New Zealand emergency clinics have just recommended its creation as an answer for the inadequacies found [7, 8]. Similarly, the "Centro Antiveleni di Pavia - Centro Nazionale di Informazione Tossicologica" made the Banca Dati Nazionale degli Antidoti (BaNdA), in light of an investigation of the accessibility of antidotes in Italian Emergency Units, among others [9–16]. It is an on-line stage that permits to discover refreshed information on the subjective and quantitative accessibility of counteractants in all the clinic units required, to look for a particular antitoxin by city or area and to get to all the contact information important to apply for an advance.

Some information on antitoxins and how they are arranged through Spanish antidote network as antitoxins are always a problem for both developing and developed countries. Particularly, some information on botulinum antitoxins and anti venoms:

Botulism Antitoxin Heptavalent—A, B, C, D, E, F, G (BAT), solution for injection: Adult dosage administration: Dilute the vial in a ratio of 1:10 and administer at a speed of 0.5 mL/min for 30 min and increase to double the speed every 30 min up to a maximum of 2 mL/min. For child dosage: Between 20 and 100% of the vial according to body weight. In children under 1 year the dose is 10% of the vial regardless of body weight. For administration: Dilute the vial in a ratio of 1:10 and administer at a speed of 0.01 mL/kg/min and increase by 0.01 mL/kg/min every 30 min to a maximum of 0.03 mL/min without exceeding adult rates. For dilution: Since the filling volume of each vial varies depending on the lot number (approximately 10–22 mL per vial), 90–200 mL of saline solution will be required for dilution. Conservation conditions: Store frozen or below ≤−15°C until used. Once thawed, it can be stored at 2–8°C for up to 36 months or up to 48 months from the date of manufacture (whichever comes first). Do not refreeze the vial. Administer the drug at room temperature. To defrost it, leave it at room temperature for 1 h and then immerse it in a bath of water at 37°C until it defrosts completely.

Snake Venom Antiserum (Bulvio® and Viperfav®): Adult and child dosage:

- Viperfav: IV Perfusion of 4 mL of serum (1 vial) in 100 mL SF at 50 ml/h.
- Snake Venom Antiserum: 100 IU (5 mL) via SC, followed by a second IM dose in the buttock. 1,2 or more IM doses may be necessary depending on the

patient's condition and on the second and third days 1 or 2 more doses may be needed. Viperfav® has a low risk of anaphylactic reactions. On the other hand, in the case of Snake Venom Antiserum® it is recommended to carry out a hypersensitivity test prior to its administration.

Building up a network of antitoxins can improve correspondence between focuses that oversee harmed patients, adjust and institutionalize antidotes assets in various focuses, and accelerate credits if essential. Eventually, it can improve the nature of consideration for harmed patients.

5. Conclusions

Antidote Network could allow improved communication between centers involved in the management of poisoned patients, help in adjusting and harmonizing antidotes stock and accelerate antidote borrowing, if required.

Furthermore, this Antidote Network provide prompt and easy access to antidotes (especially expensive and rare-use ones), to rapidly find them in the nearby hospitals or regions (avoiding lengthy and expensive transport), and it is useful also to optimize antidote stockpiles with saving of resources.

As future proposals it would be very convenient to expand the network throughout the national territory and implement it in other countries, which would allow an increase in the quality of life of the patient and an improvement in public health.

Conflict of interest

The author declares no conflict of interest.

Author details

Alberto Frutos Pérez-Surio[1,2]

1 Technological College, University of Zaragoza, Zaragoza, Spain

2 University Clinical Hospital Lozano Blesa, Zaragoza, Spain

*Address all correspondence to: ajfrutos@unizar.es

References

[1] Dart RC, Stark Y, Fulton B, Koziol-McLain J, Lowenstein SR. Insufficient stocking of poisoning antidotes in hospital pharmacies. JAMA. 1996;**276**:1508-1510

[2] Bradberry S, Vale A. Management of poisoning: Antidotes. Medicine. 2016;**44**(2):101-102

[3] Marraffa JM, Cohen V, Howland MA. Antidotes for toxicological emergencies: A practical review. American Journal of Health-System Pharmacy. 2012;**69**(3):199-212

[4] Nogué S, Munné P, Soy D, Millà J. Disponibilidad, utilidad y coste de los antídotos en Cataluña. Medicina Clínica (Barcelona). 1998;**110**:609-613

[5] Aguilar R, Soy D, Nogué S. Disponibilidad de antídotos en los ámbitos sanitarios de Cataluña. Medicina Clínica (Barcelona). 2006;**127**(20):770 773

[6] García-Martín A, Torres Santos-Olmos R. Antídotos: Guía de utilización y stock mínimo en el servicio de urgencias. Farmacia Hospitalaria. 2012;**36**:292-298

[7] Aguilar-Salmerón R, Martínez-Sánchez L, Broto-Sumalla T, Fernández deGamarra-MartínezE, Garcia-PelaezM, Nogue-Xarau S. Recomendaciones de disponibilidad y utilización de antídotos en los hospitales según el nivel de complejidad asistencial. Emergencias. 2016;**28**:45-54

[8] Nogué S, Cino J, Civeira E, Puiguriguer J, Burillo-Putze G, Dueñas A, et al. Tratamiento de la intoxicación digitálica. Bases para el uso de los anticuerpos antidigital. Emergencias. 2012;**24**:462-475

[9] Schep LJ, Slaughter RJ. Availability and quantity of antidotes in New Zealand. The New Zealand Medical Journal. 2015;**128**:20-22

[10] Fountain JS, Sly B, Holt A, MacDonell S. Availability of antidotes, antivenoms, and antitoxins in New Zealand hospital pharmacies. New Zealand Medical Journal. 2015;**128**:23-33

[11] Locatelli C, Petrolini V, Lonati D, Butera R, Bove A, Mela L, et al. Antidotes availability in Emergency Departments of the Italian National Health System and development of a national data-bank on antidotes. Annali dell'Istituto Superiore di Sanità. 2006;**42**(3):298-309

[12] Buscaglia E, Mazzoneli M, Lonati D, Giampreti A, Vecchio S, Petrolini VM, et al. Antidotes supply in emergency from Pavia Poison Control Centre. Clinical Toxicology (Philadelphia, Pa.). 2013;**51**:361

[13] Boels D, De Haro L, Harry P. Le banque de sérums antivenimeux (BSA). Bulletin de la Société de Toxicologie Clinique. 2012;**38**:1-3

[14] Mazer-Amirshahi M, Hawley KL, Zocchi M, Fox E, Pines JM, Nelson LS. Drug shortages: Implications for medical toxicology. Clinical Toxicology (Philadelphia, Pa.). 2015;**53**(6):519-524

[15] American College of Medical Toxicology. Antidote shortages in the USA: Impact and response. Journal of Medical Toxicology. 2015;**11**(1):144-146

[16] Locatelli C et al. Disponibilità di antidoti nei servizi d'urgenza del Sistema Sanitario Nazionale e realizzazione della Banca Dati Nazionale degli Antidoti (BaNdA). Annali dell'Istituto Superiore di Sanità. 2006;**42**(3):298-309